Cancer Challenges during COVID-19 Pandemic

Cancer Challenges during COVID-19 Pandemic

Editors

Franco M. Buonaguro
Attilio AM Bianchi

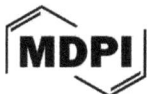

Basel • Beijing • Wuhan • Barcelona • Belgrade • Novi Sad • Cluj • Manchester

Editors

Franco M. Buonaguro
Translational Research
Ist Naz Tumori - IRCCS Fond Pascale
Napoli
Italy

Attilio AM Bianchi
Director General
Ist Naz Tumori - IRCCS Fond Pascale
Napoli
Italy

Editorial Office
MDPI
St. Alban-Anlage 66
4052 Basel, Switzerland

This is a reprint of articles from the Special Issue published online in the open access journal *Journal of Personalized Medicine* (ISSN 2075-4426) (available at: www.mdpi.com/journal/jpm/special_issues/Cancer_COVID_Pandemic).

For citation purposes, cite each article independently as indicated on the article page online and as indicated below:

Lastname, A.A.; Lastname, B.B. Article Title. *Journal Name* **Year**, *Volume Number*, Page Range.

ISBN 978-3-0365-8804-9 (Hbk)
ISBN 978-3-0365-8803-2 (PDF)
doi.org/10.3390/books978-3-0365-8803-2

© 2023 by the authors. Articles in this book are Open Access and distributed under the Creative Commons Attribution (CC BY) license. The book as a whole is distributed by MDPI under the terms and conditions of the Creative Commons Attribution-NonCommercial-NoDerivs (CC BY-NC-ND) license.

Contents

About the Editors . . . . **vii**

Preface . . . . **ix**

Lucia Mangone, Paolo Giorgi Rossi, Martina Taborelli, Federica Toffolutti, Pamela Mancuso and Luigino Dal Maso et al.
SARS-CoV-2 Infection, Vaccination and Risk of Death in People with An Oncological Disease in Northeast Italy
Reprinted from: *J. Pers. Med.* **2023**, *13*, 1333, doi:10.3390/jpm13091333 . . . . **1**

Vincenza Granata, Roberta Fusco, Alberta Villanacci, Simona Magliocchetti, Fabrizio Urraro and Nardi Tetaj et al.
Imaging Severity COVID-19 Assessment in Vaccinated and Unvaccinated Patients: Comparison of the Different Variants in a High Volume Italian Reference Center
Reprinted from: *J. Pers. Med.* **2022**, *12*, 955, doi:10.3390/jpm12060955 . . . . **12**

Roberta Fusco, Igino Simonetti, Stefania Ianniello, Alberta Villanacci, Francesca Grassi and Federica Dell'Aversana et al.
Pulmonary Lymphangitis Poses a Major Challenge for Radiologists in an Oncological Setting during the COVID-19 Pandemic
Reprinted from: *J. Pers. Med.* **2022**, *12*, 624, doi:10.3390/jpm12040624 . . . . **33**

Vincenza Granata, Stefania Ianniello, Roberta Fusco, Fabrizio Urraro, Davide Pupo and Simona Magliocchetti et al.
Quantitative Analysis of Residual COVID-19 Lung CT Features: Consistency among Two Commercial Software
Reprinted from: *J. Pers. Med.* **2021**, *11*, 1103, doi:10.3390/jpm11111103 . . . . **49**

Roberta Fusco, Roberta Grassi, Vincenza Granata, Sergio Venanzio Setola, Francesca Grassi and Diletta Cozzi et al.
Artificial Intelligence and COVID-19 Using Chest CT Scan and Chest X-ray Images: Machine Learning and Deep Learning Approaches for Diagnosis and Treatment
Reprinted from: *J. Pers. Med.* **2021**, *11*, 993, doi:10.3390/jpm11100993 . . . . **66**

Roberto Grassi, Salvatore Cappabianca, Fabrizio Urraro, Vincenza Granata, Giuliana Giacobbe and Simona Magliocchetti et al.
Evolution of CT Findings and Lung Residue in Patients with COVID-19 Pneumonia: Quantitative Analysis of the Disease with a Computer Automatic Tool
Reprinted from: *J. Pers. Med.* **2021**, *11*, 641, doi:10.3390/jpm11070641 . . . . **85**

Marino Marcic, Ljiljana Marcic, Barbara Marcic, Vesna Capkun and Katarina Vukojevic
Cerebral Vasoreactivity Evaluated by Transcranial Color Doppler and Breath-Holding Test in Patients after SARS-CoV-2 Infection
Reprinted from: *J. Pers. Med.* **2021**, *11*, 379, doi:10.3390/jpm11050379 . . . . **99**

Francesca Maio, Daniele Ugo Tari, Vincenza Granata, Roberta Fusco, Roberta Grassi and Antonella Petrillo et al.
Breast Cancer Screening during COVID-19 Emergency: Patients and Department Management in a Local Experience
Reprinted from: *J. Pers. Med.* **2021**, *11*, 380, doi:10.3390/jpm11050380 . . . . **112**

Valentina Natalucci, Milena Villarini, Rita Emili, Mattia Acito, Luciana Vallorani and Elena Barbieri et al.
Special Attention to Physical Activity in Breast Cancer Patients during the First Wave of COVID-19 Pandemic in Italy: The DianaWeb Cohort
Reprinted from: *J. Pers. Med.* **2021**, *11*, 381, doi:10.3390/jpm11050381 . . . . **122**

Vincenzo D'Agostino, Ferdinando Caranci, Alberto Negro, Valeria Piscitelli, Bernardino Tuccillo and Fabrizio Fasano et al.
A Rare Case of Cerebral Venous Thrombosis and Disseminated Intravascular Coagulation Temporally Associated to the COVID-19 Vaccine Administration
Reprinted from: *J. Pers. Med.* **2021**, *11*, 285, doi:10.3390/jpm11040285 . . . . **135**

About the Editors

Franco M. Buonaguro

Franco M. Buonaguro is an M.D. Director Emeritus of the Molecular Biology & Viral Oncology Unit at Natl Cancer Inst, Naples (IT). He graduated cum laude in 1977 at the "Federico II" Medical School, Naples (IT), and is board-certified in Endocrinology (1982) in Microbiology & Virology (1992). He was a postdoctoral fellow at the Dpt of Cell Biology, Argonne Natl Laboratory, Argonne, IL, USA (1979-81) and a WHO Fellow and research associate at the Tumor Biology Program, FHCRC Seattle USA (1983-86). Since 1987, he has been a member at the Natl Cancer Institute "Istituto Nazionale Tumori - IRCCS Fondazione Pascale", Naples (IT).

Attilio AM Bianchi

Attilio A.M. Bianchi, M.D. Director General of the Natl Cancer Inst, Naples (IT). He graduated cum laude in 1982 at the "Federico II" Medical School, Naples (IT) and is board-certified in Hygiene and Preventive Medicine (1994). He completed an Executive MSc in Health Economics, Policy and Management in 2005 at the Bocconi Univ, Milan (IT). He was a Medical Director of ex-ASL NA3, Naples, IT (2001-05); Medical Director of ASL Regione Marche, Ancona, IT (2005-07); Director General of University Hospital "S. Giovanni di Dio e Ruggi d'Aragona", Salerno, IT (2007-09); and the Director General of Salerno University, Salerno, IT (2009-16). Since 2016, he has been the Director General of the Natl Cancer Institute "Istituto Nazionale Tumori - IRCCS Fondazione Pascale", Naples (IT).

Preface

The COVID-19 pandemic, which presented a greater risk of severe morbidity in older and fragile patients, resulted in higher mortality rates in people with chronic diseases (particularly cardiovascular disease and diabetes) and cancer, highlighting the weakness of many welfare systems all over the world.

Most responsive cancer institutes have had to redesign their strategies to continue their activities. In particular, new therapeutic protocols and follow-up procedures have been implemented. Patients have had to be carefully evaluated to plan the optimal personalized treatment and to adopt the most appropriate therapeutic strategies, including telemedicine and digital monitoring. Healthcare professionals have had to be monitored for exposure to SARS-CoV-2 using genetic/antigen diagnostic kits and serological tests and, most recently, have been vaccinated with one of the several—not yet fully studied—available vaccines.

Furthermore, general management and planning aspects have also had to be reorganized, with particular attention being paid to the triage of patients for access to day hospital or day surgery sections, outpatient clinics, and clinical wards.

This Special Issue has focused on methodological issues relevant to the identification, particularly via radiological imaging, of serious clinical conditions requiring the sub intensive/intensive treatment of the acute phase and for the development/implementation of the more rigorous follow up of fragile cancer patients in the post-COVID period at highest risk of death, significantly for unvaccinated patients.

Franco M. Buonaguro and Attilio AM Bianchi
Editors

Article

SARS-CoV-2 Infection, Vaccination and Risk of Death in People with An Oncological Disease in Northeast Italy

Lucia Mangone [1], Paolo Giorgi Rossi [1,*], Martina Taborelli [2], Federica Toffolutti [2], Pamela Mancuso [1], Luigino Dal Maso [2], Michele Gobbato [3], Elena Clagnan [3], Stefania Del Zotto [3], Marta Ottone [1], Isabella Bisceglia [1], Antonino Neri [4] and Diego Serraino [2]

[1] Epidemiology Unit, AUSL-IRCCS di Reggio Emilia, 42122 Reggio Emilia, Italy; lucia.mangone@ausl.re.it (L.M.); pamela.mancuso@ausl.re.it (P.M.); isabella.bisceglia@ausl.re.it (I.B.)
[2] Unit of Cancer Epidemiology, Centro di Riferimento Oncologico di Aviano (CRO) IRCCS, 33081 Aviano, Italy; mtaborelli@cro.it (M.T.); ftoffolutti@cro.it (F.T.); dalmaso@cro.it (L.D.M.); serrainod@cro.it (D.S.)
[3] Agenzia Regionale di Coordinamento per la Salute Udine, 33100 Udine, Italy; michele.gobbato@arcs.sanita.fvg.it (M.G.); elena.clagnan@arcs.sanita.fvg.it (E.C.); stefania.delzotto@arcs.sanita.fvg.it (S.D.Z.)
[4] Scientific Directorate, AUSL-IRCCS di Reggio Emilia, 42122 Reggio Emilia, Italy; antonino.neri@ausl.re.it
* Correspondence: paolo.giorgirossi@ausl.re.it

Abstract: People with a history of cancer have a higher risk of death when infected with SARS-CoV-2. COVID-19 vaccines in cancer patients proved safe and effective, even if efficacy may be lower than in the general population. In this population-based study, we compare the risk of dying of cancer patients diagnosed with COVID-19 in 2021, vaccinated or non-vaccinated against SARS-CoV-2 and residing in Friuli Venezia Giulia or in the province of Reggio Emilia. An amount of 800 deaths occurred among 6583 patients; the risk of death was more than three times higher among unvaccinated compared to vaccinated ones [HR 3.4; 95% CI 2.9–4.1]. The excess risk of death was stronger in those aged 70–79 years [HR 4.6; 95% CI 3.2–6.8], in patients with diagnosis made <1 year [HR 8.5; 95% CI 7.3–10.5] and in all cancer sites, including hematological malignancies. The study results indicate that vaccination against SARS-CoV-2 infection is a necessary tool to be included in the complex of oncological therapies aimed at reducing the risk of death.

Keywords: COVID-19; vaccination; risk of death; tumors

1. Introduction

Since the beginning of the COVID-19 pandemic, it has been documented that people with an oncological disease, both those in active treatment and those undergoing periodic follow-up checks, are at an elevated risk of severe COVID-19 and further sequelae [1–4]. For these people, biological (related to the disease and/or anticancer treatments) and organizational factors combine to expose them to significantly higher risks of hospital admissions for COVID-19 and death as compared to corresponding people without cancer [5–7].

The relative effect of cancer on COVID-19 prognosis is stronger in younger patients [6]. Giannakoulis and colleagues confirmed that COVID-19 cancer patients are at increased risk of dying than non-cancer patients [HR 1.66; 95% CI 1.3–2.1] and that such elevated risk tends to reduce at over 65 years of age [HR 1.06; 95% CI 0.8–1.4] [8], as for other comorbidities [9]. Furthermore, haematological tumors can represent a negative prognostic factor compared to solid tumors, especially in response to therapies [10], but also for a complete immunization after vaccination [11].

On the contrary, evidence about the association between cancer and infection is less conclusive [6,12]. Consistent with this evidence of elevated health risks, people with a history of oncological disease have been included in the high-priority population groups for vaccination against SARS-CoV-2 infection [13,14]. Several studies, including national ones, have already documented the impact of SARS-CoV-2 infection on the mortality of people with cancer [6,15,16].

Most of the studies studied the efficacy of vaccination in cancer patients recruited in oncological services who do not represent the total population living after a cancer diagnosis. It is important to assess the impact of vaccination in the population of cancer patients across all the phases of the disease and cure and across all cancer sites in large population-based studies. A vaccination campaign in Italy started on December 2020, targeting initial health operators and residents in nursing homes. Older and vulnerable people were vaccinated with a high priority [17] and reached a high two-dose coverage by the end of March 2021. People with a previous diagnosis of cancer were included in the vulnerable group and were mostly vaccinated with an mRNA vaccine.

The aim of the study is to assess the risk of death in cancer patients based on their SARS-CoV-2 infection history and vaccination status.

2. Materials and Methods

2.1. Setting and Study Design

A retrospective population study was conducted in all residents of the Friuli Venezia Giulia Region and the province of Reggio Emilia living on 1 January 2021. They were therefore eligible for anti-SARs-CoV-2 vaccination and targeted to a molecular swab search for SARS-CoV-2 infection between 1 January 2021 and 31 December 2021. This study compared the risk of death for any cause in patients who tested positive for SARS-CoV-2 in 2021 at least once.

2.2. Data Sources and Linkage Procedures

To this end, the anonymised data included in the databases of the regional health information system were used for the Friuli Venezia Giulia Region, which covers the entire resident population [18]. For the province of Reggio Emilia, anonymised data from the Population Cancer Registry (CR) were used [19]. For the Friuli Venezia Giulia region, the initial population consisted of 725,475 residents who underwent a nasopharyngeal swab for the detection of SARS-CoV-2, of which 27,429 who tested positive had a previous history of cancer. For Reggio Emilia province, the corresponding population with cancer was made up of 5940 individuals (Figure 1a,b).

Persons with all negative swabs were considered SARS-CoV-2 negative on the date of the first swab while those with at least one positive result were considered SARS-CoV-2 positive on the date of the first positive swab. The history of the oncological disease was reconstructed thanks to data from the Reggio Emilia-CR and the Friuli Venezia Giulia Regional CR. For patients with multiple tumours, the most recent diagnosis, before 1 January 2021, was considered. The living status information was updated on 8 January 2022 for Friuli Venezia Giulia or on 30 March 2022 for Reggio Emilia. The study, approved by the Bioethics Committee of the Veneto Region (protocol No. 245343/2020) and by the Area Vasta Emilia Nord Ethic Committee (protocol No. 2020/0045199), was conducted through a record linkage procedure of de-identified data with the use of a semi-annually modified anonymous individual key. For this analysis, the databases of microbiology laboratories, cancer registries and mortality were used. Study subjects were categorized as vaccinated if they received at least one dose of available vaccine or unvaccinated.

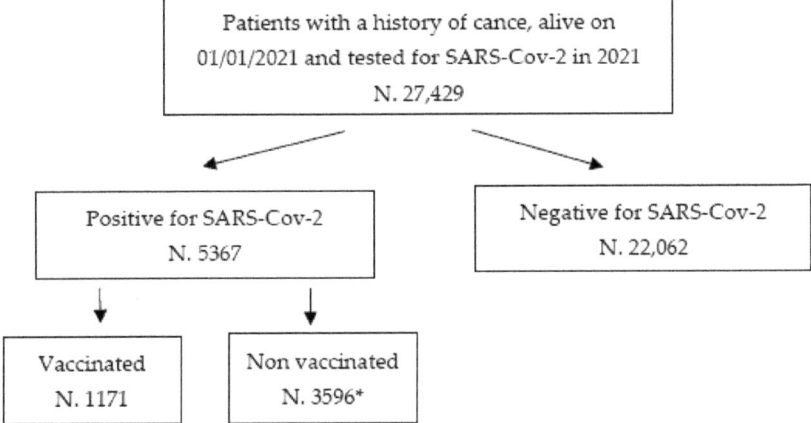

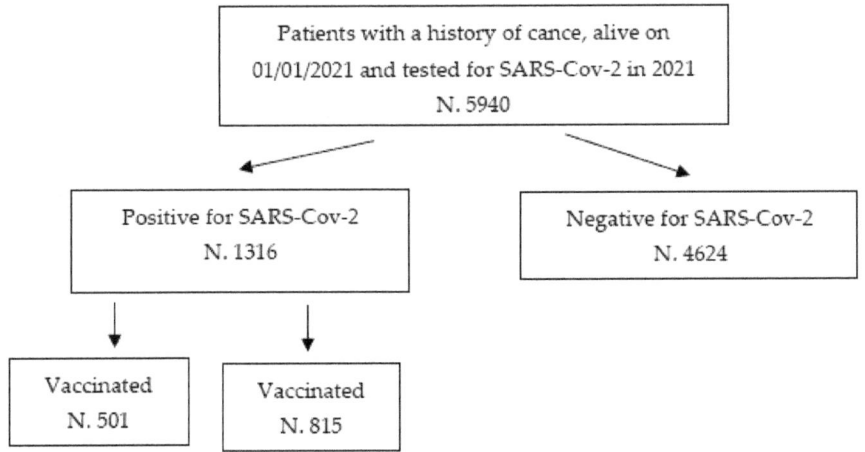

Figure 1. Description of the study population: Friuli Venezia Giulia (**1a**) and Reggio Emilia (**1b**) * It includes 2273 patients who received their first dose after SARS-CoV-2 positive test.

2.3. Data Analyses

The risk of death was assessed for unvaccinated versus vaccinated cancer patients, overall and by strata of sex, age, cancer type and time since cancer diagnosis. For the calculation of the risk of death, a multivariate analysis based on the Cox model was conducted aimed at estimating the hazard ratios (HR) and their 95% confidence intervals (CI). Models were adjusted for gender, age and time since diagnosis. The time at risk of death was calculated from the date of SARS-CoV-2 infection to the date of death or the study closure date (i.e., 31 March 2022), vaccination status was considered at the time of SARS-CoV-2 infection, as previously described [20]. To better evaluate the impact according to single tumor site, we also reported the relative survivals (adjusted by causes of death) of patients with cancer diagnoses in the years 2015–2017 and follow-up on 31 December 2021.

A descriptive analysis of the causes of death among vaccinated and unvaccinated patients and of the delay time between infection and death was possible only for the incident cases in the province of Reggio Emilia. Data are listed in the Supplementary Materials.

3. Results

An oncological history was documented in 27,429 people residing in Friuli Venezia Giulia living on 1 January 2021 and tested for SARS-CoV-2 infection during 2021. Among these oncological patients, 5367 (19.6%) tested positive at least once for SARS-CoV-2 infection during 2021 while 22,062 always tested negative (80.4%). The subsequent statistical analyses concerned the 5367 positive patients: 1171 vaccinated (21.8%) and 3596 (78.2%) unvaccinated at the time of infection (Figure 1a).

Figure 1b shows similar data documented in the province of Reggio Emilia: among 5940 patients with a previous history of cancer and tested in 2021, 1316 (22.2%) were positive and 4624 (77.8%) were negative for SARS-CoV-2 infection. Among the 1316 positives, 501 (38.1%) received at least one dose of the vaccine, and 815 (61.9%) were unvaccinated.

3.1. Frequency of Deaths among Vaccinated and Unvaccinated

In Friuli Venezia Giulia (Table 1), among those positive for the infection and vaccinated before infection, 102 died (5.8%); among those unvaccinated, there were 595 deaths (16.6%). Twenty-four deaths (4.1%) occurred among Reggio Emilia patients (Table 1) who received at least one dose of vaccine before infection. Conversely, there were 79 deaths (9.7%) among unvaccinated patients (Table 1).

As regards the study conducted in the Friuli Venezia Giulia region, particularly an elevated percentage of deaths among vaccinated people were documented in males (7.5%), in those aged 80 years or more (13.6%), in patients diagnosed with cancer in the previous 12 months (8.3%) and in patients with haematological malignancies (8.3%), bladder (10.4%) or colorectal (8.9%) among solid tumors.

In the province of Reggio Emilia (Table 1), high proportions of deaths among vaccinated patients occurred in females (5.7%), in those aged 80 or more years (16.1%) and in patients with hematological malignancies (8.2%), kidney (18.2%) or bladder cancer (8.8%), whereas no trend was observed by the time since diagnosis.

Among the unvaccinated patients in Friuli Venezia Giulia, males showed elevated death risk (20.8%); the death risk increases with age (18.4% in 70–79; 37.5% in 80+) and mainly affected patients diagnosed less than 12 months (28.8%). In addition to haematological tumours (18.7%), the lungs (37.2%) and bladder (26.9%) were among the tumour sites with elevated death percentages. Similarly, in the province of Reggio Emilia, unvaccinated males presented an elevated death risk (11.7%); the risk increased with age, especially to 80+ (35.9%), and mainly affected patients with a diagnosis made less than 12 months (21.3%) prior. Among tumor sites, a greater risk was observed for lung cancer (26.5%) and endometrium (29.6%).

Table 1. Numbers of cancer patients and deaths (all causes) in patients who tested positive for SARS-CoV-2 at least once according to vaccine status in 2021 in Friuli Venezia Giulia and Reggio Emilia areas, Italy.

	Positive for SARS-CoV-2							
	Friuli Venezia Giulia				Reggio Emilia			
	Vaccinated		Not Vaccinated		Vaccinated		Not Vaccinated	
	Total	Deaths	Total	Deaths	Total	Deaths	Total	Deaths
	N	N (Row %)	N	N (Row %)	N	N (Row %)	N	N (Row %)
All	1771	102 (5.8)	3596	595 (16.6)	501	24 (4.8)	815	79 (9.7)
Sex								
Male	858	64 (7.5)	1665	346 (20.8)	237	9 (3.8)	341	40 (11.7)
Female	913	38 (4.2)	1931	249 (12.9)	264	15 (5.7)	474	39 (8.2)
Age at infection (years)								
<40	56	0 (0.0)	145	1 (0.7)	43	0 (0.0)	67	0 (0.0)
40–59	364	3 (0.8)	869	25 (2.9)	124	1 (0.8)	289	6 (2.1)
60–69	285	6 (2.1)	710	61 (8.6)	88	2 (2.3)	149	4 (2.7)
70–79	522	19 (3.6)	1017	187 (18.4)	134	3 (2.2)	178	22 (12.4)
≥80	544	74 (13.6)	855	321 (37.5)	112	18 (16.1)	131	47 (35.9)
Time since cancer diagnosis								
<1 year	168	14 (8.3)	354	102 (28.8)	40	2 (5.0)	75	16 (21.3)
1–2 years	128	5 (3.9)	298	59 (19.8)	41	0 (0.0)	87	8 (9.2)
2–5 years	365	21 (5.8)	735	95 (12.9)	136	7 (5.2)	221	9 (4.1)
>5 years	1110	62 (5.6)	2209	339 (15.4)	284	15 (5.3)	432	46 (10.6)
Tumor site								
Solid tumors	1614	89 (5.5)	3275	535 (16.3)	440	19 (4.3)	847	130 (15.3)
Breast	415	13 (3.1)	882	84 (9.5)	118	4 (3.4)	222	14 (6.3)
Prostate	284	20 (7.0)	539	109 (20.2)	54	3 (5.6)	77	9 (11.7)
Colorectal	236	21 (8.9)	434	85 (19.6)	53	2 (3.8)	67	10 (14.9)
Skin Melanoma	148	6 (4.1)	287	18 (6.3)	42	2 (4.8)	53	2 (3.8)
Lung and larynx	73	4 (5.5)	180	67 (37.2)	12	0 (0.0)	34	9 (26.5)
Thyroid	91	1 (1.1)	155	10 (6.5)	43	0 (0.0)	74	1 (1.4)
Kidney	63	3 (4.8)	141	19 (13.5)	11	2 (18.2)	29	1 (3.4)
Bladder	48	5 (10.4)	93	25 (26.9)	34	3 (8.8)	44	5 (11.4)
Endometrium	47	1 (2.1)	107	13 (12.2)	15	0 (0.0)	27	8 (29.6)
Other solid tumours	209	15 (7.2)	457	105 (23.0)	58	3 (5.2)	109	19 (17.4)
Hematological malignancies	157	13 (8.3)	321	60 (18.7)	61	5 (8.2)	79	1 (1.3)
Non-Hodgkin lymphoma	73	5 (6.9)	165	38 (23.0)	24	2 (8.3)	38	1 (2.6)
Leukaemia	42	4 (9.5)	65	12 (18.5)	20	2 (10.0)	28	0 (0.0)
Hodgkin's lymphoma	21	2 (9.5)	51	2 (3.9)	7	0 (0.0)	7	0 (0.0)
Multiple myeloma	21	2 (9.5)	40	8 (20.0)	10	1 (10.0)	6	0 (0.0)

3.2. Multivariate Analysis of Deaths among Unvaccinated vs. Vaccinated Patients

The risks of death in unvaccinated vs. vaccinated patients are illustrated in Table 2. In Friuli Venezia Giulia, the risk of death among the unvaccinated was almost three-fold that of the vaccinated ones [HR 2.7; 95% CI 2.2–3.4]. The excess of risk was similar in males and females [HR 2.7; 95% CI 2.1–3.6; and HR 2.7; 95% CI 1.8–3.9] in the age group 70–79 [HR 3.7; 95% CI 2.3–5.9] and in subjects diagnosed between one–two years before diagnosis [HR 4.5; 95% CI 1.8–15.3]. Among solid tumours, the excess risk was particularly marked for lung [HR 5.0; 95% CI 1.8–14.1], breast [HR 3.0; 95% CI 1.6–5.3], prostate [HR 2.8; 95% CI 1.7–4.6] and colorectal [HR 2.3; 95% CI 1.4–3.7] cancers.

Table 2. Risk of death in unvaccinated vs. vaccinated patients in 2020–2021 in Friuli Venezia Giulia and in the province of Reggio Emilia, Italy.

	Friuli Venezia Giulia			Reggio Emilia			Overall		
	HR	95% CI		HR	95% CI		HR	95% CI	
All	2.7	2.2	3.4	8.2	5.1	13.2	3.4	2.9	4.1
Sex									
Male	2.7	2.1	3.6	12.1	6	24.5	3.4	2.8	4.3
Female	2.7	1.9	3.8	3.1	1.7	5.4	2.8	2.0	3.9
Age at infection (years)									
<40	-	-	-	-	-	-	-	-	-
40–59	1.8	0.52	6	4.2	0.46	37.9	2.1	0.8	6.3
60–69	2.4	1	5.6	5.9	1	33.4	2.8	1.4	6.0
70–79	3.7	2.3	5.9	19.3	5.7	65.7	4.6	3.2	6.8
≥80	2.5	2	3.3	6.5	3.6	11.6	3.1	2.6	3.9
Time since cancer diagnosis									
<1 year	2.7	1.5	4.7	20.7	4	10.7	8.5	7.3	10.5
1–2 years	4.5	1.8	11.3	Infinite	-	-	5.3	2.6	12.1
2–5 years	2.4	1.5	3.8	5	1.9	13.6	2.8	1.9	4.2
>5 years	2.7	2.1	3.6	6.6	3.6	12.1	3.3	2.7	4.2
Tumor site									
Solid tumors	2.6	2.2	3.5	9.1	5.4	15.2	3.4	3.0	4.3
Breast	3	1.6	5.3	7.5	2.1	26.6	3.6	2.2	5.9
Prostate	2.8	1.7	4.6	8.2	2	34.1	3.2	2.1	5.0
Colorectal	2.3	1.4	3.7	18.2	3.5	95.5	2.7	1.8	4.1
Skin Melanoma	1.4	0.54	3.8	1.5	0.17	13.5	1.4	0.6	3.8
Lung and larynx	5.1	1.8	14.1	Infinite	-	-	5.8	2.5	14.8
Thyroid	6.5	0.8	51	-	-	-	7.0	1.3	51.5
Kidney	2.2	0.6	7.5	0.46	0.04	5.6	1.2	0.1	6.5
Bladder	1.2	0.43	3.3	20.6	1.5	275	1.4	0.63	3.5
Endometrium	6.1	0.77	48.6	Infinite	-	-	10.0	4.67	52.5
Other solid cancers	3	1.7	5.2	12.4	3.2	48.8	3.7	2.4	5.9
Haematologic Malignancies	2.4	1.3	4.4	-	-	-	2.2	1.1	4.2

For hematologic malignancies, the excess risk was significant [HR 2.4; 95% CI 1.3–4.4].
In the province of Reggio Emilia (Table 2), the risk of death among unvaccinated was eight-fold higher than in vaccinated patients [HR 8.2; 95% CI 5.1–13.2]. The excess risk was higher in males [HR 12.1; 95% CI 6.0–24.5], in the 70–79 age group [HR 19.3; 95% CI 5.7–65] and in subjects diagnosed one year before vaccination [HR 20.7; 95% CI 4.0–10.7].

The excess risk in non-vaccinated people was appreciable for bladder [HR 20.6; 95% CI 1.5–27.5], colorectal [HR 18.2; 95% CI 3.5–95.5], prostate [HR 8.2; 95% CI 2.0–34.1] and breast tumours [HR 7.5; 95% CI 2.1–26.6]. For haematological malignancies, sparse data made it difficult to calculate the HRs.

When pooling data from the two cohorts, the general picture of a large excess risk of death in unvaccinated was confirmed with more than three-fold risks. Differences between sexes almost disappeared, while the higher excess risk in older patients was confirmed, while a clearer trend according to time since cancer diagnosis emerged with a stronger excess risk in newly diagnosed. The excess risk was appreciable for almost all cancer sites, but for skin melanoma, kidney cancer and bladder cancer, the excess was compatible with random fluctuations.

Table 3 shows the survivals one year and five years after a diagnosis of the cases recorded in the years 2015–2017. One year after diagnosis, Friuli Venezia Giulia presents an extremely low survival for lung cancer (44%) and low for leukemia (66%) and colorectal cancer and non-Hodgkin's lymphoma (82%); at five years, survival drops drastically for the sites studied, except breast, prostate, melanoma and thyroid cancer.

Table 3. One-year and five-year net survival (NS, %) of patients (men and women, all ages) with most frequent cancer types diagnosed in 2015–2017 (follow-up at 2021), in Friuli Venezia Giulia and in the province of Reggio Emilia, Italy.

	Friuli Venezia Giulia		Reggio Emilia	
	1-Year NS	5-Year NS	1-Year NS	5-Year NS
Tumor site				
Breast	97	90	99	92
Prostate	98	94	98	88
Colorectal	82	64	84	64
Skin Melanoma	97	91	99	91
Lung	44	17	41	16
Thyroid	96	94	94	92
Kidney	83	72	84	65
Bladder	90	77	90	76
Corpus Uteri	93	79	91	78
Non-Hodgkin lymphomas	82	70	88	72
Leukemias	66	42	76	57
All sites, but skin non-melanoma	77	62	78	61

Reggio Emilia confirms an extremely low survival for lung cancer (41%) and low for leukemia (76%) and colorectal cancer and kidney cancer (84%) one year after diagnosis; at five years, survival drops drastically for the sites studied, except for breast, prostate, melanoma and thyroid cancer.

Regarding the causes of death, available only for the province of Reggio Emilia (Supplementary Table S1), of the 103 deaths, 17%, 50% and 33% e 20%, 57% e 23% died from a tumor, COVID-19 or other causes among vaccinated and non-vaccinated patients, respectively. Supplementary Figure S2 instead shows the distribution over time between infection and death. Among the vaccinated, 71% and 88% die within 30 and 60 days of infection, respectively, while among the unvaccinated, the percents are 62% and 70%, respectively.

4. Discussion

The results of this longitudinal investigation from two population-based cohorts agree in indicating that unvaccinated cancer patients infected with SARS-CoV-2 have a risk of death approximately three times higher than the corresponding vaccinated cancer patients. When the vaccine was not yet available, the national and international literature demonstrated a higher COVID-19 mortality among patients with cancer compared to the general population [1–7,15,16].

Specifically, national data [16] showed that cancer patients had a higher chance of being hospitalized (56.6% vs. 34.4%) and dying (14.7% vs. 4.5%) from COVID-19 than the general population, confirmed by a subsequent study [6], which showed a higher risk of hospitalization [OR = 1.27; 95% CI 1.09–1.48] and death [OR = 1.45; 95% CI 1.12–1.89] in cancer patients compared to the general population, especially in the presence of metastases and in tumors diagnosed in the two years preceding the infection. A previous Friuli Venezia Giulia study [15] also confirmed the risk of death [OR = 1.63; 95% CI 1.49–1.78], but not an increased risk of hospitalization (in this case the data refers only to admissions to intensive care). Since their development and dissemination, lower immunogenicity of SARS-CoV-2 vaccines has been demonstrated in patients suffering from various forms of cancer compared to healthy populations, particularly in patients with haematological malignancies and in patients undergoing active treatments [21]. The safety profile was similar in cancer patients and the general population [22]. Vaccines and particularly mRNA vaccines [23] was shown to be effective in protecting cancer patients from severe COVID-19 [22]. It is also well-known that SARS-Cov-2 mRNA vaccines are more effective in the general population than in the tumor population and that among the latter, the immune response in hematological patients is significantly lower than in patients with solid tumors [24].

Following the spread of SARS-CoV-2 vaccines, some studies have analyzed their impact on clinical complications, including death [3,23]. In Europe, the results of the multicenter retrospective study "OnCovid Registry Study" showed a statistically significant 74% reduction in the risk of death 28 days after vaccination for vaccinated cancer patients [5]. Our findings indicate that those vaccinated within two years of a cancer diagnosis (and likely to receiving anti-cancer therapies) were at a higher risk of death—an observation in line with previous reports (1, 5).

In general, our study confirms an excess of death for unvaccinated people compared to vaccinated people, which increases with age and which presents a gradient inversely proportional to the time from cancer diagnosis.

Some of the results that emerged from our study deserve particular attention. To avoid overestimating the impact of the vaccine due to differences in testing and biases in the probability of reporting a diagnosis of COVID-19, we compared the risk of death in vaccinated and unvaccinated cancer patients who had at least one positive test for SARS-CoV-2. Nevertheless, with this approach, we only measure the effect of the vaccine on reducing the severity of the disease once the infection occurred and not the protection due to reducing the probability of having a detectable infection, which was probably also not negligible during 2021 when the dominant viral variants were alpha and delta [23], for which sustained efficacy at least in the 6 to 12 months after vaccination has been demonstrated [23,25–27]. In both Friuli Venezia Giulia and Reggio Emilia provinces, the excess risk in unvaccinated cancer patients was larger in elderly people aged 70 or more. Considering that the absolute risk of death and particularly of COVID-19-related death is particularly high in this group, the impact of the vaccine in terms of avoided death is more important than what could be inferred by the average protection of a three-fold reduction observed overall. As well, it is worth noting that the excess risk is highest in patients in one to two years from diagnosis, and it is also well appreciable in the first year after cancer diagnosis, the periods when cancer-related mortality is higher [28]. The stronger protection observed in the most fragile patients is probably due to the early vaccination of these groups, i.e., in January and February 2021, when the alpha peak was rising in Italy and both risks of infection, mortality and fatality rate among reported cases were particularly high [29]. A similar effect has been observed in the general population in Reggio Emilia [19]. Different timing of vaccination relative to different epidemiology of epidemic waves could explain the reason for the different protection observed in Friuli Venezia Giulia and Reggio Emilia. In fact, in Reggio Emilia the proportion of patients who were vaccinated after the infection was higher than in Friuli Venezia Giulia, suggesting that infections in early 2021 were more important than those during autumn 2021 in Reggio Emilia compared to Friuli Venezia Giulia. We know that the vaccine was more effective against alpha infections and that it partially lost its effectiveness in late autumn 2021 [19,25–27]. Nevertheless, the protection is high in both cohorts.

As far as individual tumor sites are concerned, an excess risk of death for hematological tumors compared to solid tumors is confirmed in both settings studied. As regards solid neoplasms, Friuli Venezia Giulia shows an excess of deaths among the unvaccinated for lung cancers and, subsequently, breast, prostate and colorectal cancers. For Reggio Emilia, an excess of risk for bladder, colorectal and breast is confirmed. The excess risk for lung cancer, already described in the literature [30], was evident only in Friuli Venezia Giulia, suggesting that early hospitalization in Reggio perhaps had a protective effect on mortality [6].

The effect is appreciable in almost all cancer sites, and the few exceptions are largely compatible with random fluctuations. Our data do not confirm a lower vaccine efficacy in patients with haematological patients [21]. Nevertheless, due to very few deaths, we could not assess differences for specific hematological malignancies.

Among the limitations of the study, we must point out that we have no information on the stage of the tumors or on the severity of the COVID-19 infection. Furthermore, information on comorbidities that may have played an important role in the evolution of the disease is lacking.

Among the strengths of this study is the complete observation of the resident population both in the Friuli Venezia Giulia Region and in the province of Reggio Emilia thanks to the availability of complete and accurate health databases. This allowed for all RT-PCR tests for SARS-CoV-2 to be included during the study period. Another strength of the study was the use of data from two population-based cancer registries with a long history and a high-quality standard in terms of completeness and accuracy of the data collected.

5. Conclusions

In conclusion, this investigation shows that vaccination significantly reduces the risk of death of people with cancer who are infected with SARS-CoV-2.

Supplementary Materials: The following supporting information can be downloaded at: https://www.mdpi.com/article/10.3390/jpm13091333/s1, Figure S1. Distribution of death by infection' time, by vaccination status: 79 non vaccinated and 24 vaccinated. Data from Reggio Emilia, 2021. Table S1. Distribution of causes of death between vaccinated and unvaccinated. Data from Reggio Emilia.

Author Contributions: Conceptualization, investigation, writing—original draft, visualization, supervision, L.M., P.G.R., D.S. and M.G.; formal analysis, M.T., F.T., P.M. and M.O.; writing—review and editing, and visualization, supervision L.D.M., I.B.; investigation, supervision, conceptualization, writing—original draft, investigation, and management, A.N., E.C. and S.D.Z. All authors have read and agreed to the published version of the manuscript.

Funding: This study was partially supported by the Italian Ministry of Health—Ricerca Corrente Annual Program 2024, Line 2 for CRO-IRCCS Aviano and line 3 for AUSL-IRCCS di Reggio Emilia.

Institutional Review Board Statement: The study was approved by the Bioethics Committee of the Veneto Region (protocol No. 245343/2020) and by the Area Vasta Emilia Nord Ethic Committee (protocol No. 2020/0045199), furthermore, Reggio Emilia Cancer Registry procedures and scope have been approved by the Ethics Committee of Reggio Emilia (protocol No. 2014/0019740), and was conducted through a record linkage procedure of de-identified data with the use of a semi-annually modified anonymous individual key.

Informed Consent Statement: Not applicable.

Data Availability Statement: The data presented in this study are available on request from the corresponding author. The data are not publicly available due to ethical and privacy issues; requests for data must be approved by the Ethics Committee after the presentation of a study protocol.

Conflicts of Interest: The authors declare that the research was conducted without any commercial or financial relationships construed as a potential conflict of interest.

References

1. Grivas, P.; Khaki, A.R.; Wise-Draper, T.M.; French, B.; Hennessy, C.; Hsu, C.-Y.; Shyr, Y.; Li, X.; Choueiri, T.; Painter, C.; et al. Association of clinical factors and recent anticancer therapy with COVID-19 severity among patients with cancer: A report from the COVID-19 and Cancer Consortium. *Ann. Oncol.* **2021**, *32*, 787–800. [CrossRef]
2. Kuderer, N.M.; Choueiri, T.K.; Shah, D.P.; Shyr, Y.; Rubinstein, S.M.; Rivera, D.R.; Shete, S.; Hsu, C.-Y.; Desai, A.; de Lima Lopes, G., Jr.; et al. Clinical impact of COVID-19 on patients with cancer (CCC19): A cohort study. *Lancet* **2020**, *395*, 1907–1918.e2. [CrossRef]
3. Addeo, A.; Shah, P.K.; Bordry, N.; Hudson, R.D.; Albracht, B.; Di Marco, M.; Kaklamani, V.; Dietrich, P.-Y.; Taylor, B.S.; Simand, P.-F.; et al. Immunogenicity of SARS-CoV-2 messenger RNA vaccines in patients with cancer. *Cancer Cell* **2021**, *39*, 1091–1098. [CrossRef] [PubMed]
4. Pinato, D.J.; Tabernero, J.; Bower, M.; Scotti, L.; Patel, M.; Colomba, E.; Dolly, S.; Loizidou, A.; Chester, P.J.; Mukherjee, U.; et al. Prevalence and impact of COVId-19 sequelae on treatment and survival of patients with cancer who recovered from SARS-CoV-2 infection: Evidence from the OnCovid retrospective, multicentre registry study. *Lancet Oncol.* **2021**, *22*, 1668–1680. [CrossRef]
5. Pinato, D.J.; Aguilar-Company, J.; Ferrante, D.; Hanbury, G.; Bower, M.; Salazar, R.; Mirallas, O.; Sureda, A.; Plaja, A.; Cucurull, M.; et al. Outcomes of the SARS-CoV-2 omicron (B.1.1.529) variant outbreak among vaccinated and unvaccinated patients with cancer in Europe: Results from the retrospective, multicentre, OnCovid registry study. *Lancet Oncol.* **2022**, *23*, 865–875. [CrossRef] [PubMed]
6. Mangone, L.; Gioia, F.; Mancuso, P.; Bisceglia, I.; Ottone, M.; Vicentini, M.; Pinto, C.; Rossi, P.G. CumulativeCOVID-19 incidence, mortality and prognosis in cancer survivors: A population-based study in Reggio Emilia, Northern Italy. *Int. J. Cancer* **2021**, *149*, 820–826. [CrossRef] [PubMed]
7. Tian, Y.; Qiu, X.; Wang, C.; Zhao, J.; Jiang, X.; Niu, W.; Huang, J.; Zhang, F. Cancer associates with risk and severe events of COVID-19: A systematic review and meta-analysis. *Int. J. Cancer* **2020**, *148*, 363–374. [CrossRef]
8. Giannakoulis, V.G.; Papoutsi, E.; Siempos, I.I. Effect of Cancer on Clinical Outcomes of Patients With COVID-19: A Meta-Analysis of Patient Data. *JCO Glob. Oncol.* **2020**, *6*, 799–808. [CrossRef]
9. Ferroni, E.; Rossi, P.G.; Alegiani, S.S.; Trifirò, G.; Pitter, G.; Leoni, O.; Cereda, D.; Marino, M.; Pellizzari, M.; Fabiani, M.; et al. Survival of Hospitalized COVID-19 Patients in Northern Italy: A Population-Based Cohort Study by the ITA-COVID-19 Network. *Clin. Epidemiol.* **2020**, *12*, 1337–1346. [CrossRef]
10. Fendler, A.; Shepherd, S.T.C.; Au, L.; Wilkinson, K.A.; Wu, M.; Byrne, F.; Cerrone, M.; Schmitt, A.M.; Joharatnam-Hogan, N.; Shum, B.; et al. Adaptive immunity and neutralizing antibodies against SARS-CoV-2 variants of concern following vaccination in patients with cancer: The CAPTURE study. *Nat. Cancer* **2021**, *2*, 1305–1320. [CrossRef]
11. Becerril-Gaitan, A.; Vaca-Cartagena, B.F.; Ferrigno, A.S.; Mesa-Chavez, F.; Barrientos-Gutiérrez, T.; Tagliamento, M.; Lambertini, M.; Villarreal-Garza, C. Immunogenicity and risk of Severe Acute Respiratory Syndrome Coronavirus 2 (SARS-CoV-2) infection after Coronavirus Disease 2019 (COVID-19) vaccination in patients with cancer: A systematic review and meta-analysis. *Eur. J. Cancer* **2022**, *160*, 243–260. [CrossRef] [PubMed]
12. Carle, C.; Hughes, S.; Freeman, V.; Campbell, D.; Egger, S.; Caruana, M.; Hui, H.; Yap, S.; Deandrea, S.; Onyeka, T.C.; et al. The risk of contracting SARS-CoV-2 or developing COVID-19 for people with cancer: A systematic review of the early evidence. *J. Cancer Policy* **2022**, *33*, 100338. [CrossRef] [PubMed]
13. Castelo-Branco, L.; Cervantes, A.; Curigliano, G.; Garassino, M.C.; Giesen, N.; Grivas, P.; Haanen, J.; Jordan, K.; Gerd Liebert, U.; Lordick, F.; et al. ESMO Statements on Vaccination against COVID-19 in People with Cancer. Available online: https://www.esmo.org/covid-19-and-cancer/covid-19-vaccination (accessed on 7 August 2023).
14. Mauri, D.; Kamposioras, K.; Tsali, L.; Dambrosio, M.; De Bari, B.; Hindi, N.; Salembier, C.; Nixon, J.; Dimitrios, T.; Alongi, F.; et al. COVID-19 Vaccinations: Summary Guidance for Cancer Patients in 28 Languages: Breaking Barriers to Cancer Patient Information. *Rev. Recent Clin. Trials* **2022**, *17*, 11–14. [CrossRef] [PubMed]
15. Serraino, D.; Zucchetto, A.; Maso, L.D.; Del Zotto, S.; Taboga, F.; Clagnan, E.; Fratino, L.; Tosolini, F.; Burba, I. Prevalence, determinants, and outcomes of SARS-CoV-2 infection among cancer patients. A population-based study in northern Italy. *Cancer Med.* **2021**, *10*, 7781–7792. [CrossRef]
16. Rugge, M.; Zorzi, M.; Guzzinati, S. SARS-CoV-2 infection in the Italian Veneto region: Adverse outcomes in patients with cancer. *Nat. Cancer* **2020**, *1*, 784–788. [CrossRef]
17. Available online: https://www.aiom.it/documento-aiom-cipomo-comu-vaccinazione-covid-19-per-i-pazienti-oncologici/ (accessed on 7 August 2023).

18. Calagnan, E.; Gobbato, M.; Burba, I.; Del Zotto, S.; Toffolutti, F.; Serraino, D.; Tonutti, G. COVID-19 infections in the Friuli Venezia Giulia Region (Northern Italy): A population-based retrospective analysis. *Epidemiol. Prev.* **2021**, *44* (Suppl. S2), 323–329.
19. Vicentini, M.; Venturelli, F.; Mancuso, P.; Bisaccia, E.; Zerbini, A.; Massari, M.; Cossarizza, A.; De Biasi, S.; Pezzotti, P.; Bedeschi, E.; et al. Risk of SARS-CoV-2 reinfection by vaccination status, predominant variant and time from prior infection: A cohort study, Reggio Emilia province, Italy, February 2020 to February 2022. *Eurosurveillance* **2023**, *28*, 2200494. [CrossRef]
20. Gobbato, M.; Clagnan, E.; Toffolutti, F.; Del Zotto, S.; Burba, I.; Tosolini, F.; Polimeni, J.; Serraino, D.; Taborelli, M. Vaccination against SARS-CoV-2 and risk of hospital admission and death among infected cancer patients: A population-based study in northern Italy. *Cancer Epidemiol.* **2023**, *82*, 102318. [CrossRef]
21. Li, H.-J.; Yang, Q.-C.; Yao, Y.-Y.; Huang, C.-Y.; Yin, F.-Q.; Xian-Yu, C.-Y.; Zhang, C.; Chen, S.-J. COVID-19 vaccination effectiveness and safety in vulnerable populations: A meta-analysis of 33 observational studies. *Front. Pharmacol.* **2023**, *14*, 1144824. [CrossRef]
22. Shear, S.; Shams, K.; Weisberg, J.; Hamidi, N.; Scott, S. COVID-19 Vaccination Safety Profiles in Patients With Solid Tumour Cancers: A Systematic Review. *Clin. Oncol.* **2023**, *35*, e421–e433. [CrossRef]
23. Oosting, S.F.; Van der Veldt, A.A.M.; GeurtsvanKessel, C.H.; Fehrmann, R.S.N.; van Binnendijk, R.S.; Dingemans, A.-M.C.; Smit, E.F.; Hiltermann, T.J.N.; Hartog, G.D.; Jalving, M.; et al. mRNA-1273 COVID-19 vaccination in patients receiving chemotherapy, immunotherapy, or chemoimmunotherapy for solid tumours: A prospective, multicentre, non-inferiority trial. *Lancet Oncol.* **2021**, *22*, 1681–1691. [CrossRef] [PubMed]
24. Fendler, A.; Au, L.; Shepherd, S.T.C.; Byrne, F.; Cerrone, M.; Boos, L.A.; Rzeniewicz, K.; Gordon, W.; Shum, B.; Gerard, C.L.; et al. Functional antibody and T-cell immunity following SARS-CoV-2 infection, including by variants of concern, in patients with cancer: The CAPTURE study. *Res Sq.* **2021**, *3*, rs-916427; Update in: *Nat. Cancer* **2021**, *2*, 1321–1337. [CrossRef] [PubMed]
25. Fabiani, M.; Puopolo, M.; Morciano, C.; Spuri, M.; Alegiani, S.S.; Filia, A.; D'ancona, F.; Del Manso, M.; Riccardo, F.; Tallon, M.; et al. Effectiveness of mRNA vaccines and waning of protection against SARS-CoV-2 infection and severe COVID-19 during predominant circulation of the delta variant in Italy: Retrospective cohort study. *BMJ* **2022**, *376*, e069052. [CrossRef] [PubMed]
26. Mateo-Urdiales, A.; Alegiani, S.S.; Fabiani, M.; Pezzotti, P.; Filia, A.; Massari, M.; Riccardo, F.; Tallon, M.; Proietti, V.; Del Manso, M.; et al. Risk of SARS-CoV-2 infection and subsequent hospital admission and death at different time intervals since first dose of COVID-19 vaccine administration, Italy, 27 December 2020 to mid-April 2021. *Eurosurveillance* **2021**, *26*, 2100507. [CrossRef]
27. Kahn, F.; Bonander, C.; Moghaddassi, M.; Rasmussen, M.; Malmqvist, U.; Inghammar, M.; Björk, J. Risk of severe COVID-19 from the Delta and Omicron variants in relation to vaccination status, sex, age and comorbidities—Surveillance results from southern Sweden, July 2021 to January 2022. *Eurosurveillance* **2022**, *27*, 2200121. [CrossRef] [PubMed]
28. Coviello, V.; Buzzoni, C.; Fusco, M.; Barchielli, A.; Cuccaro, F.; De Angelis, R.; Giacomin, A.; Luminari, S.; Randi, G.; Mangone, L.; et al. Survival of cancer patients in Italy. *Epidemiol. Prev.* **2017**, *41* (Suppl. S1), 1–244. [CrossRef] [PubMed]
29. Ceccarelli, E.; Dorrucci, M.; Minelli, G.; Lasinio, G.J.; Prati, S.; Battaglini, M.; Corsetti, G.; Bella, A.; Boros, S.; Petrone, D.; et al. Assessing COVID-19-Related Excess Mortality Using Multiple Approaches—Italy, 2020–2021. *Int. J. Environ. Res. Public Health* **2022**, *19*, 16998. [CrossRef]
30. Tagliamento, M.; Agostinetto, E.; Bruzzone, M.; Ceppi, M.; Saini, K.S.; de Azambuja, E.; Punie, K.; Westphalen, C.B.; Morgan, G.; Pronzato, P.; et al. Mortality in adult patients with solid or hematological malignancies and SARS-CoV-2 infection with a specific focus on lung and breast cancers: A systematic review and meta-analysis. *Crit. Rev. Oncol. Hematol.* **2021**, *163*, 103365. [CrossRef]

Disclaimer/Publisher's Note: The statements, opinions and data contained in all publications are solely those of the individual author(s) and contributor(s) and not of MDPI and/or the editor(s). MDPI and/or the editor(s) disclaim responsibility for any injury to people or property resulting from any ideas, methods, instructions or products referred to in the content.

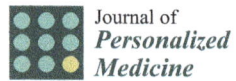

Article

Imaging Severity COVID-19 Assessment in Vaccinated and Unvaccinated Patients: Comparison of the Different Variants in a High Volume Italian Reference Center

Vincenza Granata [1], Roberta Fusco [2,*], Alberta Villanacci [3], Simona Magliocchetti [4], Fabrizio Urraro [4], Nardi Tetaj [5], Luisa Marchioni [5], Fabrizio Albarello [3], Paolo Campioni [3], Massimo Cristofaro [3], Federica Di Stefano [3], Nicoletta Fusco [3], Ada Petrone [3], Vincenzo Schininà [3], Francesca Grassi [4,6], Enrico Girardi [7] and Stefania Ianniello [3]

[1] Division of Radiology, Istituto Nazionale Tumori IRCCS Fondazione Pascale—IRCCS di Napoli, 80131 Naples, Italy; v.granata@istitutotumori.na.it
[2] Medical Oncology Division, Igea SpA, 80013 Napoli, Italy
[3] Diagnostic Imaging of Infectious Diseases, National Institute for Infectious Diseases Lazzaro Spallanzani IRCCS, 00149 Rome, Italy; alberta.villanacci@inmi.it (A.V.); fabrizio.albarello@inmi.it (F.A.); paolo.campioni@inmi.it (P.C.); massimo.cristofaro@inmi.it (M.C.); federica.distefano@inmi.it (F.D.S.); nicoletta.fusco@inmi.it (N.F.); ada.petrone@inmi.it (A.P.); vincenzo.schinina@inmi.it (V.S.); stefania.ianniello@inmi.it (S.I.)
[4] Division of Radiology, Università degli Studi della Campania Luigi Vanvitelli, 80128 Naples, Italy; simona.magliocchetti@unicampania.it (S.M.); fabrizio.urraro@unicampania.it (F.U.); francescagrassi1996@gmail.com (F.G.)
[5] Intensive Care Unit, National Institute for Infectious Diseases Lazzaro Spallanzani IRCCS, 00149 Rome, Italy; nardi.tetaj@inmi.it (N.T.); luisa.marchioni@inmi.it (L.M.)
[6] Italian Society of Medical and Interventional Radiology (SIRM), SIRM Foundation, Via Della Signora 2, 20122 Milan, Italy
[7] Department of Epidemiology and Research, National Institute for Infectious Diseases Lazzaro Spallanzani IRCCS, 00149 Rome, Italy; enrico.girardi@inmi.it
* Correspondence: r.fusco@igeamedical.com

Citation: Granata, V.; Fusco, R.; Villanacci, A.; Magliocchetti, S.; Urraro, F.; Tetaj, N.; Marchioni, L.; Albarello, F.; Campioni, P.; Cristofaro, M.; et al. Imaging Severity COVID-19 Assessment in Vaccinated and Unvaccinated Patients: Comparison of the Different Variants in a High Volume Italian Reference Center. *J. Pers. Med.* **2022**, *12*, 955. https://doi.org/10.3390/jpm12060955

Academic Editor: Franco M. Buonaguro

Received: 28 April 2022
Accepted: 9 June 2022
Published: 10 June 2022

Publisher's Note: MDPI stays neutral with regard to jurisdictional claims in published maps and institutional affiliations.

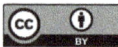

Copyright: © 2022 by the authors. Licensee MDPI, Basel, Switzerland. This article is an open access article distributed under the terms and conditions of the Creative Commons Attribution (CC BY) license (https://creativecommons.org/licenses/by/4.0/).

Abstract: Purpose: To analyze the vaccine effect by comparing five groups: unvaccinated patients with Alpha variant, unvaccinated patients with Delta variant, vaccinated patients with Delta variant, unvaccinated patients with Omicron variant, and vaccinated patients with Omicron variant, assessing the "gravity" of COVID-19 pulmonary involvement, based on CT findings in critically ill patients admitted to Intensive Care Unit (ICU). Methods: Patients were selected by ICU database considering the period from December 2021 to 23 March 2022, according to the following inclusion criteria: patients with proven Omicron variant COVID-19 infection with known COVID-19 vaccination with at least two doses and with chest Computed Tomography (CT) study during ICU hospitalization. Wee also evaluated the ICU database considering the period from March 2020 to December 2021, to select unvaccinated consecutive patients with Alpha variant, subjected to CT study, consecutive unvaccinated and vaccinated patients with Delta variant, subjected to CT study, and, consecutive unvaccinated patients with Omicron variant, subjected to CT study. CT images were evaluated qualitatively using a severity score scale of 5 levels (none involvement, mild: ≤25% of involvement, moderate: 26–50% of involvement, severe: 51–75% of involvement, and critical involvement: 76–100%) and quantitatively, using the Philips IntelliSpace Portal clinical application CT COPD computer tool. For each patient the lung volumetry was performed identifying the percentage value of aerated residual lung volume. Non-parametric tests for continuous and categorical variables were performed to assess statistically significant differences among groups. Results: The patient study group was composed of 13 vaccinated patients affected by the Omicron variant (Omicron V). As control groups we identified: 20 unvaccinated patients with Alpha variant (Alpha NV); 20 unvaccinated patients with Delta variant (Delta NV); 18 vaccinated patients with Delta variant (Delta V); and 20 unvaccinated patients affected by the Omicron variant (Omicron NV). No differences between the groups under examination were found (p value > 0.05 at Chi square test) in terms of risk factors (age, cardiovascular diseases, diabetes, immunosuppression, chronic kidney, cardiac, pulmonary, neurologic, and liver disease, etc.). A different median value of aerated residual lung volume was observed in the Delta variant groups: median value of aerated residual lung volume was 46.70% in unvaccinated patients compared to 67.10% in vaccinated patients. In addition, in patients with Delta variant every other extracted volume by automatic tool showed a statistically significant difference between vaccinated and unvaccinated group. Statistically significant differences were observed for each extracted volume by automatic tool between unvaccinated patients affected by Alpha variant and vaccinated patients affected by Delta variant of COVID-19. Good statistically significant correlations among volumes extracted by automatic tool for each lung lobe and overall radiological severity score were obtained (ICC range 0.71–0.86). GGO was the main sign of COVID-19 lesions on CT images found in 87 of the 91 (95.6%) patients. No statistically significant differences were observed in CT findings (ground glass opacities (GGO), consolidation or crazy paving sign) among patient groups. Conclusion: In our study, we showed that in critically ill patients no difference were observed in terms of severity of disease or exitus, between unvaccinated and vaccinated patients. The only statistically significant differences were observed, with regard to the severity of COVID-19 pulmonary parenchymal involvement, between unvaccinated patients affected by Alpha variant and vaccinated patients affected by Delta variant, and between unvaccinated patients with Delta variant and vaccinated patients with Delta variant.

Keywords: COVID-19; vaccination; Computed Tomography

1. Introduction

Over two years after the first described SARS-CoV-2 patient, the COVID-19 pandemic is still ongoing, with many countries undergoing new infection waves [1–12]. Extensive vaccination promotion is underway all over the world, although with extremely variable levels of population coverage [1,13–24]. In addition, the pandemic perseveres with the appearance of new variants that could compromise diagnostic tests and vaccine efficacy. Developing evidence has demonstrated that these variants are able to evade the action of neutralizing antibodies [25–43]. Evidence of declining vaccine immunity over time has also arisen: following the second dose, there is a substantial decline in efficacy against symptomatic infection; from a peak of ~90% in the weeks immediately following to a much lower 50–80% six months after vaccination [44–48]. Consequently, several nations are proposing booster vaccinations. Data from these countries have proven the benefit of a booster dose in reducing symptomatic infection and offering a significant decrease in critical outcomes [49–54]. Moreover, the protection level offered by previous SARS-CoV-2 infection, both in terms of infection and disease severity and, therefore, of outcome, is still unclear [55–61]. In this scenario, the main essential element leading to the evolution of SARS-CoV-2 infection is the interaction with the host's immune system. However, there is a need to understand how the new variants can lead to severe forms of the disease, as well as how the time elapsed since vaccination can impact the outcome. An assessment of disease severity requires tools that can objectify the data to reduce the variability between patients due to qualitative evaluation. As to the "gravity assessment" of COVID-19 infection and evaluation of pulmonary parenchymal involvement, several scores have been proposed [62,63]. The main goal of these tools is to establish a well-defined strategy for evaluation of the airways and lungs of COVID-19 positive patients from Computed Tomography (CT) scans, including detected abnormalities [64–74]. Their identification and the volumetric quantification may allow an easier classification in terms of gravity, extent and progression of the disease. Moreover, this may provide a high-impact tool to enhance awareness of the severity of COVID-19 pneumonia [75–90].

In this retrospective cohort study, we aim to analyze the vaccine effect by comparing five groups: (a) unvaccinated patients with Alpha variant; (b) unvaccinated patients with Delta variant; (c) vaccinated patients with Delta variant; (d) unvaccinated patients with Omicron variant; and (e) vaccinated patients with Omicron variant, assessing the "gravity" of COVID-19 pulmonary involvement, based on CT findings in critically ill patients admitted to Intensive Care Unit (ICU).

2. Materials and Methods

2.1. Patient Characteristics

The study was conducted according to the guidelines of the Declaration of Helsinki and approved by the Institutional Ethics Committee of IRCCS L. Spallanzani. Data acquisition and analysis were performed in compliance with protocols approved by the Ethical Committee of the National Institute for Infectious Diseases IRCCS Lazzaro Spallanzani, Rome, Italy (ethical approval number 164, 26 June 2020). The Local Ethical Committee board renounced patient informed consent, considering the ongoing epidemic emergency.

Patients were selected from the Intensive Care Unit (ICU) database considering the period from December 2021 to 23 March 2022, having COVID-19 infection variant sequencing, according to the following inclusion criteria: (1) patients with proven Omicron variant COVID-19 infection; (2) patients with known COVID-19 vaccination with at least two doses; (3) patients with chest CT study during ICU hospitalization. The exclusion criteria were: (1) no CT study, (2) patients with no data on COVID-19 vaccination status.

We also evaluated the ICU database considering the period from March 2020 to December 2021, to select unvaccinated consecutive patients with Alpha variant, subjected to CT study; consecutive unvaccinated patients with Delta variant, subjected to CT study; consecutive vaccinated patients with Delta variant, subjected to CT study; consecutive unvaccinated patients with Omicron variant, subjected to CT study.

2.2. CT Technique

Chest CT scan was performed with 128 slices using Incisive Philips CT scanners (Amsterdam, The Netherlands). CT examinations were performed with the patient in the supine position in breath-hold, and inspiration using a standard dose protocol, without contrast intravenous injection. The scanning range was from the apex to the base of the lungs. The tube voltage and the current tube were 120 kV and 100–200 mA (and if applicable, using z-axis tube current modulation), respectively. All data were reconstructed with a 0.6–1.0 mm increment. The matrix was 512 mm × 512 mm. Images were reconstructed using a sharp reconstruction kernel for parenchyma evaluation and hard reconstruction kernel for other lung evaluation. All data were reconstructed with a 0.6–1.0 mm increment. Multiplanar reconstruction (MPR) was also obtained.

2.3. CT Post Processing

DICOM data were transferred into a PACS workstation and CT images were evaluated using the Philips IntelliSpace Portal clinical application CT COPD (Philips Eindihoven, The Netherlands) computer tool.

Philips IntelliSpace Portal clinical application CT COPD software is a CE-marked medical device designed to quantify pulmonary emphysema in patients with chronic obstructive pulmonary disease. The tool provides segmentation of the lungs and of the airway tree. Moreover, the tool helps visualize and quantify the destructive process of diffuse lung disease (e.g., emphysema), providing a guided workflow for airway analysis, reviewing and measuring airway lumen, and assessing trapped air. Compared to others tools, it allows assessment consolidation. For each patient the lung volumetry was performed identifying the percentage value of aerated residual lung volume, and for each lung lobe: right upper lobe volume, right lower lobe volume, medium lobe volume, left upper lobe volume, left lower lobe volume (Figures 1 and 2).

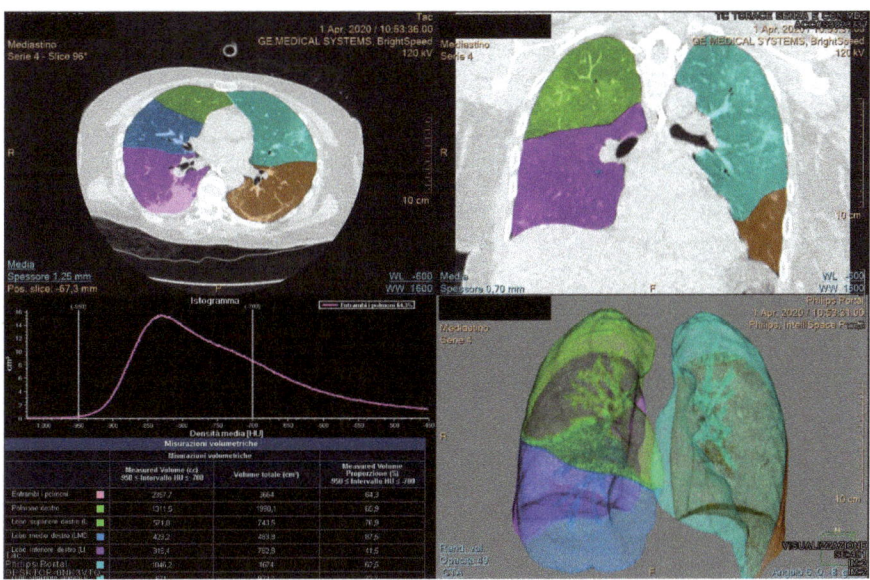

Figure 1. Example 1 of Quantitative assessment of COVID-19 pulmonary parenchymal involvement by automatic tool.

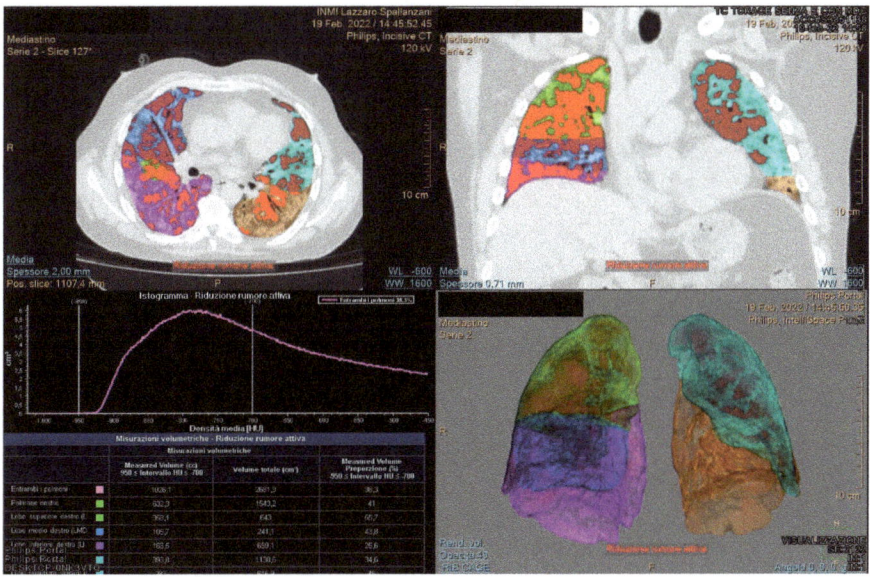

Figure 2. Example 2 of Quantitative assessment of COVID-19 pulmonary parenchymal involvement by automatic tool.

Disease severity was assessed by considering the percentage of aerated residual lung volume: patients with lower aerated residual lung volume were considered more compromised.

2.4. Radiologists' Analysis

Radiologists attributed for each lung lobe (right upper and lower lobe, medium lobe, left upper and lower lobe) a severity score using a scale of 5 levels (no involvement, mild: $\leq 25\%$ of involvement, moderate: 26–50% of involvement, severe: 51–75% of involvement and critic involvement: 76–100%) as reported in Li et al. [91]. Moreover, an overall radiological severity score was obtained summing the scores for each lung lobe and then considering a low severity ≤ 5, mild severity 6–10, moderate 11–15, severe 16–20 and critical 21–25. Two radiologists with more than 10 years of thoracic-imaging analysis experience evaluated the severity of images in a double-blind manner. Another, more experienced, radiologist resolved any disagreement between the two radiologists determining a radiological consensus.

In addition, a qualitative assessment including the evaluation of the following CT findings, ground glass opacities (GGOs), consolidation and crazy paving, was defined according to the Fleischner Society glossary [92].

2.5. Statistical Analysis

Continuous data were expressed in terms of median values and range. Chi square test, Mann Whitney test and Kruskal Wallis test were used to verify differences among groups. Intraclass correlation coefficient was used to analyze the correlations and variability among quantitative measurements generated by automatic tool and radiological severity score.

Bonferroni correction was considered for multiple comparisons.

p value < 0.05 was considered significant for all tests.

The statistical analyses were performed using the Statistics and Machine Toolbox of MATLAB R2021b (MathWorks, Natick, MA, USA).

3. Results

According to the inclusion and exclusion criteria, the patient study group was composed of 13 vaccinated patients affected by the Omicron variant (Omicron V). As control groups we identified: 20 unvaccinated patients with Alpha variant (Alpha NV); 20 unvaccinated patients with Delta variant (Delta NV); 18 vaccinated patients with Delta variant (Delta V); and 20 unvaccinated patients affected by the Omicron variant (Omicron NV). Mean age and sex distribution for each group is reported in Table 1.

Table 1. Demographic and CT findings of Patients in the Study.

Characteristic	Alpha Variant $n = 20$	Unvaccinated Delta Variant $n = 20$	Unvaccinated Delta Variant $n = 18$	Unvaccinated Omicron Variant $n = 20$	Vaccinated Omicron Variant $n = 13$	p Value
Age (y)						
Mean	62	58	64	69	75	0.07
Range	43–78	37–83	35–87	42–88	55–94	
Sex, no. (%) of patients						
Male	14	17	15	13	12	0.43
Female	6	3	3	7	1	
CT Findings						
GGO	19	20	16	19	13	0.89
Crazy Paving	17	20	14	16	11	0.10
Consolidation	15	17	11	16	11	0.70
Exitus	5	5	6	4	5	0.95

Note. p value was evaluated for continuous variable by Mann Whitney test and by Chi square test for categorical variables.

No differences between the groups under examination were found (p value > 0.05 at Chi square test) in terms of risk factors (cardiovascular diseases, diabetes, immunosuppression, chronic kidney, cardiac, pulmonary, neurologic, and liver disease, etc.).

The patient distribution with median value of aerated residual lung volume for each subgroup is reported in Table 2 and Figure 3.

Table 2. Patient distribution and median value of aerated residual lung volume for each subgroup.

		Unvaccinated	Vaccinated with 2 Doses	Vaccinated with 3 Doses	p Value
Patients with Alpha Variant	Number of patients	20	0	0	0.001
Patients with Delta variant		20	16	2	
Patients with Omicron		20	8	5	
Patients with Alpha Variant	Median value of (range) of Aerated residual lung volume [%]	39.95 (19.40–67.50)	-	-	0.05
Patients with Delta variant		46.7 (13.60–75.60)	67.10 (17.10–89.80)	52.00 (19.40–84.50)	
Patients with Omicron		48.35 (8.20–83.30)	38.30 (18.90–73.30)	61.9 (31.60–73.60)	

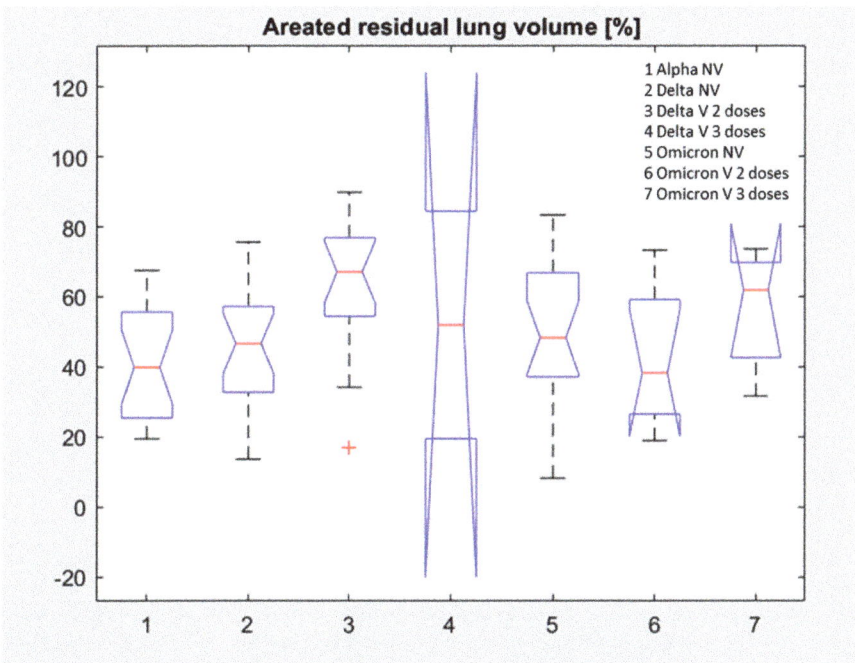

Figure 3. Distribution of aerated residual lung volume for each subgroup.

No statistically significant differences were observed between unvaccinated and vaccinated patients with Omicron variant for aerated residual lung volume, right upper lobe volume, right lower lobe volume, medium lobe volume, left upper lobe volume, or left lower lobe volume in percentage values: p value > 0.05 with Kruskal Wallis test (see boxplots in Figure 4, Table 3).

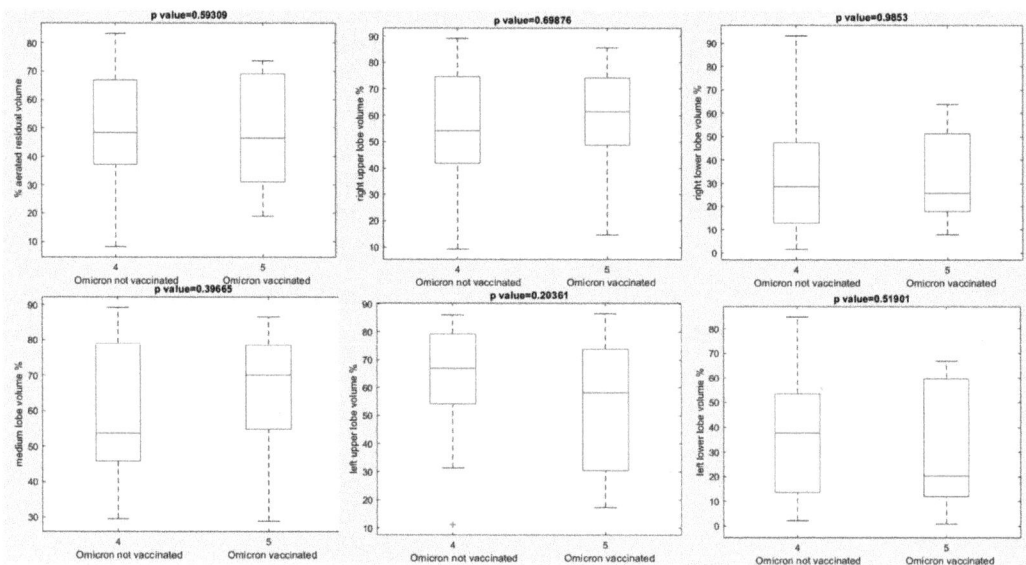

Figure 4. Boxplots of extracted volumes by automatic tool between vaccinated and unvaccinated patients affected by Omicron Variant of COVID-19.

Table 3. Median values of extracted volumes by automatic tool patients affected by Alpha, Delta or Omicron Variant of COVID-19 grouped by vaccination or no vaccination.

	Aerated Residual Volume %	Right Upper Lobe Volume %	Right Lower Lobe Volume %	Medium Lobe Volume %	Left Upper Lobe Volume %	Left Lower Lobe Volume %
Alpha	39.95	47.30	26.00	64.40	55.00	25.05
Unvaccinated	39.95	47.30	26.00	64.40	55.00	25.05
Delta	55.25	56.2	58.35	72.9	32.75	56
Unvaccinated	46.70	39.20	51.30	60.15	23.45	46.65
Vaccinated	67.10	66.50	71.55	83.50	57.00	66.80
Omicron	46.4	46.8	59	68.4	26.9	50
Unvaccinated	48.35	42.2	54.2	53.65	28.65	51.65
Vaccinated	46.4	49.8	61.4	70.1	25.7	45.1
p value at Kruskal Wallis test	0.03	0.06	0.06	0.04	0.004	0.12

A different median value of aerated residual lung volume was observed in the Delta variant groups: median value of aerated residual lung volume was 46.70% in unvaccinated patients compared to 67.10% in vaccinated patients (*p* value = 0.01 with Kruskal Wallis test). In addition, in patients with Delta variant every other extracted volume by automatic tool showed a statistically significant difference between vaccinated and unvaccinated group (see boxplots in Figure 5, Table 3): *p* value at Kruskal Wallis test = 0.02, 0.02, 0.02, 0.03, 0.03, respectively, for percentage values of right upper lobe volume, right lower lobe volume, medium lobe volume, left upper lobe volume and left lower lobe volume.

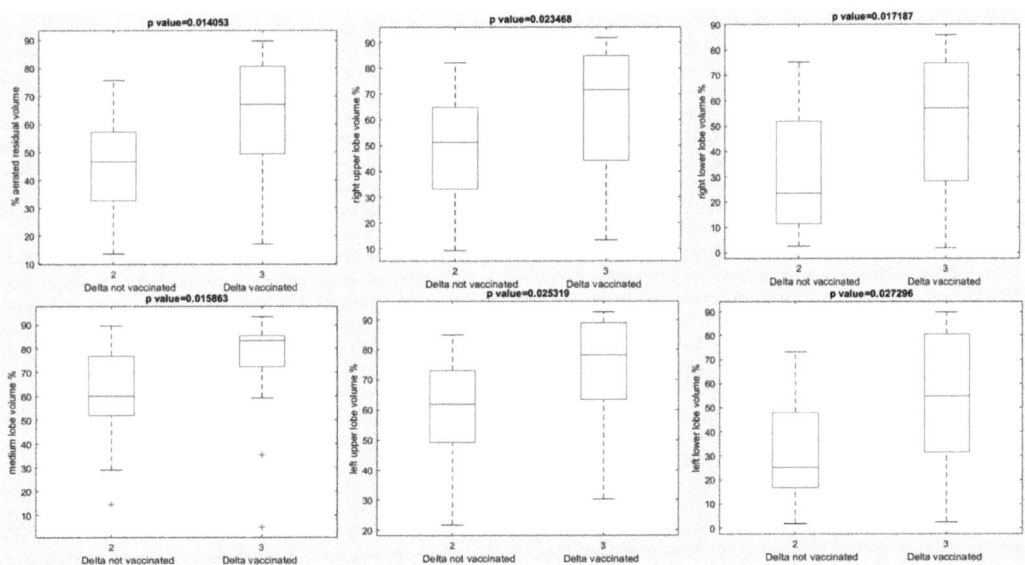

Figure 5. Boxplots of extracted volumes by automatic tool between vaccinated and unvaccinated patients affected by Delta Variant of COVID-19.

No statistically significant differences were observed in terms of aerated residual lung volume among vaccinated or unvaccinated patients with Delta and vaccinated or unvaccinated patients with Omicron variant (p value > 0.05 with Kruskal Wallis test, Figure 6). The only statistically significant differences were observed between vaccinated patients with Delta variant and vaccinated patients with Omicron variant for the right upper lobe volume, medium lobe volume and left lower lobe volume with a p value at Kruskal Wallis test, respectively, of 0.04, 0.03 and 0.01 (Figure 7) and between vaccinated patients with Delta variant and unvaccinated patients with Omicron variant for the right upper lobe volume and medium lobe volume with a p value for Kruskal Wallis test, respectively, of 0.03 and 0.02 (Figure 8).

No difference was observed in terms of each extracted volumes by automatic tool (aerated residual lung volume, right upper lobe volume, right lower lobe volume, medium lobe volume, left upper lobe volume, left lower lobe volume) between unvaccinated patients with the Alpha variant versus vaccinated or unvaccinated patients with the Omicron variant (p value > 0.05 for Kruskal Wallis test).

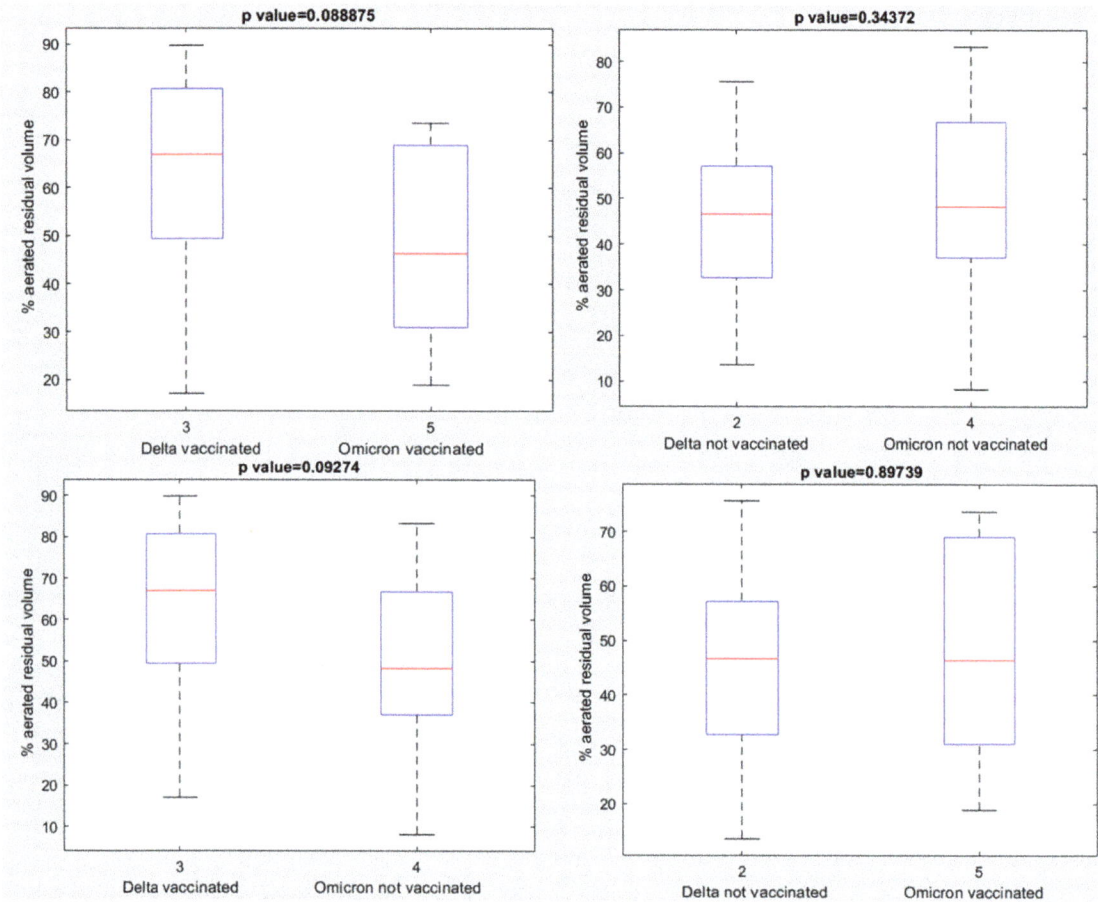

Figure 6. Boxplots of aerated residual volume between unvaccinated or vaccinated patients affected by Delta variant and vaccinated or un-vaccinated patients affected by Omicron variant.

In addition, no difference was observed in terms of each extracted volume by automatic tool between unvaccinated patients with the Alpha variant versus unvaccinated patients with the Delta variant (p value > 0.05 for Kruskal Wallis test). Instead, statistically significant differences were observed for each extracted volume by automatic tool between unvaccinated patients affected by Alpha variant and vaccinated patients affected by Delta variant of COVID-19: p value for Kruskal Wallis test = 0.003, 0.01, 0.01, 0.01, 0.001, 0.01, respectively, for percentage values of aerated residual lung volume, right upper lobe volume, right lower lobe volume, medium lobe volume, left upper lobe volume and left lower lobe volume (see boxplots in Figure 9).

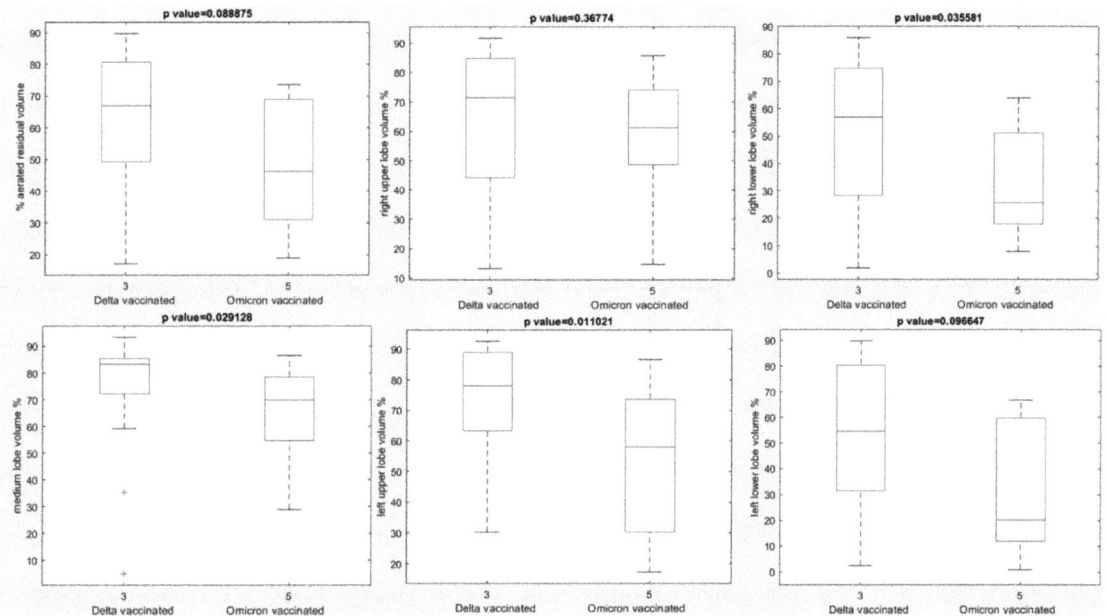

Figure 7. Boxplots of extracted volumes by automatic tool between vaccinated patients affected by Delta Variant of COVID-19 and vaccinated patients affected by Omicron Variant of COVID-19.

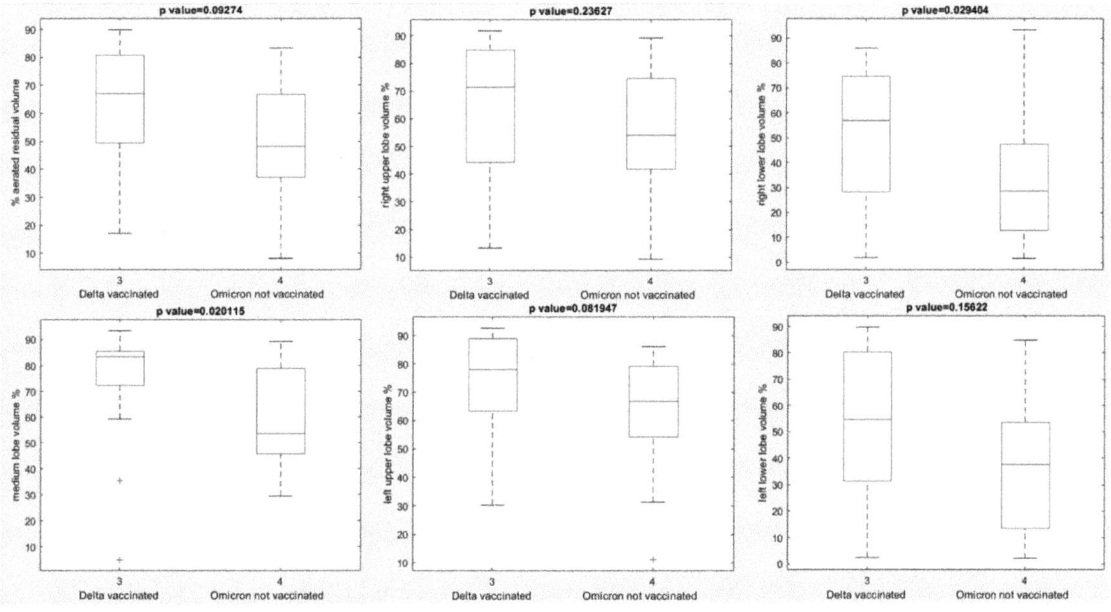

Figure 8. Boxplots of extracted volumes by automatic tool between vaccinated patients affected by Delta Variant of COVID-19 and unvaccinated patients affected by Omicron Variant of COVID-19.

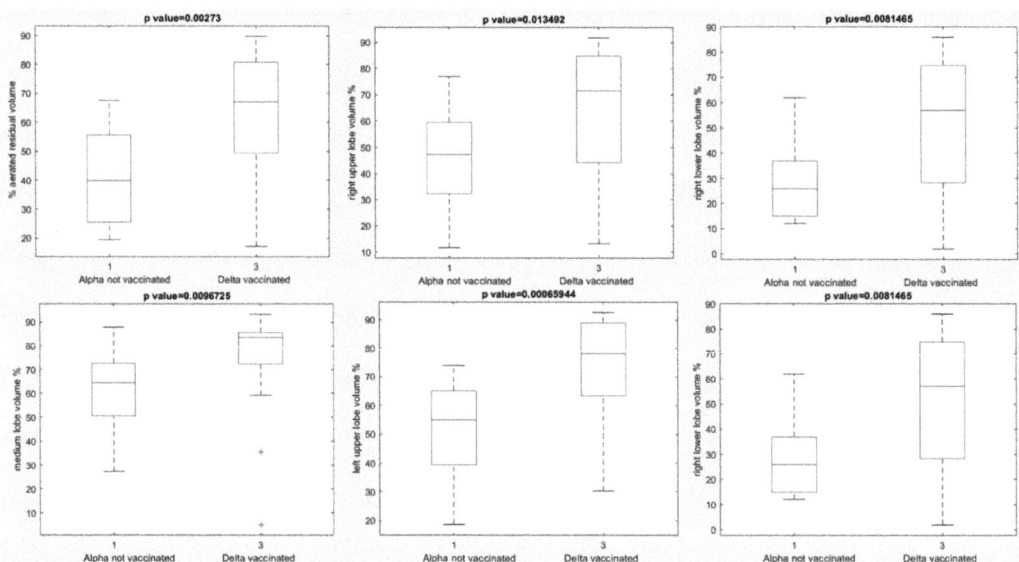

Figure 9. Boxplots of extracted volumes by automatic tool between unvaccinated patients affected by Alpha variant and vaccinated patients affected by Delta variant of COVID-19.

The highest differences were observed in median value of aerated residual lung volume (39.95% versus 67.10%) in unvaccinated patients with Alpha variant compared to vaccinated patients with Delta variant and in left upper lobe volume (55.00% versus 78.15% in unvaccinated patients with Alpha variant compared to vaccinated patients with Delta variant).

Considering all groups together to assess statistically significant differences in terms of median value of extracted volumes by automatic tool, a statistically significant difference was observed in the percentage values of the aerated residual lung volume with a p-value of 0.03 for the Kruskal Wallis test (see boxplots in Figure 10 and Table 3) due to the highest value of aerated residual volume in vaccinated patients with Delta variant compered to every other group.

No statistically significant difference was observed in the exitus number among groups (p value = 0.95 at Chi Square test).

Good statistically significant correlations among volumes extracted by automatic tool for each lung lobe and overall radiological severity score were obtained (ICC range 0.71–0.86). Boxplots of the extracted volumes with automatic tool with respect to the overall radiological severity score are reported in Figure 11: aerated residual volume, right upper lobe volume, right lower lobe volume, medium lobe volume, left upper lobe volume, left lower lobe volume in percentage values.

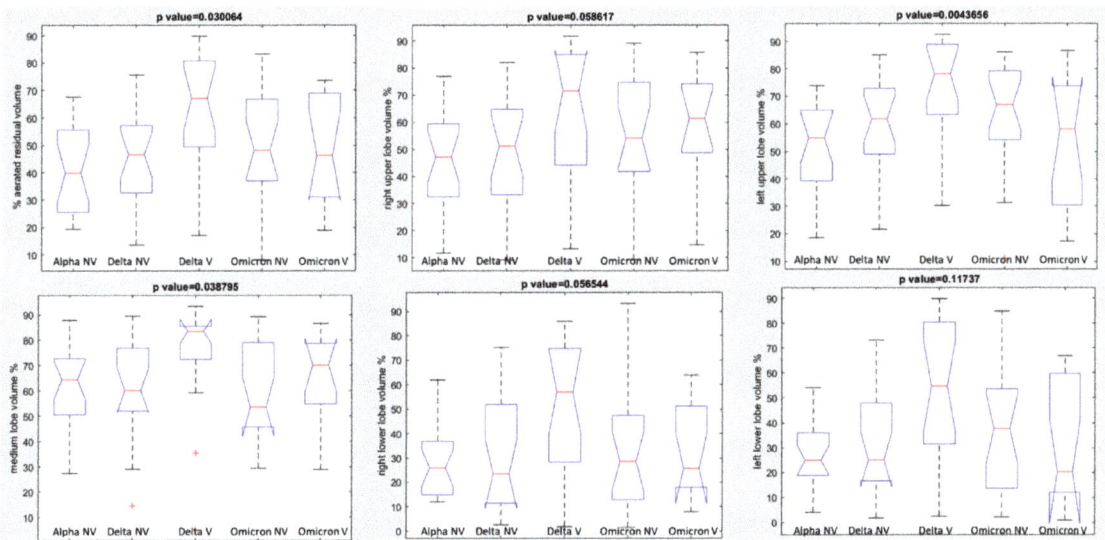

Figure 10. Boxplots of extracted volumes by automatic tool patients affected by Alpha, Delta or Omicron Variant of COVID-19.

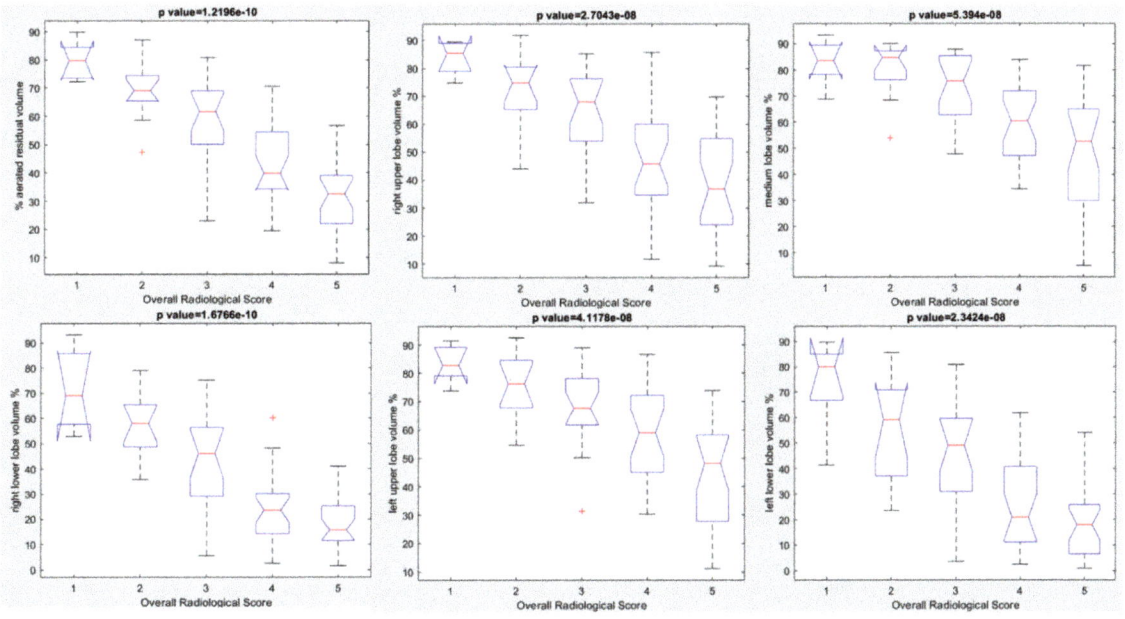

Figure 11. Boxplots of extracted volumes by automatic tool compared to Overall Radiological Severity score.

Table 4 reports the median values of extracted volumes for each patient group (Alpha, Delta and Omicron group) with respect to the overall radiological severity score (from 1 to 5). No statistically significant difference was found in the overall radiological severity score for each patient group with respect to patients age (p value > 0.05 at Chi square test, Table 5).

Table 4. Median values of extracted volumes by automatic tool for patients affected by Alpha, Delta or Omicron Variant of COVID-19 grouped by overall radiological severity score.

	Overall Radiological SCORE	Aerated Residual Volume %	Right Upper Lobe Volume %	Right Lower Lobe Volume %	Medium Lobe Volume %	Left Upper Lobe Volume %	Left Lower Lobe Volume %
Alpha	2	57.50	65.40	48.85	70.50	59.50	26.30
	3	47.37	72.07	35.27	80.50	66.67	33.03
	4	39.51	40.20	23.73	54.84	49.61	27.15
	5	36.96	39.06	23.71	57.19	44.23	25.16
Delta	1	82.17	86.83	73.63	87.37	84.87	71.67
	2	76.06	74.02	68.02	86.20	83.06	66.08
	3	65.25	68.04	54.91	75.65	72.97	56.29
	4	43.40	47.19	21.51	63.44	61.50	20.47
	5	26.86	29.34	11.54	38.18	45.60	15.18
Omicron	1	77.73	80.83	69.03	78.43	81.53	75.93
	2	67.97	72.62	51.53	78.83	75.50	57.17
	3	47.87	55.15	25.83	65.77	60.47	29.38
	4	46.64	52.84	29.56	57.07	59.79	31.39
	5	34.00	47.12	16.17	51.25	44.08	15.88
p value at Kruskal Wallis test		<0.001	<0.001	<0.001	<0.001	<0.001	<0.001

Table 5. Overall Radiological Severity Score correlated with patients' age for each group.

	Overall Radiological Severity Score	Alpha Variant $n = 20$	Delta Variant $n = 38$	Omicronvariant $n = 33$	p Value at Chi Square Test
≤65 years	≤5	0	2	3	
>65 years		0	1	0	0.55
Total		0	3	3	
≤65 years	6–10	1	2	5	
>65 years		1	3	1	0.32
Total		2	5	6	
≤65 years	11–15	0	7	4	
>65 years		3	4	2	0.11
Total		3	11	6	
≤65 years	16–20	4	3	6	
>65 years		4	8	1	0.06
Total		8	11	7	
≤65 years	21–25	3	3	8	
>65 years		4	5	3	0.25
Total		7	8	11	

GGO was the main sign of COVID-19 lesions on CT images. CT showed multiple irregular areas of GGOs in 87 of the 91 (95.6%) patients. Consolidations were found in 70/91 (76.9%) patients and crazy paving sign in 78/91 (86.6%) patients. No statistically significant differences were observed in CT findings (GGO, consolidation or crazy paving sign) among each patient group (p value > 0.05 at Chi square test, Table 1).

4. Discussion

The debate on the efficacy of the vaccine remains, unfortunately, still open, despite the clear evidence of a reduction in the number of patients admitted to ICU [93,94]. A retrospective analysis [94], based from 465 U.S. health care facilities, showed that severe COVID-19 outcomes (i.e., respiratory failure, ICU admission, or death) were rare among adults aged ≥18 years after primary vaccination. In addition, this study showed that risk for severe COVID-19 outcome after primary vaccination was higher among persons aged ≥65 years with immunosuppression, diabetes, and chronic kidney, cardiac, pulmonary, neurologic, and liver disease [94]. However, these data were obtained among persons who acquired COVID-19 after primary vaccination during periods of pre-Delta and Delta variant predominance, so that these results should not be applicable to the risk from Omicron variant or future variants [94]. In our study we showed that in critically ill patient no difference was observed in terms of severity of disease due to pulmonary parenchymal involvement, between unvaccinated and vaccinated patients with Omicron variant, between vaccinated or unvaccinated patients with Delta and vaccinated or unvaccinated patients Omicron variant, between unvaccinated patients with the Alpha variant versus vaccinated or unvaccinated patients with the Omicron variant, or between unvaccinated patients with the Alpha variant versus unvaccinated patients with the Delta variant. Instead statistically significant differences were observed between unvaccinated patients affected by Alpha variant and vaccinated patients affected by Delta variant, and between unvaccinated patients with Delta variant versus vaccinated patients with Delta variant. The highest differences were observed between unvaccinated patients with Alpha variant compared to vaccinated patients with Delta variant.

According to our results, no statistically significant difference was observed in the exitus number among groups. This result could be explained by the fact that the patients in the study were all admitted to ICU and for this reason in a serious condition regardless of vaccination. In addition, these results allow us to analyze several issues. Firstly, in critically ill patients the vaccine role is still controversial, and it could be explained by considering the evolution of the disease itself, where pulmonary impairment is also linked to a probable activation of the immune system [95]. Strong evidence indicates that critical illness caused by COVID-19 is qualitatively different from mild or moderate disease, even among hospitalized patients. Although most patients show mild clinical symptoms, about 20% of patients rapidly progress to severe illness characterized by atypical interstitial bilateral pneumonia, acute respiratory distress syndrome and multiorgan dysfunction. Almost 10% of these critically ill patients subsequently die. Insights into the pathogenic mechanisms underlying SARS-CoV-2 infection and COVID-19 progression are emerging and highlight the critical role of the immunological hyper-response in disease exacerbation [96–98].

Secondly, we found no difference between all groups considering pulmonary parenchymal involvement, except in the delta patient group. These data could be explained considering that the prevalence of the delta variant infection, in Italy, corresponds to the period in which the vaccination campaign was more intense, therefore without a decline in vaccine-related immunity, as suggested by emerging evidence [99,100]. A large observational study conducted using nationwide mass vaccination data in Israel showed that a third dose of the BNT162b2 mRNA COVID-19 vaccine is effective in preventing severe COVID-19-related outcomes. Compared with two doses of the vaccine administered at least 5 months before, adding a third dose was estimated to be 93% effective in preventing COVID-19-related admission to hospital, 92% in preventing severe disease, and 81% in preventing COVID-19-related death, as of 7 or more days after the third dose [101]. In our study group only a few patients had a booster dose; this data could explain to us why not only patients at risk, but also young people in apparent good health were hospitalized in intensive care, and why there were no statistically significant differences between the various risk factors in our sample.

Last but not least, is the tOmicron variant question. Our data do not allow us to establish whether the severity of the disease is linked to a decline in vaccine-related immunity or to the ineffectiveness of the vaccine against the omicron variant. At the present, there are four types of vaccines, i.e., virus vaccines, viral-vector vaccines, DNA/RNA vaccines, and protein-based vaccines [102]. Essentially, the current COVID-19 vaccines in use mainly target the S protein [103]. The 32 amino acid changes, including three small deletions and one small insertion in the spike protein, suggest that these mutations may dramatically enhance the Omicron variant's ability to evade current vaccines [104–106]. Although data has suggested the potential benefit of booster mRNA vaccines for protection against Omicron [107], further studies on a larger sample are necessary.

Our quantitative analysis was obtained by Philips IntelliSpace Portal clinical application CT COPD software, designed to quantify pulmonary emphysema in patients with chronic obstructive pulmonary disease. The tool provides segmentation of the lungs and of the airway tree. Moreover, the tool helps visualize and quantify the destructive process of diffuse lung disease (e.g., emphysema), providing a guided workflow for airway analysis, reviewing and measuring airway lumen, and assessing trapped ait. Compared to others tools, this allows assessment of consolidation. In fact, during our evaluation we used also two others tools, Thoracic VCAR Software (GE Healthcare, Chicago, IL, USA) and a pneumonia module of ANKE ASG-340 CT workstation (HTS Med & Anke, Naples, Italy). However, these tools were unable to identify consolidation in all patients and, to avoid excluding patients, we reported the results obtained with a single tool.

The present study has limitations, first of all the assessed sample size. However, we selected critically ill patients in intensive care who had a CT study for an evaluation of the objective "gravity" of the disease. The possibility of objectively grading the disease made the data robustly comparable, eliminating the variability associated with qualitative assessment [108–120]. Secondly is the small number of patients who had taken a booster dose, which did not allow us to assess whether the additional dose could be protective or not. Third is the selection of the control group, linked to the need to have performed a CT study, which could be responsible for bias in the results. However, we have already explained how an objective quantification of disease severity was considered crucial. Finally, since we did not know the date of the last vaccine dose for all patients, it was not possible to evaluate the severity based on the time of immunity status.

5. Conclusions

The debate on the efficacy of the vaccine remains still open, despite the clear evidence of a reduction in the number of patients admitted to Intensive Care Unit. In our study we showed that in critically ill patients no difference was observed in terms of severity of disease or exitus between unvaccinated and vaccinated patients. The only statistically significant differences were observed, with regard to the severity of COVID-19 pulmonary parenchymal involvement, between unvaccinated patients affected by Alpha variant and vaccinated patients affected by Delta variant, and between unvaccinated patients with Delta variant versus vaccinated patients with Delta variant.

Author Contributions: Each author has participated sufficiently to take public responsibility for the content of the manuscript. All authors have read and agreed to the published version of the manuscript.

Funding: This research received no external funding.

Institutional Review Board Statement: The study was conducted according to the guidelines of the Declaration of Helsin-ki and approved by the Institutional Ethics Committee of IRCCS L. Spallanzani. Data acquisition and analysis were performed in compliance with protocols approved by the Ethical

Committee of the National Institute for Infectious Diseases IRCCS Lazzaro Spallanzani, Rome, Italy (ethical approval number 164, 26 June 2020).

Informed Consent Statement: The Local Ethical Committee board renounced patient informed consent, considering the ongoing epidemic emergency.

Data Availability Statement: All data are reported in the manuscript.

Acknowledgments: The authors are grateful to Alessandra Trocino, librarian at the National Cancer Institute of Naples, Italy. Moreover, the authors are grateful to Grazia Della Valle for collaboration.

Conflicts of Interest: The authors have no conflict of interest to be disclosed.

References

1. Available online: https://covid19.who.int (accessed on 21 May 2022).
2. Stramare, R.; Carretta, G.; Capizzi, A.; Boemo, D.G.; Contessa, C.; Motta, R.; De Conti, G.; Causin, F.; Giraudo, C.; Donato, D. Radiological management of COVID-19: Structure your diagnostic path to guarantee a safe path. *Radiol. Med.* **2020**, *125*, 691–694. [CrossRef] [PubMed]
3. Granata, V.; Fusco, R.; Izzo, F.; Setola, S.V.; Coppola, M.; Grassi, R.; Reginelli, A.; Cappabianca, S.; Petrillo, A. COVID-19 infection in cancer patients: The management in a diagnostic unit. *Radiol. Oncol.* **2021**, *55*, 121–129. [CrossRef] [PubMed]
4. Ashtari, S.; Vahedian-Azimi, A.; Shojaee, S.; Pourhoseingholi, M.A.; Jafari, R.; Bashar, F.R.; Zali, M.R. Características en tomografía computarizada de la neumonía por coronavirus-2019 (COVID-19) en tres grupos de pacientes iraníes: Estudio de un solo centro [Computed tomographic features of coronavirus disease-2019 (COVID-19) pneumonia in three groups of Iranian patients: A single center study]. *Radiologia* **2021**, *63*, 314–323. (In Spanish) [CrossRef] [PubMed]
5. Gabelloni, M.; Faggioni, L.; Cioni, D.; Mendola, V.; Falaschi, Z.; Coppola, S.; Corradi, F.; Isirdi, A.; Brandi, N.; Coppola, F.; et al. Extracorporeal membrane oxygenation (ECMO) in COVID-19 patients: A pocket guide for radiologists. *Radiol. Med.* **2022**, *13*, 369–382. [CrossRef] [PubMed]
6. Giovagnoni, A. Facing the COVID-19 emergency: We can, and we do. *Radiol. Med.* **2020**, *125*, 337–338. [CrossRef] [PubMed]
7. Montesi, G.; Di Biase, S.; Chierchini, S.; Pavanato, G.; Virdis, G.E.; Contato, E.; Mandoliti, G. Radiotherapy during COVID-19 pandemic. How to create a No fly zone: A Northern Italy experience. *Radiol. Med.* **2020**, *125*, 600–603. [CrossRef]
8. Ierardi, A.M.; Wood, B.J.; Arrichiello, A.; Bottino, N.; Bracchi, L.; Forzenigo, L.; Andrisani, M.C.; Vespro, V.; Bonelli, C.; Amalou, A.; et al. Preparation of a radiology department in an Italian hospital dedicated to COVID-19 patients. *Radiol. Med.* **2020**, *125*, 894–901. [CrossRef]
9. Grassi, R.; Cappabianca, S.; Urraro, F.; Feragalli, B.; Montanelli, A.; Patelli, G.; Granata, V.; Giacobbe, G.; Russo, G.M.; Grillo, A.; et al. Chest CT Computerized Aided Quantification of PNEUMONIA Lesions in COVID-19 Infection: A Comparison among Three Commercial Software. *Int. J. Environ. Res. Public Health* **2020**, *17*, 6914. [CrossRef]
10. Pediconi, F.; Galati, F.; Bernardi, D.; Belli, P.; Brancato, B.; Calabrese, M.; Camera, L.; Carbonaro, L.A.; Caumo, F.; Clauser, P.; et al. Breast imaging and cancer diagnosis during the COVID-19 pandemic: Recommendations from the Italian College of Breast Radiologists by SIRM. *Radiol. Med.* **2020**, *125*, 926–930. [CrossRef]
11. Koç, A.; Sezgin, S.; Kayıpmaz, S. Comparing different planimetric methods on volumetric estimations by using cone beam computed tomography. *Radiol. Med.* **2020**, *125*, 398–405. [CrossRef]
12. Fusco, R.; Simonetti, I.; Ianniello, S.; Villanacci, A.; Grassi, F.; Dell'Aversana, F.; Grassi, R.; Cozzi, D.; Bicci, E.; Palumbo, P.; et al. Pulmonary Lymphangitis Poses a Major Challenge for Radiologists in an Oncological Setting during the COVID-19 Pandemic. *J. Pers. Med.* **2022**, *12*, 624. [CrossRef] [PubMed]
13. de Souza, A.S.; de Freitas Amorim, V.M.; Guardia, G.D.A.; Dos Santos, F.F.; Ulrich, H.; Galante, P.A.F.; de Souza, R.F.; Guzzo, C.R. Severe Acute Respiratory Syndrome Coronavirus 2 Variants of Concern: A Perspective for Emerging More Transmissible and Vaccine-Resistant Strains. *Viruses* **2022**, *14*, 827. [CrossRef] [PubMed]
14. Agostini, A.; Floridi, C.; Borgheresi, A.; Badaloni, M.; Pirani, P.E.; Terilli, F.; Ottaviani, L.; Giovagnoni, A. Proposal of a low-dose, long-pitch, dual-source chest CT protocol on third-generation dual-source CT using a tin filter for spectral shaping at 100 kVp for CoronaVirus Disease 2019 (COVID-19) patients: A feasibility study. *Radiol. Med.* **2020**, *125*, 365–373. [CrossRef] [PubMed]
15. Borghesi, A.; Maroldi, R. COVID-19 outbreak in Italy: Experimental chest X-ray scoring system for quantifying and monitoring disease progression. *Radiol. Med.* **2020**, *125*, 509–513. [CrossRef] [PubMed]
16. Neri, E.; Miele, V.; Coppola, F.; Grassi, R. Use of CT and artificial intelligence in suspected or COVID-19 positive patients: Statement of the Italian Society of Medical and Interventional Radiology. *Radiol. Med.* **2020**, *125*, 505–508. [CrossRef]
17. Carotti, M.; Salaffi, F.; Sarzi-Puttini, P.; Agostini, A.; Borgheresi, A.; Minorati, D.; Galli, M.; Marotto, D.; Giovagnoni, A. Chest CT features of coronavirus disease 2019 (COVID-19) pneumonia: Key points for radiologists. *Radiol. Med.* **2020**, *125*, 636–646. [CrossRef]
18. Alyasseri, Z.A.A.; Al-Betar, M.A.; Doush, I.A.; Awadallah, M.A.; Abasi, A.K.; Makhadmeh, S.N.; Alomari, O.A.; Abdulkareem, K.H.; Adam, A.; Damasevicius, R.; et al. Review on COVID-19 diagnosis models based on machine learning and deep learning approaches. *Expert Syst.* **2021**, *28*, e12759. [CrossRef]

19. Borghesi, A.; Zigliani, A.; Masciullo, R.; Golemi, S.; Maculotti, P.; Farina, D.; Maroldi, R. Radiographic severity index in COVID-19 pneumonia: Relationship to age and sex in 783 Italian patients. *Radiol. Med.* **2020**, *125*, 461–464. [CrossRef]
20. Cozzi, D.; Albanesi, M.; Cavigli, E.; Moroni, C.; Bindi, A.; Luvarà, S.; Lucarini, S.; Busoni, S.; Mazzoni, L.N.; Miele, V. Chest X-ray in new Coronavirus Disease 2019 (COVID-19) infection: Findings and correlation with clinical outcome. *Radiol. Med.* **2020**, *125*, 730–737. [CrossRef]
21. Gatti, M.; Calandri, M.; Barba, M.; Biondo, A.; Geninatti, C.; Gentile, S.; Greco, M.; Morrone, V.; Piatti, C.; Santonocito, A.; et al. Baseline chest X-ray in coronavirus disease 19 (COVID-19) patients: Association with clinical and laboratory data. *Radiol. Med.* **2020**, *125*, 1271–1279. [CrossRef]
22. Granata, V.; Fusco, R.; Vallone, P.; Setola, S.V.; Picone, C.; Grassi, F.; Patrone, R.; Belli, A.; Izzo, F.; Petrillo, A. Not only lymphadenopathy: Case of chest lymphangitis assessed with MRI after COVID 19 vaccine. *Infect. Agent Cancer* **2022**, *17*, 8. [CrossRef] [PubMed]
23. D'Agostino, V.; Caranci, F.; Negro, A.; Piscitelli, V.; Tuccillo, B.; Fasano, F.; Sirabella, G.; Marano, I.; Granata, V.; Grassi, R.; et al. A Rare Case of Cerebral Venous Thrombosis and Disseminated Intravascular Coagulation Temporally Associated to the COVID-19 Vaccine Administration. *J. Pers. Med.* **2021**, *11*, 285. [CrossRef] [PubMed]
24. Granata, V.; Fusco, R.; Setola, S.V.; Galdiero, R.; Picone, C.; Izzo, F.; D'Aniello, R.; Miele, V.; Grassi, R.; Grassi, R.; et al. Lymphadenopathy after BNT162b2 COVID-19 Vaccine: Preliminary Ultrasound Findings. *Biology* **2021**, *10*, 214. [CrossRef] [PubMed]
25. Volz, E.; Hill, V.; McCrone, J.T.; Price, A.; Jorgensen, D.; O'Toole, Á.; Southgate, J.; Johnson, R.; Jackson, B.; Nascimento, F.F.; et al. Evaluating the Effects of SARS-CoV-2 Spike Mutation D614G on Transmissibility and Pathogenicity. *Cell* **2021**, *184*, 64–75. [CrossRef]
26. Zhou, W.; Wang, W. Fast-Spreading SARS-CoV-2 Variants: Challenges to and New Design Strategies of COVID-19 Vaccines. *Signal Transduct. Target. Ther.* **2021**, *6*, 226. [CrossRef]
27. Zhang, J.; Xiao, T.; Cai, Y.; Lavine, C.L.; Peng, H.; Zhu, H.; Anand, K.; Tong, P.; Gautam, A.; Mayer, M.L.; et al. Membrane Fusion and Immune Evasion by the Spike Protein of SARS-CoV-2 Delta Variant. *Science* **2021**, *374*, 1353–1360. [CrossRef]
28. Classification of Omicron (B.1.1.529): SARS-CoV-2 Variant of Concern. Available online: https://www.who.int/news/item/26-11-2021-classification-of-omicron-(b.1.1.529)-sars-cov-2-variant-of-concern (accessed on 17 December 2021).
29. Ierardi, A.M.; Gaibazzi, N.; Tuttolomondo, D.; Fusco, S.; La Mura, V.; Peyvandi, F.; Aliberti, S.; Blasi, F.; Cozzi, D.; Carrafiello, G.; et al. Deep vein thrombosis in COVID-19 patients in general wards: Prevalence and association with clinical and laboratory variables. *Radiol. Med.* **2021**, *126*, 722–728. [CrossRef]
30. Turkahia, Y.; Thornlow, B.; Hinrichs, A.; McBroome, J.; Ayala, N.; Ye, C.; De Maio, N.; Haussler, D.; Lanfear, R.; Corbett-Detig, R. Pandemic-Scale Phylogenomics Reveals Elevated Recombination Rates in the SARS-CoV-2 Spike Region. *bioRxiv* **2021**. [CrossRef]
31. Covin, S.; Rutherford, G.W. Coinfection, Severe Acute Respiratory Syndrome Coronavirus 2 (SARS-CoV-2), and Influenza: An Evolving Puzzle. *Clin. Infect. Dis.* **2021**, *72*, e993–e994. [CrossRef]
32. Giannitto, C.; Sposta, F.M.; Repici, A.; Vatteroni, G.; Casiraghi, E.; Casari, E.; Ferraroli, G.M.; Fugazza, A.; Sandri, M.T.; Chiti, A.; et al. Chest CT in patients with a moderate or high pretest probability of COVID-19 and negative swab. *Radiol. Med.* **2020**, *125*, 1260–1270. [CrossRef]
33. Cuadrado-Payán, E.; Montagud-Marrahi, E.; Torres-Elorza, M.; Bodro, M.; Blasco, M.; Poch, E.; Soriano, A.; Piñeiro, G.J. SARS-CoV-2 and Influenza Virus Co-Infection. *Lancet* **2020**, *395*, e84. [CrossRef]
34. Moroni, C.; Cozzi, D.; Albanesi, M.; Cavigli, E.; Bindi, A.; Luvarà, S.; Busoni, S.; Mazzoni, L.N.; Grifoni, S.; Nazerian, P.; et al. Chest X-ray in the emergency department during COVID-19 pandemic descending phase in Italy: Correlation with patients' outcome. *Radiol. Med.* **2021**, *126*, 661–668. [CrossRef] [PubMed]
35. Di Serafino, M.; Notaro, M.; Rea, G.; Iacobellis, F.; Paoli, V.D.; Acampora, C.; Ianniello, S.; Brunese, L.; Romano, L.; Vallone, G. The lung ultrasound: Facts or artifacts? In the era of COVID-19 outbreak. *Radiol. Med.* **2020**, *125*, 738–753. [CrossRef]
36. Ravikanth, R. Diagnostic accuracy and false-positive rate of chest CT as compared to RT-PCR in coronavirus disease 2019 (COVID-19) pneumonia: A prospective cohort of 612 cases from India and review of literature. *Indian J. Radiol. Imaging* **2021**, *31* (Suppl. 1), S161–S169. [CrossRef] [PubMed]
37. Grassi, R.; Belfiore, M.P.; Montanelli, A.; Patelli, G.; Urraro, F.; Giacobbe, G.; Fusco, R.; Granata, V.; Petrillo, A.; Sacco, P.; et al. COVID-19 pneumonia: Computer-aided quantification of healthy lung parenchyma, emphysema, ground glass and consolidation on chest computed tomography (CT). *Radiol. Med.* **2020**, *126*, 553–560. [CrossRef] [PubMed]
38. Ippolito, D.; Giandola, T.; Maino, C.; Pecorelli, A.; Capodaglio, C.; Ragusi, M.; Porta, M.; Gandola, D.; Masetto, A.; Drago, S.; et al. Acute pulmonary embolism in hospitalized patients with SARS-CoV-2-related pneumonia: Multicentric experience from Italian endemic area. *Radiol. Med.* **2021**, *126*, 669–678. [CrossRef]
39. Mansbach, R.A.; Chakraborty, S.; Nguyen, K.; Montefiori, D.C.; Korber, B.; Gnanakaran, S. The SARS-CoV-2 Spike Variant D614G Favors an Open Conformational State. *Sci. Adv.* **2021**, *7*, eabf3671. [CrossRef]
40. Shaw, B.; Daskareh, M.; Gholamrezanezhad, A. The lingering manifestations of COVID-19 during and after convalescence: Update on long-term pulmonary consequences of coronavirus disease 2019 (COVID-19). *Radiol. Med.* **2021**, *126*, 40–46. [CrossRef]
41. Rawashdeh, M.A.; Saade, C. Radiation dose reduction considerations and imaging patterns of ground glass opacities in coronavirus: Risk of over exposure in computed tomography. *Radiol. Med.* **2021**, *126*, 380–387. [CrossRef]

42. Teruel, N.; Mailhot, O.; Najmanovich, R.J. Modelling Conformational State Dynamics and Its Role on Infection for SARS-CoV-2 Spike Protein Variants. *PLoS Comput. Biol.* **2021**, *17*, e1009286. [CrossRef]
43. Benton, D.J.; Wrobel, A.G.; Roustan, C.; Borg, A.; Xu, P.; Martin, S.R.; Rosenthal, P.B.; Skehel, J.J.; Gamblin, S.J. The Effect of the D614G Substitution on the Structure of the Spike Glycoprotein of SARS-CoV-2. *Proc. Natl. Acad. Sci. USA* **2021**, *118*, e2022586118. [CrossRef] [PubMed]
44. Chemaitelly, H.; Tang, P.; Hasan, M.R.; AlMukdad, S.; Yassine, H.M.; Benslimane, F.M.; Al Khatib, H.A.; Coyle, P.; Ayoub, H.H.; Al Kanaani, Z.; et al. Waning of BNT162b2 vaccine protection against SARS-CoV-2 infection in Qatar. *N. Engl. J. Med.* **2021**, *385*, e83. [CrossRef] [PubMed]
45. Levin, E.G.; Lustig, Y.; Cohen, C.; Fluss, R.; Indenbaum, V.; Amit, S.; Doolman, R.; Asraf, K.; Mendelson, E.; Ziv, A.; et al. Waning immune humoral response to BNT162b2 covid-19 vaccine over 6 months. *N. Engl. J. Med.* **2021**, *385*, e84. [CrossRef] [PubMed]
46. Andrews, N.; Tessier, E.; Stowe, J.; Gower, C.; Kirsebom, F.; Simmons, R.; Gallagher, E.; Chand, M.; Brown, K.; Ladhani, S.; et al. Vaccine effectiveness and duration of protection of Comirnaty, Vaxzevria and Spikevax against mild and severe COVID-19 in the UK. *medRxiv* **2021**. Available online: https://www.medrxiv.org/content/10.1101/2021.09.15.21263583v2 (accessed on 21 May 2022).
47. Goldberg, Y.; Mandel, M.; Bar-On, Y.M.; Bodenheimer, O.; Freedman, L.S.; Haas, E.; Milo, R.; Alroy-Preis, S.; Ash, N.; Huppert, A. Waning immunity of the BNT162b2 vaccine: A nationwide study from Israel. *medRxiv* **2021**. Available online: https://www.medrxiv.org/content/10.1101/2021.08.24.21262423v1 (accessed on 21 May 2022).
48. Thomas, S.J.; Moreira, E.D.; Kitchin, N.; Absalon, J.; Gurtman, A.; Lockhart, S.; Perez, J.L.; Marc, G.P.; Polack, F.P.; Zerbini, C.; et al. Six month safety and efficacy of the BNT162b2 mRNA COVID-19 vaccine. *medRxiv* **2021**. Available online: https://www.medrxiv.org/content/10.1101/2021.07.28.21261159v1 (accessed on 21 May 2022).
49. COVID-19 Vaccine Booster Doses Administered per 100 People—Our World in Data [Internet]. [Cited 2021 Nov.]. Available online: https://ourworldindata.org/grapher/covid-vaccine-booster-doses-per-capita?country=BRA~{}CHL~{}ISR~{}RUS~{}USA~{}URY~{}OWID_WRL (accessed on 21 May 2022).
50. Lombardi, A.F.; Afsahi, A.M.; Gupta, A.; Gholamrezanezhad, A. Severe acute respiratory syndrome (SARS), Middle East respiratory syndrome (MERS), influenza, and COVID-19, beyond the lungs: A review article. *Radiol. Med.* **2021**, *126*, 561–569. [CrossRef]
51. Alballa, N.; Al-Turaiki, I. Machine learning approaches in COVID-19 diagnosis, mortality, and severity risk prediction: A review. *Inform. Med. Unlocked* **2021**, *24*, 100564. [CrossRef]
52. Cozzi, D.; Bindi, A.; Cavigli, E.; Grosso, A.M.; Luvarà, S.; Morelli, N.; Moroni, C.; Piperio, R.; Miele, V.; Bartolucci, M. Exogenous lipoid pneumonia: When radiologist makes the difference. *Radiol. Med.* **2021**, *126*, 22–28. [CrossRef]
53. Palmisano, A.; Scotti, G.M.; Ippolito, D.; Morelli, M.J.; Vignale, D.; Gandola, D.; Sironi, S.; De Cobelli, F.; Ferrante, L.; Spessot, M.; et al. Chest CT in the emergency department for suspected COVID-19 pneumonia. *Radiol. Med.* **2021**, *126*, 498–502. [CrossRef]
54. Bar-On, Y.M.; Goldberg, Y.; Mandel, M.; Bodenheimer, O.; Freedman, L.; Kalkstein, N.; Mizrahi, B.; Alroy-Preis, S.; Ash, N.; Milo, R.; et al. Protection of BNT162b2 Vaccine Booster against COVID-19 in Israel. *N. Engl. J. Med.* **2021**, *385*, 1393–1400. [CrossRef]
55. Waxman, J.G.; Makov-Assif, M.; Reis, B.Y.; Netzer, D.; Balicer, R.D.; Dagan, N.; Barda, N. Comparing COVID-19-related hospitalization rates among individuals with infection-induced and vaccine-induced immunity in Israel. *Nat. Commun.* **2022**, *13*, 2202. [CrossRef] [PubMed]
56. Caruso, D.; Polici, M.; Zerunian, M.; Pucciarelli, F.; Polidori, T.; Guido, G.; Rucci, C.; Bracci, B.; Muscogiuri, E.; De Dominicis, C.; et al. Quantitative Chest CT analysis in discriminating COVID-19 from non-COVID-19 patients. *Radiol. Med.* **2020**, *126*, 243–249. [CrossRef] [PubMed]
57. Cardobi, N.; Benetti, G.; Cardano, G.; Arena, C.; Micheletto, C.; Cavedon, C.; Montemezzi, S. CT radiomic models to distinguish COVID-19 pneumonia from other interstitial pneumonias. *Radiol. Med.* **2021**, *126*, 1037–1043. [CrossRef] [PubMed]
58. Caruso, D.; Pucciarelli, F.; Zerunian, M.; Ganeshan, B.; De Santis, D.; Polici, M.; Rucci, C.; Polidori, T.; Guido, G.; Bracci, B.; et al. Chest CT texture-based radiomics analysis in differentiating COVID-19 from other interstitial pneumonia. *Radiol. Med.* **2021**, *126*, 1415–1424. [CrossRef] [PubMed]
59. Masselli, G.; Almberger, M.; Tortora, A.; Capoccia, L.; Dolciami, M.; D'Aprile, M.R.; Valentini, C.; Avventurieri, G.; Bracci, S.; Ricci, P. Role of CT angiography in detecting acute pulmonary embolism associated with COVID-19 pneumonia. *Radiol. Med.* **2021**, *126*, 1553–1560. [CrossRef] [PubMed]
60. Pecoraro, M.; Cipollari, S.; Marchitelli, L.; Messina, E.; Del Monte, M.; Galea, N.; Ciardi, M.R.; Francone, M.; Catalano, C.; Panebianco, V. Cross-sectional analysis of follow-up chest MRI and chest CT scans in patients previously affected by COVID-19. *Radiol. Med.* **2021**, *126*, 1273–1281. [CrossRef]
61. Granata, V.; Ianniello, S.; Fusco, R.; Urraro, F.; Pupo, D.; Magliocchetti, S.; Albarello, F.; Campioni, P.; Cristofaro, M.; Di Stefano, F.; et al. Quantitative Analysis of Residual COVID-19 Lung CT Features: Consistency among Two Commercial Software. *J. Pers. Med.* **2021**, *11*, 1103. [CrossRef]
62. Spinato, G.; Fabbris, C.; Conte, F.; Menegaldo, A.; Franz, L.; Gaudioso, P.; Cinetto, F.; Agostini, C.; Costantini, G.; Boscolo-Rizzo, P. COVID-Q: Validation of the first COVID-19 questionnaire based on patient-rated symptom gravity. *Int. J. Clin. Pract.* **2021**, *75*, e14829. [CrossRef]
63. Bertolini, M.; Brambilla, A.; Dallasta, S.; Colombo, G. High-quality chest CT segmentation to assess the impact of COVID-19 disease. *Int. J. Comput. Assist. Radiol. Surg.* **2021**, *16*, 1737–1747. [CrossRef]

64. Zieda, A.; Sbardella, S.; Patel, M.; Smith, R. Diagnostic Bias in the COVID-19 Pandemic: A Series of Short Cases. *Eur. J. Case Rep. Intern. Med.* **2021**, *8*, 002575. [CrossRef]
65. Giannakis, A.; Móré, D.; Erdmann, S.; Kintzelé, L.; Fischer, R.M.; Vogel, M.N.; Mangold, D.L.; von Stackelberg, O.; Schnitzler, P.; Zimmermann, S.; et al. COVID-19 pneumonia and its lookalikes: How radiologists perform in differentiating atypical pneumonias. *Eur. J. Radiol.* **2021**, *144*, 110002. [CrossRef] [PubMed]
66. Borghesi, A.; Sverzellati, N.; Polverosi, R.; Balbi, M.; Baratella, E.; Busso, M.; Calandriello, L.; Cortese, G.; Farchione, A.; Iezzi, R.; et al. Impact of the COVID-19 pandemic on the selection of chest imaging modalities and reporting systems: A survey of Italian radiologists. *Radiol. Med.* **2021**, *126*, 1258–1272. [CrossRef] [PubMed]
67. Cozzi, D.; Bicci, E.; Bindi, A.; Cavigli, E.; Danti, G.; Galluzzo, M.; Granata, V.; Pradella, S.; Trinci, M.; Miele, V. Role of Chest Imaging in Viral Lung Diseases. *Int. J. Environ. Res. Public Health* **2021**, *18*, 6434. [CrossRef] [PubMed]
68. Fusco, R.; Grassi, R.; Granata, V.; Setola, S.V.; Grassi, F.; Cozzi, D.; Pecori, B.; Izzo, F.; Petrillo, A. Artificial Intelligence and COVID-19 Using Chest CT Scan and Chest X-ray Images: Machine Learning and Deep Learning Approaches for Diagnosis and Treatment. *J. Pers. Med.* **2021**, *11*, 993. [CrossRef]
69. Reginelli, A.; Grassi, R.; Feragalli, B.; Belfiore, M.P.; Montanelli, A.; Patelli, G.; La Porta, M.; Urraro, F.; Fusco, R.; Granata, V.; et al. Coronavirus Disease 2019 (COVID-19) in Italy: Double Reading of Chest CT Examination. *Biology* **2021**, *10*, 89. [CrossRef]
70. Grassi, R.; Fusco, R.; Belfiore, M.P.; Montanelli, A.; Patelli, G.; Urraro, F.; Petrillo, A.; Granata, V.; Sacco, P.; Mazzei, M.A.; et al. Coronavirus disease 2019 (COVID-19) in Italy: Features on chest computed tomography using a structured report system. *Sci. Rep.* **2020**, *10*, 17236, Erratum in *Sci. Rep.* **2021**, *11*, 4231. [CrossRef]
71. Masci, G.M.; Iafrate, F.; Ciccarelli, F.; Pambianchi, G.; Panebianco, V.; Pasculli, P.; Ciardi, M.R.; Mastroianni, C.M.; Ricci, P.; Catalano, C.; et al. Tocilizumab effects in COVID-19 pneumonia: Role of CT texture analysis in quantitative assessment of response to therapy. *Radiol. Med.* **2021**, *126*, 1170–1180. [CrossRef]
72. Francolini, G.; Desideri, I.; Stocchi, G.; Ciccone, L.P.; Salvestrini, V.; Garlatti, P.; Aquilano, M.; Greto, D.; Bonomo, P.; Meattini, I.; et al. Impact of COVID-19 on workload burden of a complex radiotherapy facility. *Radiol. Med.* **2021**, *126*, 717–721. [CrossRef]
73. Cellini, F.; Di Franco, R.; Manfrida, S.; Borzillo, V.; Maranzano, E.; Pergolizzi, S.; Morganti, A.G.; Fusco, V.; Deodato, F.; Santarelli, M.; et al. Palliative radiotherapy indications during the COVID-19 pandemic and in future complex logistic settings: The NORMALITY model. *Radiol. Med.* **2021**, *126*, 1619–1656. [CrossRef]
74. De Felice, F.; D'Angelo, E.; Ingargiola, R.; Iacovelli, N.A.; Alterio, D.; Franco, P.; Bonomo, P.; Merlotti, A.; Bacigalupo, A.; Maddalo, M.; et al. A snapshot on radiotherapy for head and neck cancer patients during the COVID-19 pandemic: A survey of the Italian Association of Radiotherapy and Clinical Oncology (AIRO) head and neck working group. *Radiol. Med.* **2020**, *126*, 343–347. [CrossRef]
75. Ortiz, S.; Rojas, F.; Valenzuela, O.; Herrera, L.J.; Rojas, I. Determination of the Severity and Percentage of COVID-19 Infection through a Hierarchical Deep Learning System. *J. Pers. Med.* **2022**, *12*, 535. [CrossRef] [PubMed]
76. Mohiuddin Chowdhury, A.T.M.; Kamal, A.; Abbas, K.U.; Talukder, S.; Karim, M.R.; Ali, M.A.; Nuruzzaman, M.; Li, Y.; He, S. Efficacy and Outcome of Remdesivir and Tocilizumab Combination Against Dexamethasone for the Treatment of Severe COVID-19: A Randomized Controlled Trial. *Front. Pharmacol.* **2022**, *13*, 690726. [CrossRef] [PubMed]
77. Ibrahim, H.M.; Mohammad, A.A.; Fouda, E.; Abouelfotouh, K.; Habeeb, N.M.; Rezk, A.R.; Magdy, S.; Allam, A.M.; Mahmoud, S.A. Clinical Characteristics and Pulmonary Computerized Imaging Findings of Critically Ill Egyptian Patients with Multisystem Inflammatory Syndrome in Children. *Glob. Pediatr. Health* **2022**, *9*, 2333794X221085386. [CrossRef] [PubMed]
78. Lorent, N.; Vande Weygaerde, Y.; Claeys, E.; Guler Caamano Fajardo, I.; De Vos, N.; De Wever, W.; Salhi, B.; Gyselinck, I.; Bosteels, C.; Lambrecht, B.N.; et al. Prospective longitudinal evaluation of hospitalised COVID-19 survivors 3 and 12 months after discharge. *ERJ Open Res.* **2022**, *8*, 00004–2022. [CrossRef] [PubMed]
79. Ohno, Y.; Aoyagi, K.; Arakita, K.; Doi, Y.; Kondo, M.; Banno, S.; Kasahara, K.; Ogawa, T.; Kato, H.; Hase, R.; et al. Newly developed artificial intelligence algorithm for COVID-19 pneumonia: Utility of quantitative CT texture analysis for prediction of favipiravir treatment effect. *Jpn. J. Radiol.* **2022**, *9*, 1–14. [CrossRef] [PubMed]
80. Yanamandra, U.; Shobhit, S.; Paul, D.; Aggarwal, B.; Kaur, P.; Duhan, G.; Singh, A.; Srinath, R.; Saxena, P.; Menon, A.S. Relationship of Computed Tomography Severity Score with Patient Characteristics and Survival in Hypoxemic COVID-19 Patients. *Cureus* **2022**, *14*, e22847. [CrossRef]
81. Ghafuri, L.; Hamzehzadeh Alamdari, A.; Roustaei, S.; Golshani Beheshti, A.; Nayerpour, A. Predicting Severity of Novel Coronavirus (COVID-19) Pneumonia Based upon Admission Clinical, Laboratory, and Imaging Findings. *Tanaffos* **2021**, *20*, 232–239.
82. Karthik, R.; Menaka, R.; Hariharan, M.; Won, D. CT-based severity assessment for COVID-19 using weakly supervised non-local CNN. *Appl. Soft Comput.* **2022**, *121*, 108765. [CrossRef]
83. Vargas Centanaro, G.; Calle Rubio, M.; Álvarez-Sala Walther, J.L.; Martinez-Sagasti, F.; Albuja Hidalgo, A.; Herranz Hernández, R.; Rodríguez Hermosa, J.L. Long-term Outcomes and Recovery of Patients who Survived COVID-19: LUNG INJURY COVID-19 Study. *Open Forum Infect. Dis.* **2022**, *9*, ofac098. [CrossRef]
84. Küçük, M.; Ergan, B.; Yakar, M.N.; Ergün, B.; Akdoğan, Y.; Cantürk, A.; Gezer, N.S.; Kalkan, F.; Yaka, E.; Cömert, B.; et al. The Predictive Values of Respiratory Rate Oxygenation Index and Chest Computed Tomography Severity Score for High-Flow Nasal Oxygen Failure in Critically Ill Patients with Coronavirus Disease-2019. *Balkan Med. J.* **2022**, *39*, 140–147. [CrossRef]
85. Özel, M.; Aslan, A.; Araç, S. Use of the COVID-19 Reporting and Data System (CO-RADS) classification and chest computed tomography involvement score (CT-IS) in COVID-19 pneumonia. *Radiol. Med.* **2021**, *126*, 679–687. [CrossRef] [PubMed]

86. Cereser, L.; Girometti, R.; Da Re, J.; Marchesini, F.; Como, G.; Zuiani, C. Inter-reader agreement of high-resolution computed tomography findings in patients with COVID-19 pneumonia: A multi-reader study. *Radiol. Med.* **2021**, *126*, 577–584. [CrossRef] [PubMed]
87. Cappabianca, S.; Fusco, R.; de Lisio, A.; Paura, C.; Clemente, A.; Gagliardi, G.; Lombardi, G.; Giacobbe, G.; Russo, G.M.; Belfiore, M.P.; et al. Correction to: Clinical and laboratory data, radiological structured report findings and quantitative evaluation of lung involvement on baseline chest CT in COVID-19 patients to predict prognosis. *Radiol. Med.* **2021**, *126*, 643, Erratum in *Radiol. Med.* **2021**, *126*, 29–39. [CrossRef] [PubMed]
88. Cartocci, G.; Colaiacomo, M.C.; Lanciotti, S.; Andreoli, C.; De Cicco, M.L.; Brachetti, G.; Pugliese, S.; Capoccia, L.; Tortora, A.; Scala, A.; et al. Correction to: Chest CT for early detection and management of coronavirus disease (COVID-19): A report of 314 patients admitted to Emergency Department with suspected pneumonia. *Radiol. Med.* **2021**, *126*, 642, Erratum in *Radiol. Med.* **2020**, *125*, 931–942. [CrossRef] [PubMed]
89. Bianchi, A.; Mazzoni, L.N.; Busoni, S.; Pinna, N.; Albanesi, M.; Cavigli, E.; Cozzi, D.; Poggesi, A.; Miele, V.; Fainardi, E.; et al. Assessment of cerebrovascular disease with computed tomography in COVID-19 patients: Correlation of a novel specific visual score with increased mortality risk. *Radiol. Med.* **2021**, *126*, 570–576. [CrossRef] [PubMed]
90. Kovács, A.; Palásti, P.; Veréb, D.; Bozsik, B.; Palkó, A.; Kincses, Z.T. The sensitivity and specificity of chest CT in the diagnosis of COVID-19. *Eur. Radiol.* **2021**, *31*, 2819–2824. [CrossRef] [PubMed]
91. Li, K.; Wu, J.; Wu, F.; Guo, D.; Chen, L.; Fang, Z.; Li, C. The clinical and chest CT features associated with severe and critical COVID-19 pneumonia. *Investig. Radiol.* **2020**, *55*, 327–331. [CrossRef]
92. Hansell, D.M.; Bankier, A.A.; MacMahon, H.; McLoud, T.C.; Muller, N.L.; Remy, J. Fleischner Society: Glossary of terms for thoracic imaging. *Radiology* **2008**, *246*, 697–722. [CrossRef]
93. Available online: https://who.maps.arcgis.com/apps/dashboards/ead3c6475654481ca51c248d52ab9c61 (accessed on 21 May 2022).
94. Yek, C.; Warner, S.; Wiltz, J.L.; Sun, J.; Adjei, S.; Mancera, A.; Silk, B.J.; Gundlapalli, A.V.; Harris, A.M.; Boehmer, T.K.; et al. Risk Factors for Severe COVID-19 Outcomes among Persons Aged $\geq$ 18 Years Who Completed a Primary COVID-19 Vaccination Series—465 Health Care Facilities, United States, December 2020–October 2021. *MMWR Morb. Mortal. Wkly. Rep.* **2022**, *71*, 19–25. [CrossRef]
95. Pairo-Castineira, E.; Clohisey, S.; Klaric, L.; Bretherick, A.D.; Rawlik, K.; Pasko, D.; Walker, S.; Parkinson, N.; Fourman, M.H.; Russell, C.D.; et al. Genetic mechanisms of critical illness in COVID-19. *Nature* **2021**, *591*, 92–98. [CrossRef]
96. Perico, L.; Benigni, A.; Casiraghi, F.; Ng, L.F.P.; Renia, L.; Remuzzi, G. Immunity, endothelial injury and complement-induced coagulopathy in COVID-19. *Nat. Rev. Nephrol.* **2021**, *17*, 46–64. [CrossRef] [PubMed]
97. Gupta, S.; Wang, W.; Hayek, S.S.; Chan, L.; Mathews, K.S.; Melamed, M.L.; Brenner, S.K.; Leonberg-Yoo, A.; Schenck, E.J.; Radbel, J.; et al. Association Between Early Treatment with Tocilizumab and Mortality Among Critically Ill Patients with COVID-19. *JAMA Intern. Med.* **2021**, *181*, 41–51, Erratum in *JAMA Intern. Med.* **2021**, *181*, 570. [CrossRef] [PubMed]
98. Leentjens, J.; van Haaps, T.F.; Wessels, P.F.; Schutgens, R.E.G.; Middeldorp, S. COVID-19-associated coagulopathy and antithrombotic agents-lessons after 1 year. *Lancet Haematol.* **2021**, *8*, e524–e533. [CrossRef]
99. Scobie, H.M.; Johnson, A.G.; Suthar, A.B.; Severson, R.; Alden, N.B.; Balter, S.; Bertolino, D.; Blythe, D.; Brady, S.; Cadwell, B.; et al. Monitoring Incidence of COVID-19 Cases, Hospitalizations, and Deaths, by Vaccination Status—13 U.S. Jurisdictions, April 4–July 17, 2021. *MMWR Morb. Mortal. Wkly. Rep.* **2021**, *70*, 1284–1290. [CrossRef] [PubMed]
100. Mallapaty, S. China's COVID vaccines have been crucial—Now immunity is waning. *Nature* **2021**, *598*, 398–399. [CrossRef] [PubMed]
101. Barda, N.; Dagan, N.; Cohen, C.; Hernán, M.A.; Lipsitch, M.; Kohane, I.S.; Reis, B.Y.; Balicer, R.D. Effectiveness of a third dose of the BNT162b2 mRNA COVID-19 vaccine for preventing severe outcomes in Israel: An observational study. *Lancet* **2021**, *398*, 2093–2100. [CrossRef]
102. Callaway, E. The race for coronavirus vaccines: A graphical guide. *Nature* **2020**, *580*, 576–577. [CrossRef]
103. Dai, L.; Gao, G.F. Viral targets for vaccines against COVID-19. *Nat. Rev. Immunol.* **2021**, *21*, 73–82. [CrossRef]
104. Chen, J.; Wang, R.; Gilby, N.B.; Wei, G.W. Omicron (B.1.1.529): Infectivity, vaccine breakthrough, and antibody resistance. *arXiv* **2021**. Update in *J. Chem. Inf. Model.* **2022**, *62*, 412–422.
105. Ren, S.Y.; Wang, W.B.; Gao, R.D.; Zhou, A.M. Omicron variant (B.1.1.529) of SARS-CoV-2: Mutation, infectivity, transmission, and vaccine resistance. *World J. Clin. Cases.* **2022**, *10*, 1–11. [CrossRef]
106. Araf, Y.; Akter, F.; Tang, Y.D.; Fatemi, R.; Parvez, M.S.A.; Zheng, C.; Hossain, M.G. Omicron variant of SARS-CoV-2: Genomics, transmissibility, and responses to current COVID-19 vaccines. *J. Med. Virol.* **2022**, *94*, 1825–1832. [CrossRef] [PubMed]
107. Lusvarghi, S.; Pollett, S.D.; Neerukonda, S.N.; Wang, W.; Wang, R.; Vassell, R.; Epsi, N.J.; Fries, A.C.; Agan, B.K.; Lindholm, D.A.; et al. SARS-CoV-2 Omicron neutralization by therapeutic antibodies, convalescent sera, and post-mRNA vaccine booster. *bioRxiv* **2021**. [CrossRef]
108. Rampado, O.; Depaoli, A.; Marchisio, F.; Gatti, M.; Racine, D.; Ruggeri, V.; Ruggirello, I.; Darvizeh, F.; Fonio, P.; Ropolo, R. Effects of different levels of CT iterative reconstruction on low-contrast detectability and radiation dose in patients of different sizes: An anthropomorphic phantom study. *Radiol. Med.* **2021**, *126*, 55–62. [CrossRef] [PubMed]
109. Schicchi, N.; Fogante, M.; Palumbo, P.; Agliata, G.; Esposto Pirani, P.; Di Cesare, E.; Giovagnoni, A. The sub-millisievert era in CTCA: The technical basis of the new radiation dose approach. *Radiol. Med.* **2020**, *125*, 1024–1039. [CrossRef]

110. Palumbo, P.; Cannizzaro, E.; Bruno, F.; Schicchi, N.; Fogante, M.; Agostini, A.; De Donato, M.C.; De Cataldo, C.; Giovagnoni, A.; Barile, A.; et al. Coronary artery disease (CAD) extension-derived risk strati-fication for asymptomatic diabetic patients: Usefulness of low-dose coronary computed tomography angiography (CCTA) in detecting high-risk profile patients. *Radiol. Med.* **2020**, *125*, 1249–1259. [CrossRef]
111. Hussein, M.A.M.; Cafarelli, F.P.; Paparella, M.T.; Rennie, W.J.; Guglielmi, G. Phosphaturic mesenchymal tumors: Radiological aspects and suggested imaging pathway. *Radiol. Med.* **2021**, *126*, 1609–1618. [CrossRef]
112. Danti, G.; Flammia, F.; Matteuzzi, B.; Cozzi, D.; Berti, V.; Grazzini, G.; Pradella, S.; Recchia, L.; Brunese, L.; Miele, V. Gastrointestinal neuroendocrine neoplasms (GI-NENs): Hot topics in morphological, functional, and prognostic imaging. *Radiol. Med.* **2021**, *126*, 1497–1507. [CrossRef]
113. Karmazanovsky, G.; Gruzdev, I.; Tikhonova, V.; Kondratyev, E.; Revishvili, A. Computed tomography-based radiomics approach in pancreatic tumors characterization. *Radiol. Med.* **2021**, *126*, 1388–1395. [CrossRef]
114. Fusco, R.; Petrillo, M.; Granata, V.; Filice, S.; Sansone, M.; Catalano, O.; Petrillo, A. Magnetic Resonance Imaging Evaluation in Neoadjuvant Therapy of Locally Advanced Rectal Cancer: A Systematic Review. *Radiol. Oncol.* **2017**, *51*, 252–262. [CrossRef]
115. Fusco, R.; Sansone, M.; Granata, V.; Setola, S.V.; Petrillo, A. A systematic review on multiparametric MR imaging in prostate cancer detection. *Infect. Agent Cancer* **2017**, *12*, 57. [CrossRef]
116. Granata, V.; Fusco, R.; Avallone, A.; Filice, F.; Tatangelo, F.; Piccirillo, M.; Grassi, R.; Izzo, F.; Petrillo, A. Critical analysis of the major and ancillary imaging features of LI-RADS on 127 proven HCCs evaluated with functional and morphological MRI: Lights and shadows. *Oncotarget* **2017**, *8*, 51224–51237. [CrossRef] [PubMed]
117. Granata, V.; Grassi, R.; Fusco, R.; Belli, A.; Cutolo, C.; Pradella, S.; Grazzini, G.; La Porta, M.; Brunese, M.C.; De Muzio, F.; et al. Diagnostic evaluation and ablation treatments assessment in hepatocellular carcinoma. *Infect. Agent Cancer* **2021**, *16*, 53. [CrossRef]
118. Barabino, M.; Gurgitano, M.; Fochesato, C.; Angileri, S.A.; Franceschelli, G.; Santambrogio, R.; Mariani, N.M.; Opocher, E.; Carrafiello, G. LI-RADS to categorize liver nodules in patients at risk of HCC: Tool or a gadget in daily practice? *Radiol. Med.* **2021**, *126*, 5–13. [CrossRef] [PubMed]
119. Granata, V.; Fusco, R.; Filice, S.; Catalano, O.; Piccirillo, M.; Palaia, R.; Izzo, F.; Petrillo, A. The current role and future prospectives of functional parameters by diffusion weighted imaging in the assessment of histologic grade of HCC. *Infect. Agent Cancer* **2018**, *3*, 23. [CrossRef] [PubMed]
120. Orlacchio, A.; Chegai, F.; Roma, S.; Merolla, S.; Bosa, A.; Francioso, S. Degradable starch microspheres transarterial chemoembolization (DSMs-TACE) in patients with unresectable hepatocellular carcinoma (HCC): Long-term results from a single-center 137-patient cohort prospective study. *Radiol. Med.* **2020**, *125*, 98–106. [CrossRef]

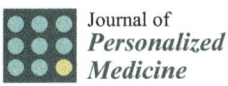

Article

Pulmonary Lymphangitis Poses a Major Challenge for Radiologists in an Oncological Setting during the COVID-19 Pandemic

Roberta Fusco [1], Igino Simonetti [2], Stefania Ianniello [3], Alberta Villanacci [3], Francesca Grassi [4], Federica Dell'Aversana [4], Roberta Grassi [4,5], Diletta Cozzi [5,6], Eleonora Bicci [5,6], Pierpaolo Palumbo [7], Alessandra Borgheresi [5,8], Andrea Giovagnoni [5,8], Vittorio Miele [5,6], Antonio Barile [9] and Vincenza Granata [2,*]

1 Medical Oncology Division, Igea SpA, 80013 Napoli, Italy; r.fusco@igeamedical.com
2 Division of Radiology, Istituto Nazionale Tumori IRCCS Fondazione Pascale—IRCCS di Napoli, 80131 Naples, Italy; igino.simonetti@istitutotumori.na.it
3 Diagnostica per Immagini nelle Malattie Infettive INMI Spallanzani IRCCS, 00161 Rome, Italy; stefania.ianniello@inmi.it (S.I.); alberta.villanacci@inmi.it (A.V.)
4 Division of Radiology, Università degli Studi della Campania Luigi Vanvitelli, 80127 Naples, Italy; francescagrassi1996@gmail.com (F.G.); federica.dellaversana@studenti.unicampania.it (F.D.); grassi.roberta89@gmail.com (R.G.)
5 Italian Society of Medical and Interventional Radiology (SIRM), SIRM Foundation, Via della Signora 2, 20122 Milan, Italy; cozzid@aou-careggi.toscana.it (D.C.); eleonora.bicci92@gmail.com (E.B.); alessandra.borgheresi@gmail.com (A.B.); a.giovagnoni@univpm.it (A.G.); vmiele@sirm.org (V.M.)
6 Department of Radiology, Azienda Ospedaliero-Universitaria Careggi, 50134 Florence, Italy
7 Abruzzo Health Unit 1, Department of Diagnostic Imaging, Area of Cardiovascular and Interventional Imaging, 67100 L'Aquila, Italy; palumbopierpaolo89@gmail.com
8 Department of Clinical, Special and Dental Sciences, Marche Polytechnic University, 60126 Ancona, Italy
9 Department of Applied Clinical Science and Biotechnology, University of L'Aquila, Via Vetoio 1, 67100 L'Aquila, Italy; antonio.barile@univaq.it
* Correspondence: v.granata@istitutotumori.na.it

Abstract: Due to the increasing number of COVID-19-infected and vaccinated individuals, radiologists continue to see patients with COVID-19 pneumonitis and recall pneumonitis, which could result in additional workups and false-positive results. Moreover, cancer patients undergoing immunotherapy may show therapy-related pneumonitis during imaging management. This is otherwise known as immune checkpoint inhibitor-related pneumonitis. Following on from this background, radiologists should seek to know their patients' COVID-19 infection and vaccination history. Knowing the imaging features related to COVID-19 infection and vaccination is critical to avoiding misleading results and alarmism in patients and clinicians.

Keywords: pulmonary lymphangitis; COVID 19; vaccination; computed tomography

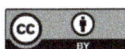

1. Background

The current coronavirus disease 2019 (COVID-19) pandemic caused by severe acute respiratory syndrome coronavirus 2 (SARS-CoV-2) has produced a worldwide public health threat with millions of people at risk [1–10]. Globally, as of 5:18 PM CET on 4 March 2022, there were 440,807,756 confirmed cases of COVID-19, including 5,978,096 deaths, reported to the World Health Organization (WHO). In Italy, from 3 January 2020 at 5:18 p.m. CET to 4 March 2022, 12,910,506 confirmed cases of COVID-19 with 155,399 deaths have been registered, reported to the WHO [11].

The symptoms of COVID-19 infection are different from patient to patient, with the most common including fever, fatigue, cough, anorexia, and shortness of breath during different phases of this disease [12–14]. Additionally, less common symptoms such as a sore throat, headache, confusion, and chest tightness have been also observed [15,16], as well as minor gastrointestinal complications such as nausea, vomiting, and diarrhoea [17]. However, there have been patients not yet symptomatic (pre-symptomatic) and there have been patients without symptoms typical of the COVID-19 disease (asymptomatic), as revealed in several reports [18–20]. Several patients with COVID-19 infection were asymptomatic throughout the infection period [21,22]. In these asymptomatic patients the diagnosis was often accidental, as they performed radiological examinations for another cause or during the follow-up periods when dealing with cancer patients [23–32].

In addition, it has been critical to develop a vaccine as soon as possible to prevent SARS-CoV-2 infection in order to safeguard persons who are at a high risk of complications. Globally, on 27 February 2022, a total of 10,585,766,316 vaccine doses had been administered [11]. The Italian government employed the subsequent vaccination policy: two vaccine doses, with a booster dose 5–6 months after the end of the vaccination cycle, in patients who have not been infected. A policy for assessing vaccine adverse events is founded on the collaboration of local and national health structures, assisted by the Italian Medicines Agency (AIFA) [33]. Since the inception of vaccine inoculation, several adverse events have been reported and shared world-wide, with different findings reported by imaging studies [34–44]. While COVID-19-vaccine-related lymphadenopathy (LAP) has been gradually reported [34], few studies have reported lymphangitis after vaccination from COVID-19, and in several patients, radiation recall pneumonitis has been reported [45–55].

Since during the imaging management of oncological patients, the lung remains as the site of metastases, with different findings, including lymphangitis pattern [56–61], as well as the site of adverse events such as pneumonitis related to such therapies as Immune Checkpoint Inhibitor-Related Pneumonitis [62–70], it is clear that radiologists should know of previous COVID-19 infection or vaccination. The knowledge of these features related to COVID-19 infection or vaccination is critical in order to not presenting misleading results in patients and clinicians by determining disease progression or an adverse treatment effect.

This narrative review aims to evaluate the different patterns of pulmonary lymphangitis to improve the knowledge.

Pulmonary Lymphangitis Carcinomatosa

Pulmonary lymphangitis carcinomatosa (PLC) is an unusual appearance of metastatic lung disease in which advanced cancers spread through pulmonary lymphatic vessels (Figure 1).

The difficult outflow of lymph from the lungs causes accumulation of interstitial fluid and disturbances in the diffusion of oxygen, which can cause respiratory dysfunction.

Imaging findings appear later than symptoms, and dyspnoea, representing the most frequent symptom, is habitually more severe than radiological findings [56–58]. The most common primary cancers that coexist with PLC are breast (17.3%), lung (10.8%) and stomach (10.8%) cancers [56]. According to Bruce et al. [70], the prevalence of PLC ranges from 6% to 8% in patients with malignant disease. Kazawa et al. [71] showed that the prevalence of PLC-related small-cell lung cancer was recognized in 8.8%. In patients with cancer and pulmonary embolism, the prevalence of PLC was 4.5% [72–77].

There are several hypotheses regarding the metastatic tumour spread, mainly limited to the lymphatics, although the precise process is still uncertain. The tumour could spread through the haematogenous route, causing obliterated endarteritis and then penetrating the vascular endothelium to reach the perivascular lymphatics, to remain stationed there. Direct entry into lymphatic circulation is possible when nearby lymph vessels are involved. Trans-diaphragmatic diffusion has also been suggested to clarify PLC due to abdominal cancers. Local obstruction and fluid accumulation follow soon after the malignant cells are trapped in the lymphatic vessels. This is followed by thickening of the bronchovascular bundles and alveolar septa due to tissue oedema and nodular thickening, suggesting local tumour cell growth.

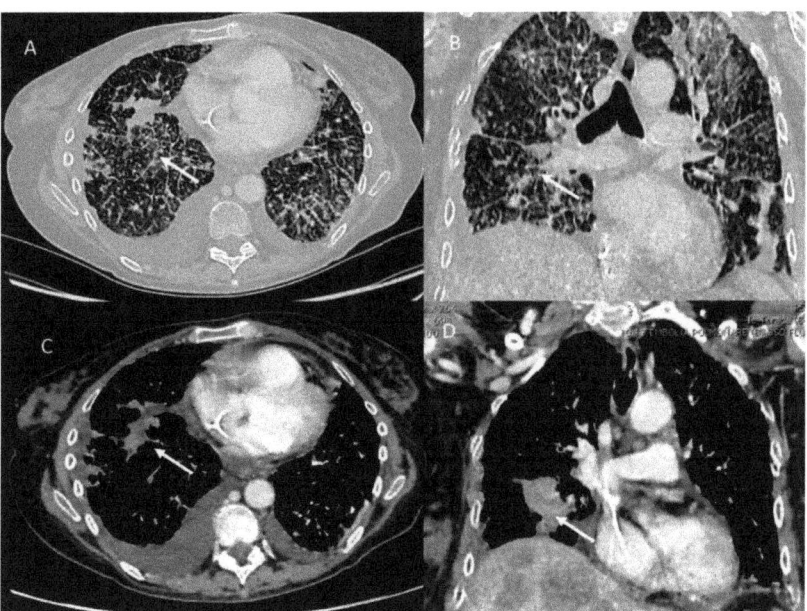

Figure 1. PLC in pancreatic cancer patient. CT (axial (**A,C**) and coronal (**B,D**)) shows comprise diffuse intrapulmonary infiltrates (arrows) with irregularly interlobular septal thickening, nodular thickening and pleural effusions.

Imaging has low specificity for PLC detection because images are often normal in initial phases. However, imaging is often performed to rule out other causes [57,78–85]. A chest radiograph (chest X-ray) may be the first approach and an association of several radiological findings could favour the diagnosis in about half the cases. However, in 30 to 50% of patients, especially in the initial phases, the X-ray may be normal [56,57]. Therefore, computed tomography (CT) and especially high-resolution CT (HRCT) are recommended techniques for studying patients with suspected PLC [55–57,86–93]. The CT results are similar to other interstitial lung diseases, so they have low diagnostic accuracy in differentiating and detecting PLC [56,57]. The usual CT findings comprise nodular or diffuse intrapulmonary infiltrates, irregularly interlobular septal thickening, smooth (early stage) or nodular thickening (late development), hilar and mediastinal lymphadenopathy, ground-glass opacity due to interstitial oedema or parenchymal extension of tumours, and pleural effusions. These features could be on one or both sides, focal or diffuse, or symmetrical or asymmetrical. Smooth or irregularly thickened interlobular septae are more conducive to PLC than to tumour embolism. Although nodular thickening of the septae is thought to differentiate PLC from other interstitial lung patterns, some conditions such as sarcoidosis or asbestosis may mimic it [57]. Another distinguishing feature of PLC is the preservation of the general and lobular architecture of the lung. [56,57].

2. Immune Checkpoint Inhibitor-Related Pneumonitis

Anti-programmed death-1 (anti-PD-1) and programmed anti-death ligand 1 (anti-PD-L1) monoclonal antibodies (mAb) for patients with multiple cancers are licensed treatments, including nivolumab and pem-brolizumab for melanoma and non-small-cell lung cancer (NSCLC), nivolumab for renal cell carcinoma and Hodgkin's lymphoma, atezolizumab for bladder cancer, and nivolumab plus ipilimumab for melanoma [94–103]. A major feature of anti-PD-1/PD-L1 mAbs is their mild toxicity, but serious immune-related adverse events can occur. Pneumonia is an immune-related adverse event defined as focal or diffuse inflammation of the lung parenchyma, and its incidence in studies with anti-PD-1/PD-L1 mAbs ranges from 0% to 10% [104]. Drug-related pneumonia can also occur with chemotherapy (docetaxel [105], gemcitabine [106], bleomycin [107]), targeted therapy (epidermal growth factor receptor inhibitors [108,109], mammalian target of rapamycin inhibitors [110]), and radiotherapy [111,112].

Compared to conventional chemotherapy for pneumonia, these patients showed a greater susceptibility to the development of treatment-related pneumonia, with an increased risk of high-grade pneumonia. Previous studies on this pneumonia have shown that clinical, radiological and pathological characterization can facilitate early diagnosis to improve patient outcomes [113–117]. The aetiology and underlying mechanisms of anti-PD-1/PD-L1 mAb-associated pneumonia are unknown [63,118–121].

Immune checkpoint inhibitor (ICI)-related pneumonia could cause significant morbidity, with possible discontinuation of therapy and possible mortality [118]. The time to onset of pneumonia ranges from 9 days to over 19 months after the initiation of therapy, with a median time of 2.8 months [118]. Imaging plays a crucial role in this effect detection. Although X-ray may be an initial tool, CT is able to detect all subtle changes in pneumonitis and help to differentiate among subtypes, as described by Delaunay et al. [122]. Investigations described 64 cases of pneumonia with the following CT patterns: (a) organized pneumonia (OP) (23%), (b) hypersensitivity pneumonitis (HP) (16%), (c) non-specific interstitial pneumonia (NSIP) (8%) and (d) bronchiolitis (6%). Some patients were diagnosed with concomitant patterns and a distinctive pattern was not identified in 36% of cases [122]. OP's pattern usually shows bilateral peribronchovascular and subpleural ground-glass and airspace opacities, with mid- to lower-lung predominance (Figure 2).

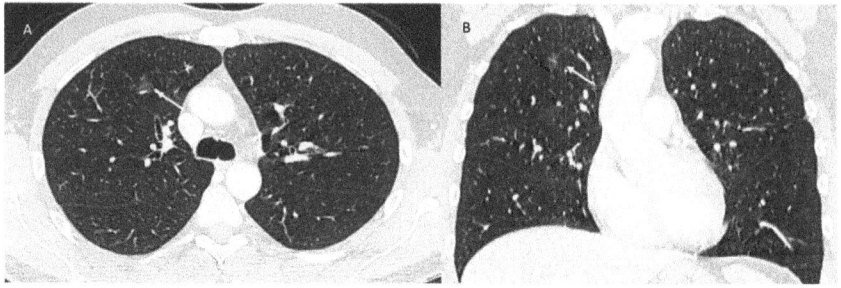

Figure 2. ICI-related pneumonitis. OP pattern on CT (axial: (**A**) and coronal: (**B**)): ground-glass and airspace opacities (arrows).

In addition, an inverted halo or atoll sign is detected. Pulmonary nodules, usually with peribroncovascular distribution and generally smaller (<10 mm) nodules, may also be detected. However, in some cases, the nodules may be nodular and massive with pointed edges, mimicking findings of malignancy [118,122]. These features should be distinguished from progression of malignancy (concurrent worsening of disease in other areas) and infection (clinical history, laboratory findings, response to appropriate therapy).

The NSIP pattern commonly manifests as ground glass and lattice opacities predominantly in the lower lobe. Airspace disease is temporally homogeneous and relatively symmetrical, with uncommon consolidation opacities, allowing NSIP patterns to be distinguished from OP patterns. Subpleural sparing of the posterior and inferior lobes has also been described as a specific feature. NSIP pattern should be distinguished from NSIP associated with autoimmune or connective tissue disease (appropriate medical history and condition-specific markers, no temporal relationship to immunotherapy course) and infection (clinical history, laboratory findings, response to appropriate therapy).

The HP pattern is associated with lower-grade symptoms. CT findings include diffuse or predominant ground-glass centrilobular nodules in the upper lobe, which may be related to air entrapment. This pattern should be distinguished from exposure-related HP (exposure and occupational history, no temporal relationship to immunotherapy course), and from respiratory and follicular bronchiolitis (smoking history or underlying connective tissue and/or autoimmune disease history) and atypical infection (clinical history, laboratory findings, response to appropriate therapy).

Acute interstitial pneumonia (AIP)–acute respiratory distress syndrome (ARDS) is not a model of ICI therapy-related pneumonia, although it is associated with a more severe clinical course and extensive pulmonary involvement with imaging. This pattern is characterized by geographic or diffuse ground-glass or consolidation opacities involving most, and sometimes all, of the lungs, although lobular sparing areas may be detected. There may also be a thickening of the interlobular septum and a "crazy pavement" pattern (Figure 3). The differential diagnosis is extensive and includes pulmonary oedema, haemorrhage, and infection. The findings of ARDS may also be due to extrapulmonary causes such as pancreatitis, sepsis and/or shock and transfusion reactions.

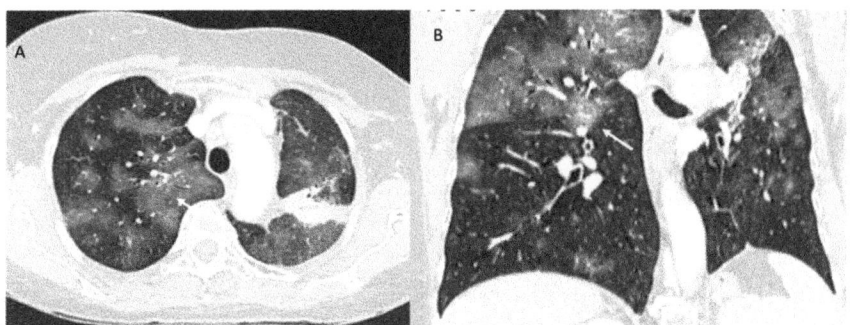

Figure 3. ICI-related pneumonitis. AIP-ARDS pattern on CT (axial: (**A**) and coronal: (**B**)): diffuse ground-glass opacities involving a majority of the lungs (arrows), although areas of lobular sparing can be detected.

The bronchiolitis pattern appears as a region of centrilobular nodularity, often ten in a tree-in-bud pattern. Thickening of the adjacent bronchial wall is frequently observed, as well as focal ground-glass and consolidation opacity, although this should not be the main feature. This pattern should be distinguished from aspiration (dependent lungs, airway and oesophageal secretion) and infection (clinical history, laboratory findings, response to appropriate therapy).

2.1. COVID-19 Vaccine Radiation Recall

Radiation recall reaction (RRR) is an infrequent but well-known event to clinicians, characterized by a late-occurring acute inflammatory reaction that develops in confined areas corresponding to previously irradiated radiation therapy (RT) treatment fields. RRP has been known to be triggered by a number of chemotherapy agents [123–132], including, recently, even COVID-19 vaccines [45]. It occurs in a variety of tissues, the commonest being skin, which accounts for two-thirds of reported cases. It is usually mild and self-limiting when the trigger drug is stopped. Re-challenge with the drug does not necessarily cause reactivation of the reaction.

This event has been reported within the lungs [52,118,133], determining radiation recall pneumonitis as acute inflammation within a previously irradiated area. The mechanism of the disease is unclear, but it seems to be related to an immune response. COVID-19 infection is known to cause immunological reactions, such as cytokine storm or multisystem inflammatory syndrome, in children [134–137]. Just like real infection, the developed vaccines are expected to induce an immune response. The inflammatory state created by the vaccine can favour the development of radiation recall. In fact, the few available papers on the topic suggest that COVID-19 vaccine can cause RRR, considering the time of vaccine administration and this event (Figure 4) [52,133]. The radioactive recall pneumonia model includes consolidated or ground-glass opacities. It should be suspected in all patients with previous radiotherapy with new airspace changes clearly demarcated from the adjacent lung. The main differential diagnosis is infection that does not respect boundaries and occurs outside of the previous radiation field.

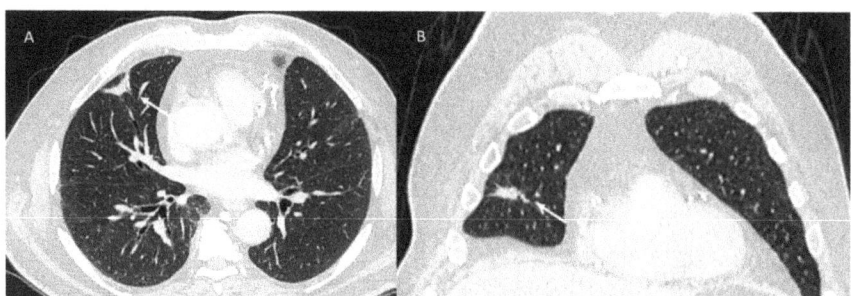

Figure 4. Radiation recall pneumonitis (CT scan axial: (**A**) and coronal: (**B**)) pattern includes consolidative opacities limited (arrows) to a prior radiation field.

2.2. Pneumonitis COVID-19

Typical chest CT imaging findings for COVID-19 patients are ground-glass opacity with bilateral multifocal patches or consolidation with the interlobular septum and vascular thickening in peripheral areas of the lungs [134–142]. These manifestations may also be compatible with other viral pneumonias [143]. In this scenario, the current gold standard for diagnosing COVID-19 is based on a molecular reverse transcription polymerase chain reaction (RT-PCR) test, aimed at detecting virus RNA in respiratory samples such as nasopharynx swabs or bronchial aspirate [144].

Compared to RT-PCR, the specificity of CT in detecting COVID-19 is lower, with an overall reported specificity of 46–80% [145–147]. This is due to the fact that the typical pattern of COVID-19 pneumonia shows a partial overlap with that of other lung diseases: ground-glass opacity (GGO), consolidation, crazy pavement, and enlargement of subsegmental vessels (diameter greater than 3 mm) in the GGO areas [148–150]. The temporal course of these anomalies was described by Pan et al., reporting four phases of the disease: initial stage (0–4 days after the onset of symptoms) with GGO as the main finding (Figure 5), progressive stage (5–8 days after onset of symptoms) with widespread GGO, mad pattern and consolidation, peak stage (9–13 days after onset of symptoms) with consolidation becoming more prevalent (Figure 6) and advanced stage ($\geq$14 days after the onset of symptoms) with gradual absorption of anomalies (Figure 7) [151]. A recent study examined the performance of radiologists in differentiating COVID-19 from non-COVID-19 viral pneumonia, revealing an accuracy of between 60 and 83% [152].

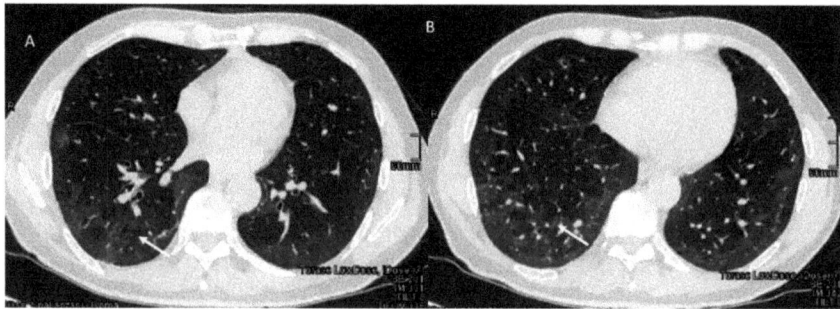

Figure 5. COVID-19 patient. CT (axial plane: (**A**,**B**)) shows early stage with GGO (arrow) as main finding.

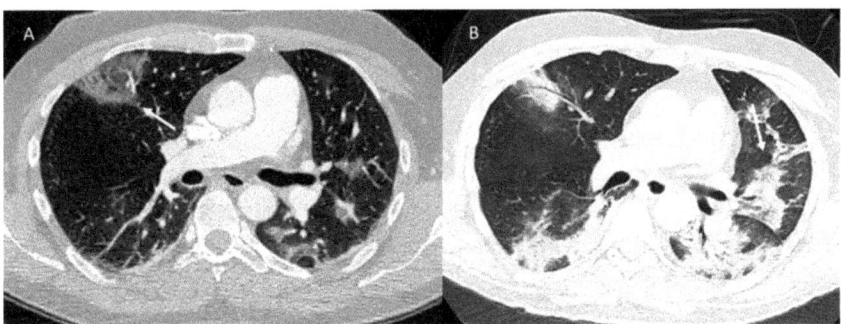

Figure 6. COVID-19 patient at peak stage. CT (axial plane: (**A**,**B**)) shows consolidation (arrow).

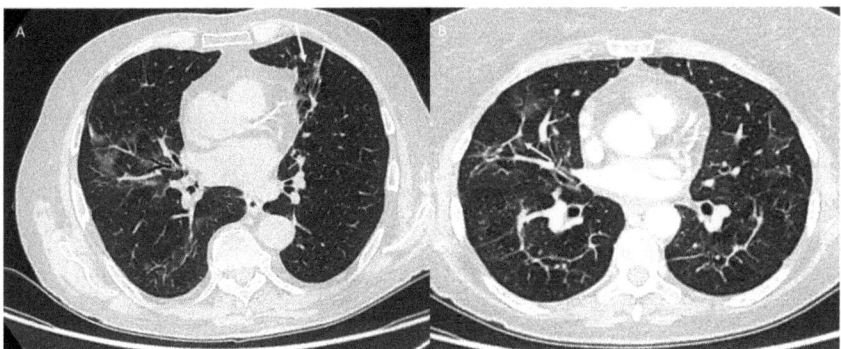

Figure 7. COVID-19 patient at late stage. CT (axial plane: (**A**,**B**)) shows fibrotic-like changes (arrow).

COVID-19 pneumonia may be misdiagnosed as non-COVID-19 lung disease in the early and late stages, reflecting the fact that the typical early-stage pattern and the absorption of late features are commonly linked to signs of organizational pneumonia or signs of early fibrosis. These characteristics can be found in different conditions and, therefore, this aspect should be considered non-specific [148–152].

3. Discussion

Since the population continues to be infected or vaccinated in larger numbers, COVID-19 pneumonitis and RRR pneumonitis caused by COVID-19 vaccination will be increasingly seen by radiologists and could result in imaging test call-backs, additional workups, and false-positive results. In addition, considering oncological patients who could develop drug-related pneumonitis or a pattern of PLC as a progressive disease, it is clear as these conditions should be taken into account for a correct diagnosis. Therefore, a correct medical history is essential to ruling out the possibility of a recent infection as well as recent vaccine administration.

RRR and SARS-CoV-2 interstitial pneumonia, so non-COVID-19-related pneumonia, show overlapping clinical features. In fact, the most common symptoms are dyspnoea and dry non-productive cough and fever. Additionally, chest CT findings are also very similar, as the radiological characteristics of COVID-19 and non-COVID-19-related pneumonia are GGO in the initial phase, patchy areas of consolidation in the peak phase and fibrotic changes in the dissipative phase [8,14].

Where the cause of the lung abnormalities is unclear, due to radiological CT findings being unspecific, multidisciplinary management would be correct to establish the main proper treatment. Although the management of oncological patients should consider the probability of malignant lung involvement with disease progression or adverse effects of specific therapies, it is clear that in pandemic conditions, several unspecific features may be related to an undiagnosed infection. Although the typical pattern of COVID-19 pneumonitis should be identified with high accuracy in symptomatic patients, this could be complicated if infection has been not diagnosed, especially in the post-infection phase. Therefore, we should consider several features, such as that the typical RRR pattern is usually strictly related to the target volume and to the dose distribution of the treatment plan, while during COVID-19 infection, the parenchymal involvement is not limited to a single lobe, although this is possible during the first phase. Additionally, PLC and ICI-related pneumonitis show diffuse parenchymal involvement. Additionally, in PLC, we find an irregularly interlobular septal thickening or nodular thickening, while in COVID-19 pneumonitis and RRR, septal thickening is more regular. These differences in chest CT patterns are the main factors that should help lead to a proper diagnosis (Table 1). However, distinguishing COVID-19 lung involvement or vaccine RRR from other lung pathologies such as cancer on chest CT may be straightforward, differentiation between COVID-19 and other pneumonias can be particularly troublesome for physicians because of the radiographic similarities, and this is particularly evident during the early or late phases of these pathologies. Inaccurate imaging interpretation makes it harder for patient management strategies to work efficiently.

Table 1. Lung involvement and CT pattern for pneumonia type.

Type of Pneumonia	Lung Involvement	CT-Patter
COVID-19 Pneumonia	Diffuse (related to the phase of disease)	ground-glass opacity, crazy-paving pattern, consolidative opacities, interlobular septal thickening (according to the phase of disease)
RRR-Related Vaccine	Target Area	Consolidative opacities
Pulmonary lymphangitis carcinomatosa	Diffuse (related to the phase of disease)	Irregularly interlobular septal thickening, smooth (early stage), or nodular thickening (late development), ground-glass opacity, pleural effusions.
ICI-Related Pneumonitis	Diffuse (related to the phase of disease)	ground-glass and reticular opacities, consolidative opacities, interlobular septal thickening, "crazy-paving" pattern

Interestingly, COVID-19 pneumonia and ICI-related pneumonitis have been suggested to share critical biological mechanisms, including the hyperactivation of immune cells associated with a significant increase in pro-inflammatory cytokines. Distinguishing between COVID-19 pneumonia and ICI-related pneumonitis is a diagnostic challenge. ICI-related pneumonitis might present with several patterns. These patterns seemingly overlap the CT features of COVID-19 pneumonia, possibly due to overlapped biological mechanisms.

Recently, the progressive integration of radiomics approaches and artificial intelligence (AI)-based solutions could be of help. To date, the application of AI in medical imaging has improved the assessment and early diagnosis of neurodegenerative diseases and heart disease, with a particularly high impact on breast and lung cancer [153–162]. A cutting-edge research direction leverages deep learning (DL) and machine learning (ML) to understand COVID-19. AI could be used for the detection and quantification of COVID-19 disease from X-ray and CT images [163–165], enabling correct patient diagnosis and management. Deep learning (DL), a form of AI, has been successfully applied to chest CT imaging to distinguish COVID-19 pneumonia from community-acquired infections, as well as to provide qualitative and quantitative analyses for disease burden estimation and facilitating and expediting imaging interpretation [166]. However, deep learning algorithms based only on CT images cannot distinguish COVID-19 pneumonia from other lung interstitial diseases with overlapping CT features with high specificity; thus, adding clinical/laboratory findings to the algorithm can improve the diagnostic performance based on binary classification [167,168].

4. Conclusions

Knowing the chest imaging features related to COVID-19 infection or vaccine is critical to avoid misleading results in patients and clinicians and determine the idea of a disease progression or an adverse treatment effect. In this context, we should consider several features, as the typical RRR pattern is usually strictly related to the target volume and the dose distribution of the treatment plan. At the same time, during COVID-19 infection, parenchymal involvement is not limited to a single lobe, although this is possible during the first phase. Additionally, PLC and ICI-related pneumonitis show a diffuse parenchymal involvement. The PLC shows an irregularly interlobular septal thickening or nodular thickening, while septal thickening is common in COVID-19 pneumonitis and RRR. These differences in chest CT patterns are the main factors that should help for proper diagnosis. However, distinguishing COVID-19 lung involvement or vaccine RRR from other lung pathologies on chest CT may be straightforward, particularly during the early or late phases of these pathologies.

Author Contributions: Conceptualization, S.I., V.M. and V.G.; Investigation, R.F., I.S., A.V., F.G., F.D., R.G., D.C., E.B., P.P., A.B. (Alessandra Borgheresi), A.G., A.B. (Antonio Barile) and V.G.; Methodology, R.F., I.S., A.V., F.G., F.D., R.G., D.C., E.B., P.P., A.B. (Alessandra Borgheresi), A.G., V.M., A.B. (Alessandra Borgheresi) and V.G. Each author has participated sufficiently to take public responsibility for the content of the manuscript. All authors have read and agreed to the published version of the manuscript.

Funding: This research received no external funding.

Institutional Review Board Statement: The study was conducted according to the guidelines of the Declaration of Helsinki. Approval by the Institutional Review Board was not needed considering the nature of the study: the findings are a description of a single case report.

Informed Consent Statement: Informed consent was obtained from the patient.

Data Availability Statement: Data are available at https://zenodo.org/record/6393020#.YkgKdhBy3A (accessed on 21 January 2022).

Acknowledgments: The authors are grateful to Alessandra Trocino, librarian at the National Cancer Institute of Naples, Italy. Moreover, for their collaboration, the authors are grateful for the research support of Paolo Pariante, Martina Totaro and Andrea Esposito of Radiology Division, "Istituto Nazionale Tumori IRCCS Fondazione Pascale—IRCCS di Napoli", Naples, I-80131, Italy.

Conflicts of Interest: The authors have no conflict of interest to disclose.

References

1. Stramare, R.; Carretta, G.; Capizzi, A.; Boemo, D.G.; Contessa, C.; Motta, R.; De Conti, G.; Causin, F.; Giraudo, C.; Donato, D. Radiological management of COVID-19: Structure your diagnostic path to guarantee a safe path. *Radiol. Med.* **2020**, *125*, 691–694. [CrossRef] [PubMed]
2. Granata, V.; Fusco, R.; Izzo, F.; Setola, S.V.; Coppola, M.; Grassi, R.; Reginelli, A.; Cappabianca, S.; Petrillo, A. COVID-19 infection in cancer patients: The management in a diagnostic unit. *Radiol. Oncol.* **2021**, *55*, 121–129. [CrossRef] [PubMed]
3. Gaia, C.; Chiara, C.M.; Silvia, L.; Chiara, A.; Luisa, D.C.M.; Giulia, B.; Silvia, P.; Lucia, C.; Alessandra, T.; Annarita, S.; et al. Chest CT for early detection and management of coronavirus disease (COVID-19): A report of 314 patients admitted to Emergency Department with suspected pneumonia. *Radiol. Med.* **2020**, *125*, 931–942. [CrossRef] [PubMed]
4. Gabelloni, M.; Faggioni, L.; Cioni, D.; Mendola, V.; Falaschi, Z.; Coppola, S.; Corradi, F.; Isirdi, A.; Brandi, N.; Coppola, F.; et al. Extracorporeal membrane oxygenation (ECMO) in COVID-19 patients: A pocket guide for radiologists. *Radiol. Med.* **2022**, *13*, 369–382. [CrossRef] [PubMed]
5. Giovagnoni, A. Facing the COVID-19 emergency: We can, and we do. *Radiol. Med.* **2020**, *125*, 337–338. [CrossRef]
6. Montesi, G.; Di Biase, S.; Chierchini, S.; Pavanato, G.; Virdis, G.E.; Contato, E.; Mandoliti, G. Radiotherapy during COVID-19 pandemic. How to create a No fly zone: A Northern Italy experience. *Radiol. Med.* **2020**, *125*, 600–603. [CrossRef]
7. Ierardi, A.M.; Wood, B.J.; Arrichiello, A.; Bottino, N.; Bracchi, L.; Forzenigo, L.; Andrisani, M.C.; Vespro, V.; Bonelli, C.; Amalou, A.; et al. Preparation of a radiology department in an Italian hospital dedicated to COVID-19 patients. *Radiol. Med.* **2020**, *125*, 894–901. [CrossRef]

8. Grassi, R.; Cappabianca, S.; Urraro, F.; Feragalli, B.; Montanelli, A.; Patelli, G.; Granata, V.; Giacobbe, G.; Russo, G.M.; Grillo, A.; et al. Chest CT Computerized Aided Quantification of PNEUMONIA Lesions in COVID-19 Infection: A Comparison among Three Commercial Software. *Int. J. Environ. Res. Public Health* **2020**, *17*, 6914. [CrossRef]
9. Pediconi, F.; Galati, F.; Bernardi, D.; Belli, P.; Brancato, B.; Calabrese, M.; Camera, L.; Carbonaro, L.A.; Caumo, F.; Clauser, P.; et al. Breast imaging and cancer diagnosis during the COVID-19 pandemic: Recommendations from the Italian College of Breast Radiologists by SIRM. *Radiol. Med.* **2020**, *125*, 926–930. [CrossRef]
10. Koç, A.; Sezgin, S.; Kayıpmaz, S. Comparing different planimetric methods on volumetric estimations by using cone beam computed tomography. *Radiol. Med.* **2020**, *125*, 398–405. [CrossRef]
11. WHO Coronavirus (COVID-19) Dashboard. Available online: https://covid19.who.int (accessed on 21 January 2022).
12. Xu, X.W.; Wu, X.X.; Jiang, X.G.; Xu, K.J.; Ying, L.J.; Ma, C.L.; Li, S.B.; Wang, H.Y.; Zhang, S.; Gaon, H.N.; et al. Clinical findings in a group of patients infected with the 2019 novel coronavirus (SARS-CoV-2) outside of Wuhan, China: Retrospective case series. *BMJ* **2020**, *368*, m606. [CrossRef] [PubMed]
13. Chen, N.; Zhou, M.; Dong, X.; Qu, J.; Gong, F.; Han, Y.; Qui, Y.; Wang, J.; Liu, Y.; Wei, Y.; et al. Epidemiological and clinical characteristics of 99 cases of 2019 novel coronavirus pneumonia in Wuhan, China: A descriptive study. *Lancet* **2020**, *395*, 507–513. [CrossRef]
14. Wu, Z.; McGoogan, J.M. Characteristics of and important lessons from the coronavirus disease 2019 (COVID-19) outbreak in China: Summary of a report of 72 314 cases from the Chinese center for disease control and prevention. *JAMA* **2020**, *323*, 1239–1242. [CrossRef] [PubMed]
15. Han, C.; Duan, C.; Zhang, S.; Spiegel, B.; Shi, H.; Wang, W.; Zhang, L.; Lin, R.; Liu, J.; Ding, Z.; et al. Digestive Symptoms in COVID-19 Patients with Mild Disease Severity: Clinical Presentation, Stool Viral RNA Testing, and Outcomes. *Am. J. Gastroenterol.* **2020**, *115*, 916–923. [CrossRef] [PubMed]
16. Pan, L.; Mu, M.; Yang, P.; Sun, Y.; Wang, R.; Yan, J.; Li, P.; Hu, B.; Wang, J.; Hu, C.; et al. Clinical characteristics of COVID-19 patients with digestive symptoms in Hubei, China: A descriptive, cross-sectional, multicenter study. *Am. J. Gastroenterol.* **2020**, *115*, 766–773. [CrossRef] [PubMed]
17. Liu, W.; Zhang, Q.; Chen, J.; Xiang, R.; Song, H.; Shu, S.; Chen, L.; Liang, L.; Zhou, J.; You, L.; et al. Detection of COVID-19 in children in early January 2020 in Wuhan, China. *N. Engl. J. Med.* **2020**, *382*, 1370–1371. [CrossRef]
18. Lu, X.; Zhang, L.; Du, H.; Zhang, J.; Li, Y.Y.; Qu, J.; Zhang, W.; Wang, Y.; Bao, S.; Li, Y.; et al. SARS-CoV-2 Infection in Children. *N. Engl. J. Med.* **2020**, *382*, 1663–1665. [CrossRef]
19. Hu, Z.; Song, C.; Xu, C.; Jin, G.; Chen, Y.; Xu, X.; Ma, X.; Chen, W.; Lin, Y.; Zheng, Y.; et al. Clinical characteristics of 24 asymptomatic infections with COVID-19 screened among close contacts in Nanjing. China. *Sci. China Life Sci.* **2020**, *63*, 706–711. [CrossRef]
20. Wang, Y.; Liu, Y.; Liu, L.; Wang, X.; Luo, N.; Li, L. Clinical Outcomes in 55 Patients with Severe Acute Respiratory Syndrome Coronavirus 2 Who Were Asymptomatic at Hospital Admission in Shenzhen, China. *J. Infect. Dis.* **2020**, *221*, 1770–1774. [CrossRef]
21. Mizumoto, K.; Kagaya, K.; Zarebski, A.; Chowell, G. Estimating the asymptomatic proportion of coronavirus disease 2019 (COVID-19) cases on board the Diamond Princess cruise ship, Yokohama, Japan, 2020. *Euro Surveill.* **2020**, *25*, 2000180. [CrossRef]
22. Pan, X.; Chen, D.; Xia, Y.; Wu, X.; Li, T.; Ou, X.; Zhou, L.; Liu, J. Asymptomatic cases in a family cluster with SARS-CoV-2 infection. *Lancet Infect Dis.* **2020**, *20*, 410–411. [CrossRef]
23. Agostini, A.; Floridi, C.; Borgheresi, A.; Badaloni, M.; Pirani, P.E.; Terilli, F.; Ottaviani, L.; Giovagnoni, A. Proposal of a low-dose, long-pitch, dual-source chest CT protocol on third-generation dual-source CT using a tin filter for spectral shaping at 100 kVp for CoronaVirus Disease 2019 (COVID-19) patients: A feasibility study. *Radiol. Med.* **2020**, *125*, 365–373. [CrossRef] [PubMed]
24. Borghesi, A.; Maroldi, R. COVID-19 outbreak in Italy: Experimental chest X-ray scoring system for quantifying and monitoring disease progression. *Radiol. Med.* **2020**, *125*, 509–513. [CrossRef] [PubMed]
25. Neri, E.; Miele, V.; Coppola, F.; Grassi, R. Use of CT and artificial intelligence in suspected or COVID-19 positive patients: Statement of the Italian Society of Medical and Interventional Radiology. *Radiol. Med.* **2020**, *125*, 505–508. [CrossRef]
26. Carotti, M.; Salaffi, F.; Sarzi-Puttini, P.; Agostini, A.; Borgheresi, A.; Minorati, D.; Galli, M.; Marotto, D.; Giovagnoni, A. Chest CT features of coronavirus disease 2019 (COVID-19) pneumonia: Key points for radiologists. *Radiol. Med.* **2020**, *125*, 636–646. [CrossRef]
27. Fusco, R.; Grassi, R.; Granata, V.; Setola, S.V.; Grassi, F.; Cozzi, D.; Pecori, B.; Izzo, F.; Petrillo, A. Artificial Intelligence and COVID-19 Using Chest CT Scan and Chest X-ray Images: Machine Learning and Deep Learning Approaches for Diagnosis and Treatment. *J. Pers. Med.* **2021**, *11*, 993. [CrossRef] [PubMed]
28. Borghesi, A.; Zigliani, A.; Masciullo, R.; Golemi, S.; Maculotti, P.; Farina, D.; Maroldi, R. Radiographic severity index in COVID-19 pneumonia: Relationship to age and sex in 783 Italian patients. *Radiol. Med.* **2020**, *125*, 461–464. [CrossRef]
29. Cozzi, D.; Albanesi, M.; Cavigli, E.; Moroni, C.; Bindi, A.; Luvarà, S.; Lucarini, S.; Busoni, S.; Mazzoni, L.N.; Miele, V. Chest X-ray in new Coronavirus Disease 2019 (COVID-19) infection: Findings and correlation with clinical outcome. *Radiol. Med.* **2020**, *125*, 730–737. [CrossRef]
30. Gatti, M.; Calandri, M.; Barba, M.; Biondo, A.; Geninatti, C.; Gentile, S.; Greco, M.; Morrone, V.; Piatti, C.; Santonocito, A.; et al. Baseline chest X-ray in coronavirus disease 19 (COVID-19) patients: Association with clinical and laboratory data. *Radiol. Med.* **2020**, *125*, 1271–1279. [CrossRef]

31. Giannitto, C.; Sposta, F.M.; Repici, A.; Vatteroni, G.; Casiraghi, E.; Casari, E.; Ferraroli, G.M.; Fugazza, A.; Sandri, M.T.; Chiti, A.; et al. Chest CT in patients with a moderate or high pretest probability of COVID-19 and negative swab. *Radiol. Med.* **2020**, *125*, 1260–1270. [CrossRef]
32. Machitori, A.; Noguchi, T.; Kawata, Y.; Horioka, N.; Nishie, A.; Kakihara, D.; Ishigami, K.; Aoki, S.; Imai, Y. Computed tomography surveillance helps tracking COVID-19 outbreak. *Jpn. J. Radiol.* **2020**, *38*, 1169–1176. [CrossRef] [PubMed]
33. Available online: https://www.aifa.gov.it (accessed on 21 January 2022).
34. Granata, V.; Fusco, R.; Setola, S.V.; Galdiero, R.; Picone, C.; Izzo, F.; D'Aniello, R.; Miele, V.; Grassi, R.; Grassi, R.; et al. Lymphadenopathy after BNT162b2 COVID-19 Vaccine: Preliminary Ultrasound Findings. *Biology* **2021**, *10*, 214. [CrossRef] [PubMed]
35. Moderna COVID-19 Vaccine. 2021. Available online: https://www.fda.gov/emergency-preparedness-and-response/coronavirus-disease-2019-covid-19/moderna-covid-19-vaccine (accessed on 8 April 2021).
36. Pfizer-BioNTech COVID-19 Vaccine. 2021. Available online: https://www.fda.gov/emergency-preparedness-and-response/coronavirus-disease-2019-covid-19/pfizer-biontech-covid-19-vaccine (accessed on 21 January 2022).
37. Janssen COVID-19 Vaccine. 2021. Available online: https://www.fda.gov/emergency-preparedness-and-response/coronavirus-disease-2019-covid-19/janssen-covid-19-vaccine (accessed on 21 January 2022).
38. Baden, L.R.; El Sahly, H.M.; Essink, B.; Kotloff, K.; Frey, S.; Novak, R.; Diemert, D.; Spector, S.A.; Rouphael, N.; Creech, C.B.; et al. Efficacy and safety of the mRNA-1273 SARS-CoV-2 vaccine. *N. Engl. J. Med.* **2021**, *384*, 403–416. [CrossRef] [PubMed]
39. Polack, F.P.; Thomas, S.J.; Kitchin, N.; Absalon, J.; Gurtman, A.; Lockhart, S.; Perez, J.L.; Pérez Marc, G.; Moreira, E.D.; Zerbini, C.; et al. Safety and efficacy of the BNT162b2 mRNA COVID-19 Vaccine. *N. Engl. J. Med.* **2020**, *383*, 2603–2615. [CrossRef]
40. Local Reactions, Systemic Reactions, Adverse Events, and Serious Adverse Events: Pfizer-BioNTech COVID-19 Vaccine. 2021. Available online: https://www.cdc.gov/vaccines/covid-19/info-by-product/pfizer/reactogenicity.html (accessed on 4 August 2021).
41. Di Serafino, M.; Notaro, M.; Rea, G.; Iacobellis, F.; Paoli, V.D.; Acampora, C.; Ianniello, S.; Brunese, L.; Romano, L.; Vallone, G. The lung ultrasound: Facts or artifacts? In the era of COVID-19 outbreak. *Radiol. Med.* **2020**, *125*, 738–753. [CrossRef]
42. Reginelli, A.; Grassi, R.; Feragalli, B.; Belfiore, M.; Montanelli, A.; Patelli, G.; La Porta, M.; Urraro, F.; Fusco, R.; Granata, V.; et al. Coronavirus Disease 2019 (COVID-19) in Italy: Double Reading of Chest CT Examination. *Biology* **2021**, *10*, 89. [CrossRef]
43. Grassi, R.; Belfiore, M.P.; Montanelli, A.; Patelli, G.; Urraro, F.; Giacobbe, G.; Fusco, R.; Granata, V.; Petrillo, A.; Sacco, P.; et al. COVID-19 pneumonia: Computer-aided quantification of healthy lung parenchyma, emphysema, ground glass and consolidation on chest computed tomography (CT). *Radiol. Med.* **2020**, *126*, 553–560. [CrossRef]
44. Özel, M.; Aslan, A.; Araç, S. Use of the COVID-19 Reporting and Data System (CO-RADS) classification and chest computed tomography involvement score (CT-IS) in COVID-19 pneumonia. *Radiol. Med.* **2021**, *126*, 679–687. [CrossRef]
45. Soyfer, V.; Gutfeld, O.; Shamai, S.; Schlocker, A.; Merimsky, O. COVID-19 Vaccine-Induced Radiation Recall Phenomenon. *Int. J. Radiat. Oncol.* **2021**, *110*, 957–961. [CrossRef]
46. Marples, R.; Douglas, C.; Xavier, J.; Collins, A.-J. Breast Radiation Recall Phenomenon After Astra-Zeneca COVID-19 Vaccine: A Case Series. *Cureus* **2022**, *14*, e21499. [CrossRef]
47. Ishikawa, Y.; Umezawa, R.; Yamamoto, T.; Takahashi, N.; Takeda, K.; Suzuki, Y.; Jingu, K. Radiation recall phenomenon after administration of the mRNA-1273 SARS-CoV-2 vaccine. *Int. Cancer Conf. J.* **2022**, *11*, 91–95. [CrossRef] [PubMed]
48. Shinada, K.; Murakami, S.; Yoshida, D.; Saito, H. Radiation recall pneumonitis after COVID-19 vaccination. *Thorac. Cancer* **2021**, *13*, 144–145. [CrossRef]
49. Ierardi, A.M.; Gaibazzi, N.; Tuttolomondo, D.; Fusco, S.; La Mura, V.; Peyvandi, F.; Aliberti, S.; Blasi, F.; Cozzi, D.; Carrafiello, G.; et al. Deep vein thrombosis in COVID-19 patients in general wards: Prevalence and association with clinical and laboratory variables. *Radiol. Med.* **2021**, *126*, 722–728. [CrossRef] [PubMed]
50. Ippolito, D.; Giandola, T.; Maino, C.; Pecorelli, A.; Capodaglio, C.; Ragusi, M.; Porta, M.; Gandola, D.; Masetto, A.; Drago, S.; et al. Acute pulmonary embolism in hospitalized patients with SARS-CoV-2-related pneumonia: Multicentric experience from Italian endemic area. *Radiol. Med.* **2021**, *126*, 669–678. [CrossRef] [PubMed]
51. Hughes, N.M.; Hammer, M.M.; Awad, M.M.; Jacene, H.A. Radiation Recall Pneumonitis on FDG PET/CT Triggered by COVID-19 Vaccination. *Clin. Nucl. Med.* **2021**, *47*, e281–e283. [CrossRef] [PubMed]
52. Steber, C.R.; Ponnatapura, J.; Hughes, R.T.; Farris, M.K. Rapid Development of Clinically Symptomatic Radiation Recall Pneumonitis Immediately Following COVID-19 Vaccination. *Cureus* **2021**, *13*, e14303. [CrossRef]
53. Moroni, C.; Cozzi, D.; Albanesi, M.; Cavigli, E.; Bindi, A.; Luvarà, S.; Busoni, S.; Mazzoni, L.N.; Grifoni, S.; Nazerian, P.; et al. Chest X-ray in the emergency department during COVID-19 pandemic descending phase in Italy: Correlation with patients' outcome. *Radiol. Med.* **2021**, *126*, 661–668. [CrossRef]
54. Cereser, L.; Girometti, R.; Da Re, J.; Marchesini, F.; Como, G.; Zuiani, C. Inter-reader agreement of high-resolution computed tomography findings in patients with COVID-19 pneumonia: A multi-reader study. *Radiol. Med.* **2021**, *126*, 577–584. [CrossRef]
55. McKay, M.J.; Foster, R. Radiation recall reactions: An oncologic enigma. *Crit. Rev. Oncol.* **2021**, *168*, 103527. [CrossRef]
56. Klimek, M. Pulmonary lymphangitis carcinomatosis: Systematic review and meta-analysis of case reports, 1970–2018. *Postgrad. Med.* **2019**, *131*, 309–318. [CrossRef]
57. Kumar, A.K.; Mantri, S.N. *Lymphangitic Carcinomatosis*; StatPearls Publishing: Treasure Island, FL, USA, 2021. Available online: https://www.ncbi.nlm.nih.gov/books/NBK560921/ (accessed on 21 January 2022).

58. Lin, W.-R.; Lai, R.-S. Pulmonary lymphangitic carcinomatosis. *QJM* **2014**, *107*, 935–936. [CrossRef] [PubMed]
59. Liguori, C.; Farina, D.; Vaccher, F.; Ferrandino, G.; Bellini, D.; Carbone, I. Myocarditis: Imaging up to date. *Radiol. Med.* **2020**, *125*, 1124–1134. [CrossRef] [PubMed]
60. Shaw, B.; Daskareh, M.; Gholamrezanezhad, A. The lingering manifestations of COVID-19 during and after convalescence: Update on long-term pulmonary consequences of coronavirus disease 2019 (COVID-19). *Radiol. Med.* **2021**, *126*, 40–46. [CrossRef] [PubMed]
61. Rawashdeh, M.A.; Saade, C. Radiation dose reduction considerations and imaging patterns of ground glass opacities in coronavirus: Risk of over exposure in computed tomography. *Radiol. Med.* **2021**, *126*, 380–387. [CrossRef] [PubMed]
62. Gomatou, G.; Tzilas, V.; Kotteas, E.; Syrigos, K.; Bouros, D. Immune Checkpoint Inhibitor-Related Pneumonitis. *Respiration* **2020**, *99*, 932–942. [CrossRef]
63. Naidoo, J.; Wang, X.; Woo, K.M.; Iyriboz, T.; Halpenny, D.; Cunningham, J.; Chaft, J.E.; Segal, N.H.; Callahan, M.K.; Lesokhin, A.M.; et al. Pneumonitis in Patients Treated With Anti–Programmed Death-1/Programmed Death Ligand 1 Therapy. *J. Clin. Oncol.* **2017**, *35*, 709–717. [CrossRef]
64. Suresh, K.; Naidoo, J.; Lin, C.T.; Danoff, S. Immune Checkpoint Immunotherapy for Non-Small Cell Lung Cancer: Benefits and Pulmonary Toxicities. *Chest* **2018**, *154*, 1416–1423. [CrossRef]
65. Zhong, L.; Altan, M.; Shannon, V.R.; Sheshadri, A. Immune-Related Adverse Events: Pneumonitis. *Adv. Exp. Med. Biol.* **2020**, *1244*, 255–269. [CrossRef]
66. Lombardi, A.F.; Afsahi, A.M.; Gupta, A.; Gholamrezanezhad, A. Severe acute respiratory syndrome (SARS), Middle East respiratory syndrome (MERS), influenza, and COVID-19, beyond the lungs: A review article. *Radiol. Med.* **2021**, *126*, 561–569. [CrossRef]
67. Cozzi, D.; Bindi, A.; Cavigli, E.; Grosso, A.M.; Luvarà, S.; Morelli, N.; Moroni, C.; Piperio, R.; Miele, V.; Bartolucci, M. Exogenous lipoid pneumonia: When radiologist makes the difference. *Radiol. Med.* **2021**, *126*, 22–28. [CrossRef]
68. Palmisano, A.; Scotti, G.M.; Ippolito, D.; Morelli, M.J.; Vignale, D.; Gandola, D.; Sironi, S.; De Cobelli, F.; Ferrante, L.; Spessot, M.; et al. Chest CT in the emergency department for suspected COVID-19 pneumonia. *Radiol. Med.* **2021**, *126*, 498–502. [CrossRef] [PubMed]
69. Jain, A.; Shannon, V.R.; Sheshadri, A. Immune-Related Adverse Events: Pneumonitis. *Immunotherapy* **2018**, *995*, 131–149. [CrossRef]
70. Suresh, K.; Naidoo, J.; Zhong, Q.; Xiong, Y.; Mammen, J.; De Flores, M.V.; Cappelli, L.; Balaji, A.; Palmer, T.; Forde, P.M.; et al. The alveolar immune cell landscape is dysregulated in checkpoint inhibitor pneumonitis. *J. Clin. Investig.* **2019**, *129*, 4305–4315. [CrossRef] [PubMed]
71. Bruce, D.M.; Heys, S.D.; Eremin, O. Lymphangitis carcinomatosa: A literature review. *J. R. Coll. Surg. Edinb.* **1996**, *41*, 7–13. [PubMed]
72. Kazawa, N.; Kitaichi, M.; Hiraoka, M.; Togashi, K.; Mio, N.; Mishima, M.; Wada, H. Small cell lung carcinoma: Eight types of extension and spread on computed tomography. *J. Comput. Assist. Tomogr.* **2006**, *30*, 653–661. [CrossRef] [PubMed]
73. Jiménez-Fonseca, P.; On behalf of the EPIPHANY study investigators and the Asociación de Investigación de la Enfermedad Tromboembólica de la Región de Murcia; Carmona-Bayonas, A.; Font, C.; Plasencia-Martínez, J.; Calvo-Temprano, D.; Otero, R.; Beato, C.; Biosca, M.; Sánchez, M.; et al. The prognostic impact of additional intrathoracic findings in patients with cancer-related pulmonary embolism. *Clin. Transl. Oncol.* **2018**, *20*, 230–242. [CrossRef]
74. Caruso, D.; Polici, M.; Zerunian, M.; Pucciarelli, F.; Polidori, T.; Guido, G.; Rucci, C.; Bracci, B.; Muscogiuri, E.; De Dominicis, C.; et al. Quantitative Chest CT analysis in discriminating COVID-19 from non-COVID-19 patients. *Radiol. Med.* **2020**, *126*, 243–249. [CrossRef] [PubMed]
75. Cardobi, N.; Benetti, G.; Cardano, G.; Arena, C.; Micheletto, C.; Cavedon, C.; Montemezzi, S. CT radiomic models to distinguish COVID-19 pneumonia from other interstitial pneumonias. *Radiol. Med.* **2021**, *126*, 1037–1043. [CrossRef]
76. Caruso, D.; Pucciarelli, F.; Zerunian, M.; Ganeshan, B.; De Santis, D.; Polici, M.; Rucci, C.; Polidori, T.; Guido, G.; Bracci, B.; et al. Chest CT texture-based radiomics analysis in differentiating COVID-19 from other interstitial pneumonia. *Radiol. Med.* **2021**, *126*, 1415–1424. [CrossRef]
77. Masselli, G.; Almberger, M.; Tortora, A.; Capoccia, L.; Dolciami, M.; D'Aprile, M.R.; Valentini, C.; Avventurieri, G.; Bracci, S.; Ricci, P. Role of CT angiography in detecting acute pulmonary embolism associated with COVID-19 pneumonia. *Radiol. Med.* **2021**, *126*, 1553–1560. [CrossRef]
78. Pecoraro, M.; Cipollari, S.; Marchitelli, L.; Messina, E.; Del Monte, M.; Galea, N.; Ciardi, M.R.; Francone, M.; Catalano, C.; Panebianco, V. Cross-sectional analysis of follow-up chest MRI and chest CT scans in patients previously affected by COVID-19. *Radiol. Med.* **2021**, *126*, 1273–1281. [CrossRef] [PubMed]
79. Granata, V.; Ianniello, S.; Fusco, R.; Urraro, F.; Pupo, D.; Magliocchetti, S.; Albarello, F.; Campioni, P.; Cristofaro, M.; Di Stefano, F.; et al. Quantitative Analysis of Residual COVID-19 Lung CT Features: Consistency among Two Commercial Software. *J. Pers. Med.* **2021**, *11*, 1103. [CrossRef]
80. Granata, V.; Fusco, R.; Bicchierai, G.; Cozzi, D.; Grazzini, G.; Danti, G.; De Muzio, F.; Maggialetti, N.; Smorchkova, O.; D'Elia, M.; et al. Diagnostic protocols in oncology: Workup and treatment planning: Part 1: The optimization of CT protocol. *Eur. Rev. Med. Pharmacol. Sci.* **2021**, *25*, 6972–6994. [PubMed]

81. Rampado, O.; Depaoli, A.; Marchisio, F.; Gatti, M.; Racine, D.; Ruggeri, V.; Ruggirello, I.; Darvizeh, F.; Fonio, P.; Ropolo, R. Effects of different levels of CT iterative reconstruction on low-contrast detectability and radiation dose in patients of different sizes: An anthropomorphic phantom study. *Radiol. Med.* **2020**, *126*, 55–62. [CrossRef] [PubMed]
82. Schicchi, N.; Fogante, M.; Palumbo, P.; Agliata, G.; Pirani, P.E.; Di Cesare, E.; Giovagnoni, A. The sub-millisievert era in CTCA: The technical basis of the new radiation dose approach. *Radiol. Med.* **2020**, *125*, 1024–1039. [CrossRef]
83. Palumbo, P.; Cannizzaro, E.; Bruno, F.; Schicchi, N.; Fogante, M.; Agostini, A.; De Donato, M.C.; De Cataldo, C.; Giovagnoni, A.; Barile, A.; et al. Coronary artery disease (CAD) extension-derived risk stratification for asymptomatic diabetic patients: Usefulness of low-dose coronary computed tomography angiography (CCTA) in detecting high-risk profile patients. *Radiol. Med.* **2020**, *125*, 1249–1259. [CrossRef] [PubMed]
84. Agostini, A.; Borgheresi, A.; Carotti, M.; Ottaviani, L.; Badaloni, M.; Floridi, C.; Giovagnoni, A. Third-generation iterative reconstruction on a dual-source, high-pitch, low-dose chest CT protocol with tin filter for spectral shaping at 100 kV: A study on a small series of COVID-19 patients. *Radiol. Med.* **2021**, *126*, 388–398. [CrossRef]
85. Esposito, A.; Gallone, G.; Palmisano, A.; Marchitelli, L.; Catapano, F.; Francone, M. The current landscape of imaging recommendations in cardiovascular clinical guidelines: Toward an imaging-guided precision medicine. *Radiol. Med.* **2020**, *125*, 1013–1023. [CrossRef]
86. Cicero, G.; Ascenti, G.; Albrecht, M.H.; Blandino, A.; Cavallaro, M.; D'Angelo, T.; Carerj, M.L.; Vogl, T.J.; Mazziotti, S. Extra-abdominal dual-energy CT applications: A comprehensive overview. *Radiol. Med.* **2020**, *125*, 384–397. [CrossRef]
87. Leone, A.; Criscuolo, M.; Gullì, C.; Petrosino, A.; Bianco, N.C.; Colosimo, C. Systemic mastocytosis revisited with an emphasis on skeletal manifestations. *Radiol. Med.* **2021**, *126*, 585–598. [CrossRef]
88. Chalayer, E.; Tavernier-Tardy, E.; Clavreul, G.; Bay, J.-O.; Cornillon, J. Carcinomatosis lymphangitis and pleurisy after allo-SCT in two patients with secondary leukemia after breast cancer. *Bone Marrow Transplant.* **2012**, *47*, 155–156. [CrossRef] [PubMed]
89. Quigley, D.; Donnell, R.O.; McDonnell, C. Pulmonary lymphangitis sarcomatosis: A rare cause of severe progressive dyspnoea. *BMJ Case Rep.* **2022**, *15*, e246128. [CrossRef] [PubMed]
90. Souza, B.D.S.; Bonamigo, R.R.; Viapiana, G.L.; Cartell, A. Signet ring cells in carcinomatous lymphangitis due to gastric adenocarcinoma. *An. Bras. Dermatol.* **2020**, *95*, 490–492. [CrossRef] [PubMed]
91. Zieda, A.; Sbardella, S.; Patel, M.; Smith, R. Diagnostic Bias in the COVID-19 Pandemic: A Series of Short Cases. *Eur. J. Case Rep. Intern. Med.* **2021**, *8*, 002575. [CrossRef] [PubMed]
92. Giannakis, A.; Móré, D.; Erdmann, S.; Kintzelé, L.; Fischer, R.M.; Vogel, M.N.; Mangold, D.L.; von Stackelberg, O.; Schnitzler, P.; Zimmermann, S.; et al. COVID-19 pneumonia and its lookalikes: How radiologists perform in differentiating atypical pneumonias. *Eur. J. Radiol.* **2021**, *144*, 110002. [CrossRef] [PubMed]
93. Borghesi, A.; Sverzellati, N.; Polverosi, R.; Balbi, M.; Baratella, E.; Busso, M.; Calandriello, L.; Cortese, G.; Farchione, A.; Iezzi, R.; et al. Impact of the COVID-19 pandemic on the selection of chest imaging modalities and reporting systems: A survey of Italian radiologists. *Radiol. Med.* **2021**, *126*, 1258–1272. [CrossRef]
94. Weber, J.S.; D'Angelo, S.P.; Minor, D.; Hodi, S.F.; Gutzmer, R.; Neyns, B.; Hoeller, C.; Khushalani, N.I.; Miller, W.H., Jr.; Lao, C.D.; et al. Nivolumab versus chemotherapy in patients with advanced melanoma who progressed after anti-CTLA-4 treatment (CheckMate 037): A randomised, controlled, open-label, phase 3 trial. *Lancet Oncol.* **2015**, *16*, 375–384. [CrossRef]
95. Robert, C.; Ribas, A.; Wolchok, J.D.; Hodi, S.F.; Hamid, O.; Kefford, R.; Weber, J.S.; Joshua, A.M.; Hwu, W.-J.; Gangadhar, T.C.; et al. Anti-programmed-death-receptor-1 treatment with pembrolizumab in ipilimumab-refractory advanced melanoma: A randomised dose-comparison cohort of a phase 1 trial. *Lancet* **2014**, *384*, 1109–1117. [CrossRef]
96. Brahmer, J.; Reckamp, K.L.; Baas, P.; Crinò, L.; Eberhardt, W.E.E.; Poddubskaya, E.; Antonia, S.; Pluzanski, A.; Vokes, E.; Holgado, E.; et al. Nivolumab versus docetaxel in advanced squamous-cell non-small-cell lung cancer. *N. Engl. J. Med.* **2015**, *373*, 123–135. [CrossRef]
97. Borghaei, H.; Paz-Ares, L.; Horn, L.; Spigel, D.R.; Steins, M.; Ready, N.E.; Chow, L.Q.; Vokes, E.E.; Felip, E.; Holgado, E.; et al. Nivolumab versus docetaxel in advanced nonsquamous non-small-cell lung cancer. *N. Engl. J. Med.* **2015**, *373*, 1627–1639. [CrossRef]
98. Garon, E.B.; Rizvi, N.A.; Hui, R.; Leighl, N.; Balmanoukian, A.S.; Eder, J.P.; Patnaik, A.; Aggarwal, C.; Gubens, M.; Horn, L.; et al. Pembrolizumab for the treatment of non-small-cell lung cancer. *N. Engl. J. Med.* **2015**, *372*, 2018–2028. [CrossRef]
99. Herbst, R.S.; Baas, P.; Kim, D.W.; Felip, E.L.; Pérez-Gracia, J.L.; Han, J.-Y.; Molina, J.; Kim, J.-H.; Dubos Arvis, C.; Ahn, M.-J.; et al. Pembrolizumab versus docetaxel for previously treated, PD-L1-positive, advanced non-small-cell lung cancer (KEYNOTE-010): A randomised controlled trial. *Lancet* **2015**, *387*, 1540–1550. [CrossRef]
100. Motzer, R.J.; Escudier, B.; McDermott, D.F.; George, S.; Hammers, H.J.; Srinivas, S.; Tykodi, S.S.; Sosman, J.A.; Procopio, G.; Plimack, E.R.; et al. Nivolumab versus everolimus in advanced renal-cell carcinoma. *N. Engl. J. Med.* **2015**, *373*, 1803–1813. [CrossRef] [PubMed]
101. Ansell, S.M.; Lesokhin, A.M.; Borrello, I.; Halwani, A.; Scott, E.C.; Gutierrezz, M.; Schuster, S.J.; Millenson, M.M.; Cattry, D.; Freeman, G.J.; et al. PD-1 blockade with nivolumab in relapsed or refractory Hodgkin's lymphoma. *N. Engl. J. Med.* **2015**, *372*, 311–319. [CrossRef] [PubMed]
102. Rosenberg, J.E.; Hoffman-Censits, J.; Powles, T.; van der Heijden, M.S.; Balar, A.V.; Necchi, A.; Dawson, N.; O'Donnel, P.H.; Balmanoukian, A.; Loriot, Y.; et al. Atezolizumab in patients with locally advanced and metastatic urothelial carcinoma who have progressed following treatment with platinum-based chemotherapy: A single-arm, multicentre, phase 2 trial. *Lancet* **2016**, *387*, 1909–1920. [CrossRef]

103. Larkin, J.; Chiarion-Sileni, V.; Gonzalez, R.; Grob, J.J.; Cowey, L.; Lao, C.D.; Schadendorf, D.; Dummer, R.; Smylie, M.; Rutkowwski, P.; et al. Combined nivolumab and ipilimumab or monotherapy in untreated melanoma. *N. Engl. J. Med.* **2015**, *373*, 23–34. [CrossRef] [PubMed]
104. Naidoo, J.; Page, D.B.; Li, B.T.; Connel, L.C.; Schindler, K.; Lacouture, M.E.; Postow, M.A.; Wolchok, J.D. Toxicities of the anti-PD-1 and anti-PD-L1 immune checkpoint antibodies. *Ann. Oncol.* **2015**, *26*, 2375–2391. [CrossRef]
105. Genestreti, G.; Di Battista, M.; Trisolini, R.; Denicolo, F.; Valli, M.; Agli, L.A.; dal Piaz, G.; de Biase, D.; Bartolotti, M.; Cavallo, G.; et al. A commentary on interstitial pneumonitis induced by docetaxel: Clinical cases and systematic review of the literature. *Tumori* **2015**, *101*, e92–e95. [CrossRef]
106. Poole, B.B.; Hamilton, L.A.; Brockman, M.M.; Brockman, M.M.; Byrd, D.C. Interstitial pneumonitis from treatment with gemcitabine. *Hosp. Pharm.* **2014**, *49*, 847–850. [CrossRef]
107. Comis, R.L. Bleomycin pulmonary toxicity: Current status and future directions. *Semin. Oncol.* **1992**, *19*, 64–70.
108. Ando, M.; Okamoto, I.; Yamamoto, N.; Takeda, K.; Tamura, K.; Seto, T.; Ariyoshi, Y.; Fukuoka, M. Predictive factors for interstitial lung disease, antitumor response, and survival in non-small-cell lung cancer patients treated with gefitinib. *J. Clin. Oncol.* **2006**, *24*, 2549–2556. [CrossRef] [PubMed]
109. Liu, V.; White, D.A.; Zakowski, M.F.; Travis, W.; Kris, M.G.; Ginsberg, M.S.; Miller, V.A.; Azzoli, C.G. Pulmonary toxicity associated with erlotinib. *Chest* **2007**, *132*, 1042–1044. [CrossRef] [PubMed]
110. White, D.A.; Camus, P.; Endo, M.; Escudier, B.; Calvo, E.; Akaza, H.; Uemura, H.; Kpamegan, E.; Kay, A.; Robson, M.; et al. Noninfectious pneumonitis after everolimus therapy for advanced renal cell carcinoma. *Am. J. Respir. Crit. Care Med.* **2010**, *182*, 396–403. [CrossRef] [PubMed]
111. Bradley, J.; Movsas, B. Radiation pneumonitis and esophagitis in thoracic irradiation. *Cancer Treat. Res.* **2006**, *128*, 43–64.
112. Weshler, Z.; Breuer, J.; Or, R.; Naparste, E.; Pfefer, M.R.; Lowental, E.; Slavin, S. Interstitial pneumonitis after total body irradiation: Effect of partial lung shielding. *Br. J. Haematol.* **1990**, *74*, 61–64. [CrossRef]
113. Palmucci, S.; Roccasalva, F.; Puglisi, S.; Torrisi, S.E.; Vindigni, V.; Mauro, L.A.; Ettorre, G.C.; Piccoli, M.; Vancheri, C. Clinical and radiological features of idiopathic interstitial pneumonias (IIPs): A pictorial review. *Insights Imaging* **2014**, *5*, 347–364. [CrossRef]
114. Khunger, M.; Rakshit, S.; Pasupuleti, V.; Hernandez, A.V.; Mazzone, P.; Stevenson, J.; Pennell, N.; Velcheti, V. Incidence of Pneumonitis with Use of Programmed Death 1 and Programmed Death-Ligand 1 Inhibitors in Non-Small Cell Lung Cancer: A Systematic Review and Meta-Analysis of Trials. *Chest* **2017**, *152*, 271–281. [CrossRef]
115. Khoja, L.; Day, D.; Chen, T.W.-W.; Siu, L.L.; Hansen, A.R. Tumour- and class-specific patterns of immune-related adverse events of immune checkpoint inhibitors: A systematic review. *Ann. Oncol.* **2017**, *28*, 2377–2385. [CrossRef]
116. Suresh, K.; Voong, K.R.; Shankar, B.; Forde, P.M.; Ettinger, D.S.; Marrone, K.A.; Kelly, R.J.; Hann, C.L.; Levy, B.; Feliciano, J.L.; et al. Pneumonitis in Non–Small Cell Lung Cancer Patients Receiving Immune Checkpoint Immunotherapy: Incidence and Risk Factors. *J. Thorac. Oncol.* **2018**, *13*, 1930–1939. [CrossRef]
117. Tay, R.Y.; Califano, R. Checkpoint Inhibitor Pneumonitis—Real-World Incidence and Risk. *J. Thorac. Oncol.* **2018**, *13*, 1812–1814. [CrossRef]
118. Kalisz, K.R.; Ramaiya, N.H.; Laukamp, K.R.; Gupta, A. Immune Checkpoint Inhibitor Therapy–related Pneumonitis: Patterns and Management. *RadioGraphics* **2019**, *39*, 1923–1937. [CrossRef] [PubMed]
119. Bianchi, A.; Mazzoni, L.N.; Busoni, S.; Pinna, N.; Albanesi, M.; Cavigli, E.; Cozzi, D.; Poggesi, A.; Miele, V.; Fainardi, E.; et al. Assessment of cerebrovascular disease with computed tomography in COVID-19 patients: Correlation of a novel specific visual score with increased mortality risk. *Radiol. Med.* **2021**, *126*, 570–576. [CrossRef] [PubMed]
120. Cartocci, G.; Colaiacomo, M.C.; Lanciotti, S.; Andreoli, C.; De Cicco, M.L.; Brachetti, G.; Pugliese, S.; Capoccia, L.; Tortora, A.; Scala, A.; et al. Correction to: Chest CT for early detection and management of coronavirus disease (COVID-19): A report of 314 patients admitted to Emergency Department with suspected pneumonia. *Radiol. Med.* **2020**, *126*, 642. [CrossRef] [PubMed]
121. Zompatori, M.; Poletti, V.; Battista, G.; Schiavina, M.; Fadda, E.; Tetta, C. Diffuse cystic lung disease in the adult patient. *Radiol. Med.* **2000**, *99*, 12–21.
122. Delaunay, M.; Cadranel, J.; Lusque, A.; Meyer, N.; Gounaut, V.; Moro-Sibilot, D.; Michot, J.-M.; Raimbourg, J.; Girard, N.; Guisier, F.; et al. Immune-checkpoint inhibitors associated with interstitial lung disease in cancer patients. *Eur. Respir. J.* **2017**, *50*, 1700050. [CrossRef]
123. Teng, F.; Li, M.; Yu, J. Radiation recall pneumonitis induced by PD-1/PD-L1 blockades: Mechanisms and therapeutic implications. *BMC Med.* **2020**, *18*, 275. [CrossRef]
124. Cousin, F.; Desir, C.; Ben Mustapha, S.; Mievis, C.; Coucke, P.; Hustinx, R. Incidence, risk factors, and CT characteristics of radiation recall pneumonitis induced by immune checkpoint inhibitor in lung cancer. *Radiother. Oncol.* **2021**, *157*, 47–55. [CrossRef]
125. D'Agostino, V.; Caranci, F.; Negro, A.; Piscitelli, V.; Tuccillo, B.; Fasano, F.; Sirabella, G.; Marano, I.; Granata, V.; Grassi, R.; et al. A Rare Case of Cerebral Venous Thrombosis and Disseminated Intravascular Coagulation Temporally Associated to the COVID-19 Vaccine Administration. *J. Pers. Med.* **2021**, *11*, 285. [CrossRef]
126. Girometti, R.; Linda, A.; Conte, P.; Lorenzon, M.; De Serio, I.; Jerman, K.; Londero, V.; Zuiani, C. Multireader comparison of contrast-enhanced mammography versus the combination of digital mammography and digital breast tomosynthesis in the preoperative assessment of breast cancer. *Radiol. Med.* **2021**, *126*, 1407–1414. [CrossRef]

127. Gerasia, R.; Mamone, G.; Amato, S.; Cucchiara, A.; Gallo, G.S.; Tafaro, C.; Fiorello, G.; Caruso, C.; Miraglia, R. COVID-19 safety measures at the Radiology Unit of a Transplant Institute: The non-COVID-19 patient's confidence with safety procedures. *Radiol. Med.* **2022**, *13*, 426–432. [CrossRef]
128. McGovern, K.; Ghaly, M.; Esposito, M.; Barnaby, K.; Seetharamu, N. Radiation recall pneumonitis in the setting of immunotherapy and radiation: A focused review. *Futur. Sci. OA* **2019**, *5*, FSO378. [CrossRef] [PubMed]
129. Cellini, F.; Di Franco, R.; Manfrida, S.; Borzillo, V.; Maranzano, E.; Pergolizzi, S.; Morganti, A.G.; Fusco, V.; Deodato, F.; Santarelli, M.; et al. Palliative radiotherapy indications during the COVID-19 pandemic and in future complex logistic settings: The NORMALITY model. *Radiol. Med.* **2021**, *126*, 1619–1656. [CrossRef] [PubMed]
130. De Felice, F.; Boldrini, L.; Greco, C.; Nardone, V.; Salvestrini, V.; Desideri, I. ESTRO vision 2030: The young Italian Association of Radiotherapy and Clinical Oncology (yAIRO) commitment statement. *Radiol. Med.* **2021**, *126*, 1374–1376. [CrossRef] [PubMed]
131. Bellardita, L.; Colciago, R.R.; Frasca, S.; De Santis, M.C.; Gay, S.; Palorini, F.; La Rocca, E.; Valdagni, R.; Rancati, T.; Lozza, L. Breast cancer patient perspective on opportunities and challenges of a genetic test aimed to predict radio-induced side effects before treatment: Analysis of the Italian branch of the REQUITE project. *Radiol. Med.* **2021**, *126*, 1366–1373. [CrossRef]
132. Merlotti, A.; Bruni, A.; Borghetti, P.; Ramella, S.; Scotti, V.; Trovò, M.; Chiari, R.; Lohr, F.; Ricardi, U.; Bria, E.; et al. Sequential chemo-hypofractionated RT versus concurrent standard CRT for locally advanced NSCLC: GRADE recommendation by the Italian Association of Radiotherapy and Clinical Oncology (AIRO). *Radiol. Med.* **2021**, *126*, 1117–1128. [CrossRef]
133. Afacan, E.; Öğüt, B.; Üstün, P.; Şentürk, E.; Yazıcı, O.; Adışen, E. Radiation recall dermatitis triggered by inactivated COVID-19 vaccine. *Clin. Exp. Dermatol.* **2021**, *46*, 1582–1584. [CrossRef]
134. Masci, G.M.; Iafrate, F.; Ciccarelli, F.; Pambianchi, G.; Panebianco, V.; Pasculli, P.; Ciardi, M.R.; Mastroianni, C.M.; Ricci, P.; Catalano, C.; et al. Tocilizumab effects in COVID-19 pneumonia: Role of CT texture analysis in quantitative assessment of response to therapy. *Radiol. Med.* **2021**, *126*, 1170–1180. [CrossRef]
135. Francolini, G.; Desideri, I.; Stocchi, G.; Ciccone, L.P.; Salvestrini, V.; Garlatti, P.; Aquilano, M.; Greto, D.; Bonomo, P.; Meattini, I.; et al. Impact of COVID-19 on workload burden of a complex radiotherapy facility. *Radiol. Med.* **2021**, *126*, 717–721. [CrossRef]
136. Rivera, D.T.; Misra, A.; Sanil, Y.; Sabzghabaei, N.; Safa, R.; Garcia, R.U. Vitamin D and morbidity in children with Multisystem inflammatory syndrome related to COVID-19. *Prog. Pediatr. Cardiol.* **2022**, 101507. [CrossRef]
137. Chua, G.T.; Wong, J.S.; Chung, J.; Lam, I.; Kwong, J.; Leung, K.; Law, C.; Lam, C.; Kwok, J.; Chu, P.W.; et al. Paediatric multisystem inflammatory syndrome temporally associated with SARS-CoV-2: A case report. *Hong Kong Med. J.* **2022**, *28*, 76–78. [CrossRef]
138. Barrezueta, L.B.; Raposo, M.B.; Fernández, I.S.; Casillas, P.L.; Francisco, C.V.; Vázquez, A.P. Impact of the COVID-19 pandemic on admissions for respiratory infections in the Pediatric Intensive Care Unit. *Med. Intensiv.* **2022**. [CrossRef] [PubMed]
139. Kovács, A.; Palásti, P.; Veréb, D.; Bozsik, B.; Palkó, A.; Kincses, Z.T. The sensitivity and specificity of chest CT in the diagnosis of COVID-19. *Eur. Radiol.* **2021**, *31*, 2819–2824. [CrossRef] [PubMed]
140. De Felice, F.; D'Angelo, E.; Ingargiola, R.; Iacovelli, N.A.; Alterio, D.; Franco, P.; Bonomo, P.; Merlotti, A.; Bacigalupo, A.; Maddalo, M.; et al. A snapshot on radiotherapy for head and neck cancer patients during the COVID-19 pandemic: A survey of the Italian Association of Radiotherapy and Clinical Oncology (AIRO) head and neck working group. *Radiol. Med.* **2020**, *126*, 343–347. [CrossRef] [PubMed]
141. Katal, S.; Johnston, S.K.; Johnston, J.H.; Gholamrezanezhad, A. Imaging Findings of SARS-CoV-2 Infection in Pediatrics: A Systematic Review of Coronavirus Disease 2019 (COVID-19) in 850 Patients. *Acad. Radiol.* **2020**, *27*, 1608–1621. [CrossRef] [PubMed]
142. Fichera, G.; Stramare, R.; De Conti, G.; Motta, R.; Giraudo, C. It's not over until it's over: The chameleonic behavior of COVID-19 over a six-day period. *Radiol. Med.* **2020**, *125*, 514–516. [CrossRef]
143. Moroni, C.; Bindi, A.; Cavigli, E.; Cozzi, D.; Luvarà, S.; Smorchkova, O.; Zantonelli, G.; Miele, V.; Bartolucci, M. CT findings of non-neoplastic central airways diseases. *Jpn. J. Radiol.* **2021**, *40*, 107–119. [CrossRef]
144. Boger, B.; Fachi, M.M.; Vilhena, R.O.; Cobre, A.F.; Tonin, F.; Pontarolo, R. Systematic review with meta-analysis of the accuracy of diagnostic tests for COVID-19. *Am. J. Infect. Control* **2020**, *49*, 21–29. [CrossRef]
145. Khatami, F.; Saatchi, M.; Zadeh, S.S.T.; Aghamir, Z.S.; Shabestari, A.N.; Reis, L.O.; Aghamir, S.M.K. A meta-analysis of accuracy and sensitivity of chest CT and RT-PCR in COVID-19 diagnosis. *Sci. Rep.* **2020**, *10*, 22402. [CrossRef]
146. Waller, J.V.; Allen, I.E.; Lin, K.K.; Diaz, M.J.; Henry, T.S.; Hope, M.D. The Limited Sensitivity of Chest Computed Tomography Relative to Reverse Transcription Polymerase Chain Reaction for Severe Acute Respiratory Syndrome Coronavirus-2 Infection: A systematic review on COVID-19 diagnostics. *Investig. Radiol.* **2020**, *55*, 754–761. [CrossRef]
147. Islam, N.; Ebrahimzadeh, S.; Salameh, J.-P.; Kazi, S.; Fabiano, N.; Treanor, L.; Absi, M.; Hallgrimson, Z.; Leeflang, M.M.; Hooft, L.; et al. Thoracic imaging tests for the diagnosis of COVID-19. *Cochrane Database Syst. Rev.* **2021**, *2021*, CD013639. [CrossRef]
148. Bernheim, A.; Mei, X.; Huang, M.; Yang, Y.; Fayad, Z.A.; Zhang, N.; Diao, K.; Lin, B.; Zhu, X.; Li, K.; et al. Chest CT Findings in Coronavirus Disease-19 (COVID-19): Relationship to Duration of Infection. *Radiology* **2020**, *295*, 200463. [CrossRef] [PubMed]
149. Caruso, D.; Zerunian, M.; Polici, M.; Pucciarelli, F.; Polidori, T.; Rucci, C.; Guido, G.; Bracci, B.; De Dominicis, C.; Laghi, A. Chest CT Features of COVID-19 in Rome, Italy. *Radiology* **2020**, *296*, E79–E85. [CrossRef] [PubMed]
150. Ye, Z.; Zhang, Y.; Wang, Y.; Huang, Z.; Song, B. Chest CT manifestations of new coronavirus disease 2019 (COVID-19): A pictorial review. *Eur. Radiol.* **2020**, *30*, 4381–4389. [CrossRef] [PubMed]

151. Pan, F.; Ye, T.; Sun, P.; Gui, S.; Liang, B.; Li, L.; Zheng, D.; Wang, J.; Hesketh, R.L.; Yang, L.; et al. Time Course of Lung Changes at Chest CT during Recovery from Coronavirus Disease 2019 (COVID-19). *Radiology* **2020**, *295*, 715–721. [CrossRef]
152. Bai, H.X.; Hsieh, B.; Xiong, Z.; Halsey, K.; Choi, J.W.; Tran, T.M.L.; Pan, I.; Shi, L.-B.; Wang, D.-C.; Mei, J.; et al. Performance of Radiologists in Differentiating COVID-19 from Non-COVID-19 Viral Pneumonia at Chest CT. *Radiology* **2020**, *296*, 200823. [CrossRef]
153. Neri, E.; Coppola, F.; Miele, V.; Bibbolino, C.; Grassi, R. Artificial intelligence: Who is responsible for the diagnosis? *Radiol. Med.* **2020**, *125*, 517–521. [CrossRef]
154. van Assen, M.; Muscogiuri, G.; Caruso, D.; Lee, S.J.; Laghi, A.; De Cecco, C.N. Artificial intelligence in cardiac radiology. *Radiol. Med.* **2020**, *125*, 1186–1199. [CrossRef]
155. Hu, H.-T.; Shan, Q.-Y.; Chen, S.-L.; Li, B.; Feng, S.-T.; Xu, E.-J.; Li, X.; Long, J.-Y.; Xie, X.-Y.; Lu, M.-D.; et al. CT-based radiomics for preoperative prediction of early recurrent hepatocellular carcinoma: Technical reproducibility of acquisition and scanners. *Radiol. Med.* **2020**, *125*, 697–705. [CrossRef]
156. Loffi, M.; Regazzoni, V.; Toselli, M.; Cereda, A.; Palmisano, A.; Vignale, D.; Moroni, F.; Pontone, G.; Andreini, D.; Mancini, E.M.; et al. Incidence and characterization of acute pulmonary embolism in patients with SARS-CoV-2 pneumonia: A multicenter Italian experience. *PLoS ONE* **2021**, *22*, e0245565. [CrossRef]
157. Zhang, L.; Kang, L.; Li, G.; Zhang, X.; Ren, J.; Shi, Z.; Li, J.; Yu, S. Computed tomography-based radiomics model for discriminating the risk stratification of gastrointestinal stromal tumors. *Radiol. Med.* **2020**, *125*, 465–473. [CrossRef]
158. Bracci, S.; Dolciami, M.; Trobiani, C.; Izzo, A.; Pernazza, A.; D'Amati, G.; Manganaro, L.; Ricci, P. Quantitative CT texture analysis in predicting PD-L1 expression in locally advanced or metastatic NSCLC patients. *Radiol. Med.* **2021**, *126*, 1425–1433. [CrossRef] [PubMed]
159. Qin, H.; Que, Q.; Lin, P.; Li, X.; Wang, X.-R.; He, Y.; Chen, J.-Q.; Yang, H. Magnetic resonance imaging (MRI) radiomics of papillary thyroid cancer (PTC): A comparison of predictive performance of multiple classifiers modeling to identify cervical lymph node metastases before surgery. *Radiol. Med.* **2021**, *126*, 1312–1327. [CrossRef] [PubMed]
160. Kirienko, M.; Ninatti, G.; Cozzi, L.; Voulaz, E.; Gennaro, N.; Barajon, I.; Ricci, F.; Carlo-Stella, C.; Zucali, P.; Sollini, M.; et al. Computed tomography (CT)-derived radiomic features differentiate prevascular mediastinum masses as thymic neoplasms versus lymphomas. *Radiol. Med.* **2020**, *125*, 951–960. [CrossRef] [PubMed]
161. Farchione, A.; Larici, A.R.; Masciocchi, C.; Cicchetti, G.; Congedo, M.T.; Franchi, P.; Gatta, R.; Cicero, S.L.; Valentini, V.; Bonomo, L.; et al. Exploring technical issues in personalized medicine: NSCLC survival prediction by quantitative image analysis—Usefulness of density correction of volumetric CT data. *Radiol. Med.* **2020**, *125*, 625–635. [CrossRef]
162. D'Angelo, A.; Orlandi, A.; Bufi, E.; Mercogliano, S.; Belli, P.; Manfredi, R. Automated breast volume scanner (ABVS) compared to handheld ultrasound (HHUS) and contrast-enhanced magnetic resonance imaging (CE-MRI) in the early assessment of breast cancer during neoadjuvant chemotherapy: An emerging role to monitoring tumor response? *Radiol. Med.* **2021**, *126*, 517–526. [CrossRef]
163. Kassania, S.H.; Kassanib, P.H.; Wesolowskic, M.J.; Schneidera, K.A.; Detersa, R. Automatic Detection of Coronavirus Disease (COVID-19) in X-ray and CT Images: A Machine Learning Based Approach. *Biocybern. Biomed. Eng.* **2021**, *41*, 867–879. [CrossRef]
164. Barbosa, E.J.M.; Georgescu, B.; Chaganti, S.; Aleman, G.B.; Cabrero, J.B.; Chabin, G.; Flohr, T.; Grenier, P.; Grbic, S.; Gupta, N.; et al. Machine learning automatically detects COVID-19 using chest CTs in a large multicenter cohort. *Eur. Radiol.* **2021**, *31*, 8775–8785. [CrossRef]
165. Giordano, F.; Ippolito, E.; Quattrocchi, C.; Greco, C.; Mallio, C.; Santo, B.; D'Alessio, P.; Crucitti, P.; Fiore, M.; Zobel, B.; et al. Radiation-Induced Pneumonitis in the Era of the COVID-19 Pandemic: Artificial Intelligence for Differential Diagnosis. *Cancers* **2021**, *13*, 1960. [CrossRef]
166. Bai, H.X.; Wang, R.; Xiong, Z.; Hsieh, B.; Chang, K.; Halsey, K.; Tran, T.M.L.; Choi, J.W.; Wang, D.-C.; Shi, L.-B.; et al. Artificial Intelligence Augmentation of Radiologist Performance in Distinguishing COVID-19 from Pneumonia of Other Origin at Chest CT. *Radiology* **2020**, *296*, E156–E165. [CrossRef]
167. Granata, V.; Fusco, R.; Vallone, P.; Setola, S.V.; Picone, C.; Grassi, F.; Patrone, R.; Belli, A.; Izzo, F.; Petrillo, A. Not only lymphadenopathy: Case of chest lymphangitis assessed with MRI after COVID 19 vaccine. *Infect. Agents Cancer* **2022**, *17*, 8. [CrossRef]
168. Ozsahin, I.; Sekeroglu, B.; Musa, M.S.; Mustapha, M.T.; Ozsahin, D.U. Review on Diagnosis of COVID-19 from Chest CT Images Using Artificial Intelligence. *Comput. Math. Methods Med.* **2020**, *2020*, 9756518. [CrossRef] [PubMed]

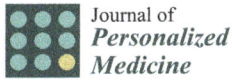

Article

Quantitative Analysis of Residual COVID-19 Lung CT Features: Consistency among Two Commercial Software

Vincenza Granata [1], Stefania Ianniello [2], Roberta Fusco [3,*], Fabrizio Urraro [4], Davide Pupo [4], Simona Magliocchetti [4], Fabrizio Albarello [2], Paolo Campioni [2], Massimo Cristofaro [2], Federica Di Stefano [2], Nicoletta Fusco [2], Ada Petrone [2], Vincenzo Schininà [2], Alberta Villanacci [2], Francesca Grassi [4], Roberta Grassi [4,5] and Roberto Grassi [4,5]

[1] Division of Radiology, Istituto Nazionale Tumori IRCCS Fondazione Pascale-IRCCS di Napoli, 80131 Naples, Italy; v.granata@istitutotumori.na.it
[2] Radiology Unit, National Institute for Infectious Diseases Lazzaro Spallanzani IRCCS, 00149 Rome, Italy; stefianni66@gmail.com (S.I.); Fabrizio.albarello@inmi.it (F.A.); paolo.campioni@inmi.it (P.C.); massimo.cristofaro@inmi.it (M.C.); federica.distefano@inmi.it (F.D.S.); nicoletta.fusco@inmi.it (N.F.); ada.petrone@inmi.it (A.P.); vincenzo.schinina@inmi.it (V.S.); alberta.villanacci@inmi.it (A.V.)
[3] Medical Oncology Division, Igea SpA, 80013 Naples, Italy
[4] Division of Radiology, Università degli Studi della Campania Luigi Vanvitelli, 80125 Naples, Italy; fabrizio.urraro@unicampania.it (F.U.); dave.dp93@gmail.com (D.P.); simonamag7@gmail.com (S.M.); francescagrassi1996@gmail.com (F.G.); grassi.roberta89@gmail.com (R.G.); roberto.grassi@unicampania.it (R.G.)
[5] Italian Society of Medical and Interventional Radiology (SIRM), SIRM Foundation, Via della Signora 2, 20122 Milan, Italy
* Correspondence: r.fusco@igeamedical.com

Abstract: Objective: To investigate two commercial software and their efficacy in the assessment of chest CT sequelae in patients affected by COVID-19 pneumonia, comparing the consistency of tools. Materials and Methods: Included in the study group were 120 COVID-19 patients (56 women and 104 men; 61 years of median age; range: 21–93 years) who underwent chest CT examinations at discharge between 5 March 2020 and 15 March 2021 and again at a follow-up time (3 months; range 30–237 days). A qualitative assessment by expert radiologists in the infectious disease field (experience of at least 5 years) was performed, and a quantitative evaluation using thoracic VCAR software (GE Healthcare, Chicago, Illinois, United States) and a pneumonia module of ANKE ASG-340 CT workstation (HTS Med & Anke, Naples, Italy) was performed. The qualitative evaluation included the presence of ground glass opacities (GGOs) consolidation, interlobular septal thickening, fibrotic-like changes (reticular pattern and/or honeycombing), bronchiectasis, air bronchogram, bronchial wall thickening, pulmonary nodules surrounded by GGOs, pleural and pericardial effusion, lymphadenopathy, and emphysema. A quantitative evaluation included the measurements of GGOs, consolidations, emphysema, residual healthy parenchyma, and total lung volumes for the right and left lung. A chi-square test and non-parametric test were utilized to verify the differences between groups. Correlation coefficients were used to analyze the correlation and variability among quantitative measurements by different computer tools. A receiver operating characteristic (ROC) analysis was performed. Results: The correlation coefficients showed great variability among the quantitative measurements by different tools when calculated on baseline CT scans and considering all patients. Instead, a good correlation (≥ 0.6) was obtained for the quantitative GGO, as well as the consolidation volumes obtained by two tools when calculated on baseline CT scans, considering the control group. An excellent correlation (≥ 0.75) was obtained for the quantitative residual healthy lung parenchyma volume, GGO, consolidation volumes obtained by two tools when calculated on follow-up CT scans, and for residual healthy lung parenchyma and GGO quantification when the percentage change of these volumes were calculated between a baseline and follow-up scan. The highest value of accuracy to identify patients with RT-PCR positive compared to the control group was obtained by a GGO total volume quantification by thoracic VCAR (accuracy = 0.75). Conclusions: Computer aided quantification could be an easy and feasible way to assess chest CT sequelae due

Citation: Granata, V.; Ianniello, S.; Fusco, R.; Urraro, F.; Pupo, D.; Magliocchetti, S.; Albarello, F.; Campioni, P.; Cristofaro, M.; Di Stefano, F.; et al. Quantitative Analysis of Residual COVID-19 Lung CT Features: Consistency among Two Commercial Software. *J. Pers. Med.* **2021**, *11*, 1103. https://doi.org/10.3390/jpm11111103

Academic Editor: Pierluigi Maria Rinaldi

Received: 3 October 2021
Accepted: 25 October 2021
Published: 28 October 2021

Publisher's Note: MDPI stays neutral with regard to jurisdictional claims in published maps and institutional affiliations.

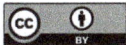

Copyright: © 2021 by the authors. Licensee MDPI, Basel, Switzerland. This article is an open access article distributed under the terms and conditions of the Creative Commons Attribution (CC BY) license (https://creativecommons.org/licenses/by/4.0/).

to COVID-19 pneumonia; however, a great variability among measurements provided by different tools should be considered.

Keywords: COVID-19; post COVID-19 sequelae; computed tomography; quantitative analysis; artificial intelligence

1. Introduction

A new coronavirus (severe acute respiratory syndrome coronavirus 2, SARS-CoV-2) is the pathogen responsible for the SARS-CoV-2 disease (COVID-19), which has spread throughout the world since December 2019 [1–9]. COVID-19 was defined as a pandemic by the World Health Organization on 11 March 2020 [10]. The clinical expressions of COVID-19 range from flu-like symptoms to respiratory failure, the management of which demands advanced respiratory assistance and artificial ventilation [11–21]. The clinical spectrum of COVID-19 pneumonia ranges from mild to critical cases, among which the diagnosis of ordinary, severe, and critical cases was related to chest computed tomography (CT) findings [22,23]. CT imaging allows for the early detection of lung abnormalities in patients with SARS-CoV-2 pneumonia [24,25], representing a useful diagnostic tool, with pooled sensitivity and a specificity of 94% and 37%, respectively [26]. Additionally, approximately one-third of COVID-19 survivors showed pulmonary fibrotic-like changes at a six-month follow-up chest CT [27]; there is speculation that some of these findings will resolve over time, and are therefore not fibrosis [27]. Although a visual method allows the assessment of these findings, a quantitative evaluation based on software systems, not dependent on the experience of the reader, allows for a greater accuracy of analysis and facilitates the evaluation of the data over time, reducing the error of the qualitative evaluation alone [8]. While several artificial intelligence (AI) models have been developed to facilitate the automation of COVID-19 diagnosis [11,13,17], there has been little study of COVID-19 lesion segmentation. To detect regions of interest (ROIs) from CT scans is an interesting and challenging task for several reasons: (a) a large divergence in the characteristics of lesions in terms of scope, location, shape, and quality makes them difficult to classify; (b) small, inter-class divergence means that the margins of ground-glass opacity (GGO) predominantly exhibit clouded manifestation and low contrast, which complicates the detection process; (c) noisy annotation is inevitable for rare or new diseases (e.g., COVID-19), which decreases segmentation efficiency. However, the quantitative assessment of infection and longitudinal changes in CT findings could offer useful and vital information in fighting against COVID-19.

The aim of this retrospective study is to investigate the efficacy of two commercial software in the assessment of chest CT sequelae in patients affected by COVID-19 pneumonia, comparing the consistency of these two tools.

2. Materials and Methods

2.1. Patient Selection

This retrospective study included patients enrolled by the National Institute of Infectious Diseases Lazzaro Spallanzani Hospital, Rome, Italy.

Considering the emergency period, the local institutional review board waived informed consent for included patients in this retrospective study.

In order to homogenize the sample under examination, only patients who were subjected to CT at discharge and at a 3-month follow-up (range 30–237 days) were included.

The study group included 120 patients (56 women and 104 men; median age: 61 years; range: 21–93 years) who were confirmed to be infected with COVID-19 using the nucleic acid amplification test in the respiratory tract with a reverse transcription real-time fluorescence polymerase chain reaction test (RT-PCR) between 5 March 2020 and 15 March 2021.

As a control group, we selected 40 patients (median age: 60 years; range: 38–90) without lung disease who underwent chest CT at the same institute that was staging an examination for colorectal cancer.

2.2. CT Technique

We performed 128 slices of chest CT scans with Incisive Philips CT scanners (Amsterdam, The Netherlands). CT examinations were performed with the patient in the supine position in breath-hold, and inspiration using a standard dose protocol, without contrast intravenous injection. The scanning range was from the apex to the base of the lungs. The tube voltage and the current tube were 120 kV and 100–200 mA (and if applicable, using z-axis tube current modulation), respectively. All data were reconstructed with a 0.6–1.0 mm increment. The matrix was 512 mm × 512 mm. Images were reconstructed using a sharp reconstruction kernel for parenchyma evaluation and hard reconstruction kernel for other lung evaluation. All data were reconstructed with a 0.6–1.0 mm increment. Multiplanar reconstruction was also calculated. Details are provided in previous papers [8,11].

2.3. Qualitative Assessment

Four expert radiologists in the infectious disease field (with experience of at least 5 years) were working independently on the same CT series of studies, and in addition, discrepant findings were recorded and evaluated in consensus. A qualitative evaluation included the presence of the following CT findings: (a) GGOs, (b) consolidation, (c) interlobular septal thickening, (d) fibrotic-like changes (reticular pattern and/or honeycombing), (e) bronchiectasis, (d) air bronchogram, (e) bronchial wall thickening, (f) pulmonary nodules surrounded by GGOs, (g) pleural and (h) pericardial effusion, (i) lymphadenopathy (defined as lymph node with short axis > 10 mm), and (j) emphysema.

All chest CT findings were defined according to the Fleischner Society glossary [28].

For each of them, they reported (1) location, (2) multilobe involvement, (3) total lobar involvement, and (4) bilateral distribution.

2.4. CT Post-Processing

Primary image data sets (0.6–1.0 mm) were transferred to the PACS workstation and the same CT images were evaluated using two clinically available computer tools by the same 4 readers in consensus (no discrepant data can be obtained with automatic computerized quantification). The tools used were thoracic VCAR software (GE Healthcare, Chicago, IL, USA) and a pneumonia module of ANKE ASG-340 CT workstation (HTS Med & Anke, Naples, Italy). Table 1 reports a comparison among evaluated commercial software based on the provided functionalities.

Table 1. Description of computed based tool functionalities.

Functionalities	Thoracic VCAR	ANKE ASG-340 CT Workstation
Quantitative data for each lobe	no	yes
Manually segmentation	yes	no
Preliminary possibility to exclude airways	yes	no
CE marking for lung study	yes	no
Evaluation separately pleural effusion	no	no
Unstructured report	yes	yes
Combined structured report	no	yes
Proportion of pneumonia lesion measurement	no	yes
Comparison among exams	no	yes

2.4.1. Post-Processing with Thoracic VCAR Software

Thoracic VCAR software is a CE-marked medical device designed to quantify pulmonary emphysema in patients with chronic obstructive pulmonary disease. The tool provides segmentation of the lungs and of the airway tree. Moreover, the tools provided the quantification of the emphysema, healthy residual lung parenchyma, GGO, and consolidation based on a Hounsfield unit. Details are provided in previous papers [8,11]. The total volumes for both the right and left lung were also calculated (Figure 1).

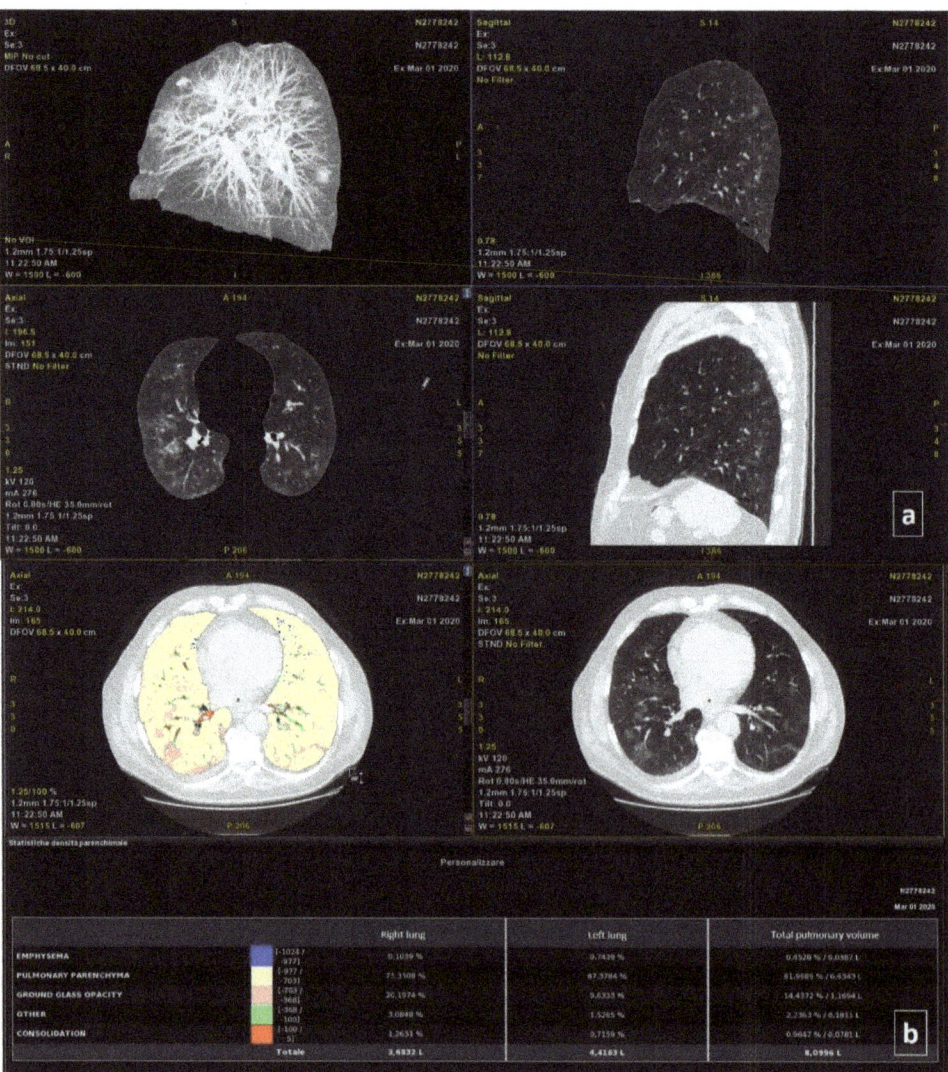

Figure 1. Automatic segmentation of thoracic disease by COVID-19 using the Thoracic VCAR Tool of General Electric Healthcare: (**a**) 3D axial and sagittal plane reconstruction; (**b**) density analysis of parenchyma. This case had bilateral and diffuse, and consolidations in multiple lobes.

2.4.2. Post-Processing with ANKE ASG-340 CT Workstation

The ANKE ASG-340 CT workstation from HTS Med & ANKE is a comprehensive CT workstation that uses lung nodules analysis, pneumonia analysis, dental pack, vascular analysis cerebral hemorrhage analysis, and so on. The pneumonia module is designed to quantify pneumonia patients. The software provides automatic segmentation of the lungs and lung lobs and automatic location and measurement pneumonia including volume, CT value, and component analysis. It provides the classification of voxels based on Hounsfield Units (Figure 2), as was previously described for the thoracic VCAR Tool.

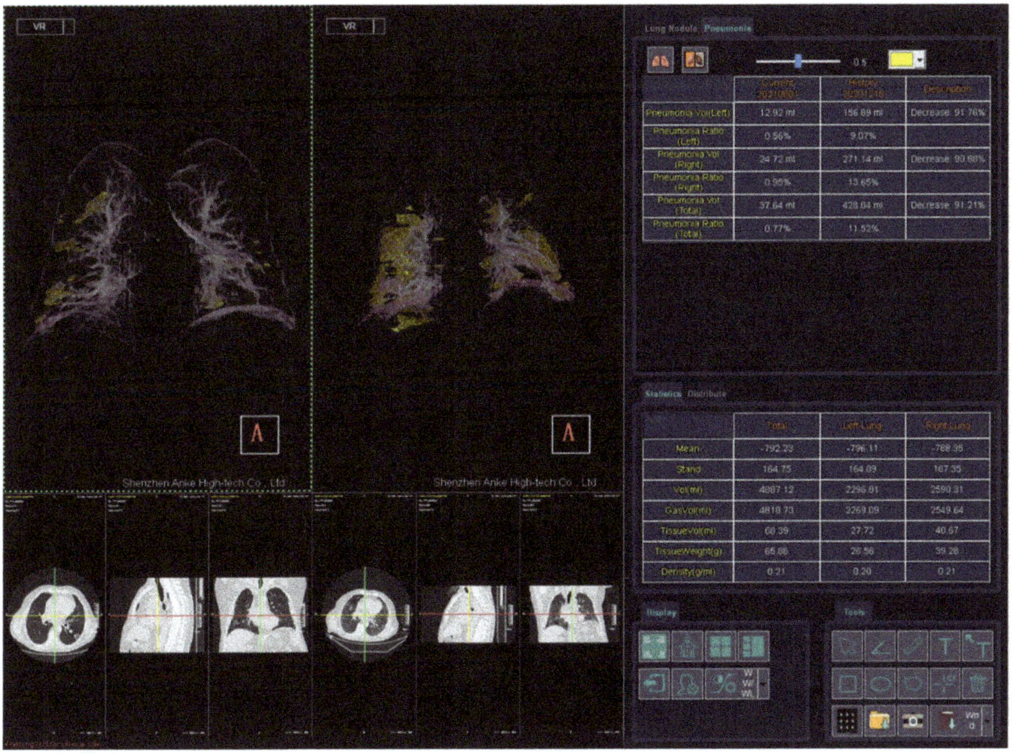

Figure 2. Automatic Segmentation of Thoracic Disease by COVID-19 using the pneumonia tool of ANKE ASG-340 CT workstation.

2.5. Statistical Analysis

The median value and range were calculated. A chi-square test, Mann–Whitney test, and Kruskal–Wallis test were used to verify the differences between groups. The Pearson correlation coefficient and intraclass correlation coefficient were used to analyze the correlation and variability among the quantitative measurements generated by different tools [3].

A receiver operating characteristic (ROC) analysis was performed. The area under curve (AUC), sensitivity, specificity, positive predictive value, negative predictive value, and accuracy were obtained. A p value of <0.05 was considered significant for all tests.

The statistical analyses were performed using the Statistics Toolbox of MATLAB R2007a (MathWorks, Natick, MA, USA).

3. Results

In the study group, 240 chest CT examinations (at discharge/baseline and follow-up time; range: 30–237 days) were analyzed.

3.1. Qualitative Assessment

At baseline, the patients had: GGOs (120; 100%); consolidation (108; 90.0%); interlobular septal thickening (120; 100%); fibrotic-like changes (reticular pattern and/or honeycombing) (116; 96.7%); bronchiectasis (80; 66.7%); air bronchogram (10; 8.3%); bronchial wall thickening (120; 100%); pulmonary nodules surrounded by GGOs (40; 33.3%); pleural (45; 37.5%) and pericardial effusion (6; 5%); lymphadenopathy (0; 0%), and emphysema (107; 89.2%).

All patients had a multilobe and bilateral distribution.

At follow-up, the patients had: GGOs (120; 100%); consolidation (120; 100%); interlobular septal thickening (120; 100%); fibrotic-like changes (reticular pattern and/or honeycombing) (120; 100%); bronchiectasis (120; 100%); air bronchogram (40; 33.3%); bronchial wall thickening (120; 100%); pulmonary nodules surrounded by GGOs (0; 0%); pleural (4; 3.3%) and pericardial effusion (0; 0%), and emphysema (107; 89.2%).

A statistically significant difference was found considering the presence in the percentage value of pulmonary nodules surrounded by GGOs pleural effusion between the two groups ($p < 0.01$ at Chi square test).

All patients had a bilateral distribution with multilobe involvement.

In the control group, we evaluated 40 chest CT examinations in 12 patients (30%), and the only features identified was emphysema.

3.2. Quantitative Assessment

The thoracic VCAR software was not able to perform volume segmentation in 12/280 (4.3%) cases, while the pneumonia module of the ANKE ASG-340 CT workstation performed in 19/280 (6.8%) patients.

The ICC showed great variability among the quantitative measurements of the emphysema, residual healthy lung parenchyma volume, GGO, and consolidations volumes obtained by different tools when calculated on baseline CT scans (Table 2), and considering all patients.

A good ICC (≥ 0.6) was obtained for the quantitative GGO and consolidations volumes obtained by two tools when calculated on baseline CT scans (Table 2), and considering the control group (Table 2).

An excellent ICC (≥ 0.75) was obtained for the quantitative residual healthy lung parenchyma, GGO, and consolidations volumes obtained by two tools when calculated on follow-up CT scans (Table 3).

In addition, an excellent ICC (≥ 0.75) was obtained for the residual healthy lung parenchyma volume and GGO quantifications when the percentage change of these volumes was calculated between the baseline and follow-up examination.

The lowest variability in the quantification was obtained for the GGO volume quantification (ICC = 0.94). The Pearson correlation analyses (Table 4) showed a low correlation for each of the quantitative volume measurements determined by the thoracic VCAR tool and ANKE ASG-340 CT workstation pneumonia tool; exclusively, the GGO measurement showed a moderate correlation (Pearson correlation coefficient = 0.682, $p < 0.01$).

The lung volumes quantified using the thoracic VCAR tool on baseline CT scans were significantly different between RT-PCR positive and the control group ($p < 0.05$) for all volumes, except that for the quantification of the emphysema volume (Table 5, Figure 3).

Instead, using ANKE ASG-340 CT pneumonia software baseline CT scans, GGO and consolidation volumes exclusively showed statistically significant differences among patients with RT-PCR positive and the control group ($p < 0.05$) (Table 6, Figure 4).

Table 7 shows the volumes percentage change between baseline and follow-up time in patients with positive RT-PCR in terms of median, minimum, and maximum values.

The lung volumes quantified by two tools in terms of median, minimum, and maximum values obtained on follow-up CT scans are reported in the Table 8.

Table 9 showed ROC analysis results for volumes obtained on baseline CT scans for both tools. The highest value of accuracy to identify patients with RT-PCR positive was obtained by GGO total volume quantification by the thoracic VCAR (accuracy = 0.75).

Considering the results obtained by the ANKE ASG-340 CT pneumonia tool, the consolidation volume of the left lung obtained the highest accuracy, equal to 0.

Table 2. The intraclass coefficient (ICC) among quantitative volumes obtained using different commercial computerized tools on baseline CT scans.

	Variability	EMP DX (%)	EMP SX (%)	EMP TOT (%/L)	HP DX (%)	HP SX (%)	HP TOT (%/L)	GGO DX (%)	GGO SX (%)	GGO TOT (%/L)	OTHER DX (%)	OTHER SX (%)	OTHER TOT (%/L)	CONSOL DX (%)	CONSOL SX (%)	CONSOL TOT (%/L)	VOLUME DX (L)	VOLUME SX (L)	VOLUME TOT (L)
All patients	ICC	0.04	0.04	0.04	0.11	0.08	0.08	0.07	0.05	0.07	0.05	0.05	0.05	0.05	0.05	0.05	0.00	0.00	0.00
	Lower Bound	−0.04	−0.04	−0.04	−0.03	−0.04	−0.04	−0.07	−0.09	−0.07	−0.10	−0.09	−0.09	−0.11	−0.10	−0.10	−0.02	−0.02	−0.02
	Upper Bound	0.14	0.14	0.15	0.25	0.21	0.21	0.22	0.19	0.21	0.19	0.20	0.19	0.20	0.21	0.21	0.03	0.03	0.03
RT-PCR positive	ICC	0.04	0.02	0.03	0.06	0.04	0.04	0.03	0.01	0.02	0.00	0.00	−0.01	0.00	0.00	0.00	0.00	0.00	0.00
	Lower Bound	−0.05	−0.05	−0.05	−0.08	−0.10	−0.10	−0.15	−0.17	−0.15	−0.17	−0.17	−0.18	−0.18	−0.18	−0.18	−0.03	−0.03	−0.02
	Upper Bound	0.14	0.11	0.13	0.21	0.18	0.18	0.20	0.17	0.19	0.17	0.17	0.16	0.18	0.18	0.18	0.03	0.03	0.03
Control group	ICC	0.06	0.09	0.08	0.06	0.04	0.05	0.60	0.68	0.60	0.51	0.10	0.11	0.68	0.66	0.68	0.00	0.00	0.00
	Lower Bound	−0.06	−0.07	−0.07	−0.05	−0.06	−0.06	−0.07	−0.08	−0.07	−0.08	−0.09	−0.08	0.09	0.06	0.09	−0.03	−0.02	−0.03
	Upper Bound	0.23	0.31	0.27	0.23	0.18	0.20	0.77	0.74	0.76	0.53	0.32	0.33	0.81	0.80	0.81	0.05	0.04	0.04

Note. EMP = emphysema; HP = health parenchyma; GGO = ground-glass opacity; CONSOL = consolidations; ICC = intraclass coefficient.

Table 3. The intraclass coefficient (ICC) among quantitative volumes obtained using different commercial computerized tools on follow-up CT scans.

Variability	EMP DX (%)	EMP SX (%)	EMP TOT (%/L)	HP DX (%)	HP SX (%)	HP TOT (%/L)	GGO DX (%)	GGO SX (%)	GGO TOT (%/L)	OTHER DX (%)	OTHER SX (%)	OTHER TOT (%/L)	CONSOL DX (%)	CONSOL SX (%)	CONSOL TOT (%/L)	VOLUME DX (L)	VOLUME SX (L)	VOLUME TOT (L)
							In follow-up CT scans											
ICC	0.18	0.20	0.19	0.87	0.87	0.85	0.82	0.83	0.94	0.63	0.71	0.68	0.02	0.90	0.91	0.00	0.00	0.00
Lower Bound	−0.06	−0.06	−0.06	0.46	0.60	0.40	0.62	0.66	0.63	0.14	0.18	0.14	−0.14	0.85	0.85	−0.05	−0.05	−0.05
Upper Bound	0.39	0.43	0.42	0.95	0.94	0.94	0.90	0.90	0.92	0.82	0.87	0.85	0.17	0.93	0.94	0.06	0.06	0.06
							Considering percentage change of volume measurements calculated between baseline and follow-up.											
ICC	0.01	0.02	0.01	0.75	0.75	0.78	0.75	0.75	0.76	0.34	0.30	0.31	0.02	0.06	0.37	0.61	0.35	0.61
Lower Bound	−0.15	−0.13	−0.14	0.63	0.61	0.02	0.21	0.16	0.19	0.19	0.15	0.16	−0.15	−0.10	0.23	0.49	0.20	0.49
Upper Bound	0.17	0.18	0.17	0.79	0.77	0.33	0.79	0.80	0.87	0.47	0.44	0.45	0.18	0.22	0.50	0.70	0.48	0.70

Note. EMP = emphysema; HP = health parenchyma; GGO = ground-glass opacity; CONSOL = consolidations; ICC = intraclass coefficient.

Table 4. Pearson correlation coefficient among quantitative volumes obtained using different tools.

		Thoracic VCAR EMP TOT (%/L)	Thoracic VCAR HP TOT (%/L)	Thoracic VCAR GGO TOT (%/L)	Thoracic VCAR OTHER TOT (%/L)	Thoracic VCAR CONSOL TOT (%/L)	Thoracic VCAR VOLUME TOT (L)	ANKE ASG-340 CT EMP TOT (%/L)	ANKE ASG-340 CT HP TOT (%/L)	ANKE ASG-340 CT GGO TOT (%/L)	ANKE ASG-340 CT OTHER TOT (%/L)	ANKE ASG-340 CT CONSOL TOT (%/L)	ANKE ASG-340 CT VOLUME TOT (L)
Thoracic VCAR EMP TOT (%/L)	Pearson Correlation Coefficient	1	0.056	−0.278**	−0.208**	−0.202**	0.311**	0.437**	−0.076	−0.183**	−0.124*	−0.067	0.127*
	p value		0.362	0.000	0.001	0.001	0.000	0.000	0.222	0.003	0.048	0.288	0.043
Thoracic VCAR HP TOT (%/L)	Pearson Correlation Coefficient	0.056	1	−0.959**	−0.895**	−0.806**	0.589**	0.098	0.217**	−0.336**	−0.254**	−0.154*	0.253**
	p value	0.362		0.000	0.000	0.000	0.000	0.119	0.000	0.000	0.000	0.013	0.000
Thoracic VCAR GGO TOT (%/L)	Pearson Correlation Coefficient	−0.278**	−0.959**	1	0.826**	0.724**	−0.645**	−0.208**	−0.192**	0.682**	0.267**	0.151*	−0.284**
	p value	0.000	0.000		0.000	0.000	0.000	0.001	0.002	0.000	0.000	0.015	0.000
Thoracic VCAR OTHER TOT (%/L)	Pearson Correlation Coefficient	−0.208**	−0.895**	0.826**	1	0.924**	−0.526**	−0.098	−0.164**	0.250**	0.236**	0.163**	−0.191**

Table 4. Cont.

		Thoracic VCAR EMP TOT (%/L)	Thoracic VCAR HP TOT (%/L)	Thoracic VCAR GGO TOT (%/L)	Thoracic VCAR OTHER TOT (%/L)	Thoracic VCAR CONSOL TOT (%/L)	Thoracic VCAR VOLUME TOT (L)	ANKE ASG-340 CT EMP TOT (%/L)	ANKE ASG-340 CT HP TOT (%/L)	ANKE ASG-340 CT GGO TOT (%/L)	ANKE ASG-340 CT OTHER TOT (%/L)	ANKE ASG-340 CT CONSOL TOT (%/L)	ANKE ASG-340 CT VOLUME TOT (L)
Thoracic VCAR CONSOL TOT (%/L)	p value	0.001	0.000	0.000	0.000		0.000	0.117	0.009	0.000	0.000	0.009	0.002
	Pearson Correlation Coefficient	−0.202**	−0.806**	0.724**	0.924**	1	−0.485**	−0.144*	−0.157*	0.257**	0.248**	0.184**	−0.197**
Thoracic VCAR VOLUME TOT (L)	p value	0.001	0.000	0.000	0.000	0.000		0.021	0.012	0.000	0.000	0.003	0.001
	Pearson Correlation Coefficient	0.311**	0.569**	−0.645**	−0.526**	−0.485**	1	0.197**	0.122	−0.341**	−0.231**	−0.121	0.523**
ANKE ASG-340 CT EMP TOT (%/L)	p value	0.000	0.000	0.000	0.000	0.000	0.000		0.050	0.000	0.000	0.054	0.000
	Pearson Correlation Coefficient	0.437**	0.098	−0.208**	−0.098	−0.144*	0.197**	1	−0.053	−0.484**	−0.426**	−0.335**	0.372**
ANKE ASG-340 CT HP TOT (%/L)	p value	0.000	0.119	0.001	0.117	0.021	0.001			0.000	0.000	0.000	0.000
	Pearson Correlation Coefficient	−0.076	0.217**	−0.192**	−0.164**	−0.157*	0.122	−0.053	1	−0.705**	−0.701**	−0.583**	0.422**
ANKE ASG-340 CT GGO TOT (%/L)	p value	0.222	0.000	0.002	0.009	0.012	0.050	0.391			0.000	0.000	0.000
	Pearson Correlation Coefficient	−0.183**	−0.336**	0.682**	0.250**	0.257**	−0.341**	−0.484**	−0.705**	1	0.839**	0.625**	−0.666**
ANKE ASG-340 CT OTHER TOT (%/L)	p value	0.003	0.000	0.000	0.000	0.000	0.000	0.000	0.000			0.000	0.000
	Pearson Correlation Coefficient	−0.124*	−0.254**	0.267**	0.236**	0.248**	−0.231**	−0.426**	−0.701**	0.839**	1	0.895**	−0.572**
ANKE ASG-340 CT CONSOL TOT (%/L)	p value	0.048	0.000	0.000	0.000	0.000	0.000	0.000	0.000	0.000			0.000
	Pearson Correlation Coefficient	−0.067	−0.154*	0.151**	0.163**	0.184**	−0.121	−0.335**	−0.583**	0.625**	0.895**	1	−0.437*
ANKE ASG-340 CT VOLUME TOT (L)	p value	0.288	0.013	0.015	0.009	0.003	0.054	0.000	0.000	0.000	0.000	0.000	
	Pearson Correlation Coefficient	0.127*	0.253**	−0.284**	−0.191**	−0.197**	0.523**	0.372**	0.422**	−0.666**	−0.572**	−0.437**	1
	p value	0.043	0.000	0.000	0.002	0.001	0.000	0.000	0.000	0.000	0.000	0.000	

Note. EMP = Emphysema; HP = health parenchyma; GGO = ground–glass opacity; CONSOL = consolidations. ** The correlation is significant at the 0.01 level (two−tailed). * The correlation is significant at 0.05 level (two-tailed).

Table 5. Lung volumes quantified using the thoracic VCAR tool in terms of median, minimum, and maximum values obtained on baseline CT scans.

		EMP DX (%)	EMP SX (%)	EMP TOT (%/L)	HP DX (%)	HP X (%)	HP TOT (%/L)	GGO DX (%)	GGO SX (%)	GGO TOT (%/L)	OTHER DX (%)	OTHER SX (%)	OTHER TOT (%/L)	CONSOL DX (%)	CONSOL SX (%)	CONSOL TOT (%/L)	VOLUME DX (L)	VOLUME SX (L)	VOLUME TOT (L)
All Patients	Median	0.91	1.10	1.03	88.21	87.69	87.54	7.62	8.14	7.81	1.40	1.61	1.56	0.48	0.54	0.52	2.20	2.00	4.22
	Minimum	0.00	0.00	0.00	34.80	16.54	36.39	2.00	2.53	2.15	0.59	0.68	0.65	0.17	0.01	0.19	0.84	0.65	1.60
	Maximum	34.29	15.95	26.04	95.68	95.43	95.58	43.25	56.76	43.03	14.77	19.48	14.70	7.73	7.50	7.20	4.72	4.08	8.81
RT-PCR positive	Median	0.89	1.09	0.96	84.04	84.16	84.44	10.25	11.08	10.59	1.92	2.16	2.15	0.59	0.61	0.64	2.09	1.86	3.96
	Minimum	0.00	0.00	0.00	34.80	16.54	36.39	2.53	2.70	2.61	0.59	0.68	0.65	0.20	0.01	0.23	0.84	0.65	1.60
	Maximum	34.29	15.95	26.04	95.51	94.57	95.09	43.25	56.76	43.03	14.77	19.48	14.70	7.73	7.50	7.20	4.27	3.72	7.66
Control group	Median	0.91	1.11	1.08	92.38	91.62	92.01	4.52	4.59	4.62	1.03	1.11	1.07	0.34	0.42	0.39	2.32	2.19	4.65
	Minimum	0.00	0.04	0.05	75.40	69.80	73.75	2.00	2.53	2.15	0.60	0.70	0.65	0.17	0.21	0.19	1.25	1.05	2.30
	Maximum	4.06	5.57	4.76	95.68	95.43	95.58	21.87	27.25	23.58	2.45	2.94	2.60	0.77	0.93	0.84	4.72	4.08	8.81
p Value at Kruskal Wallis test		0.278	0.270	0.229	0.000	0.000	0.000	0.000	0.000	0.000	0.000	0.000	0.000	0.000	0.000	0.000	0.025	0.002	0.003

Note. EMP = emphysema; HP = health parenchyma; GGO = ground–glass opacity; CONSOL = consolidations.

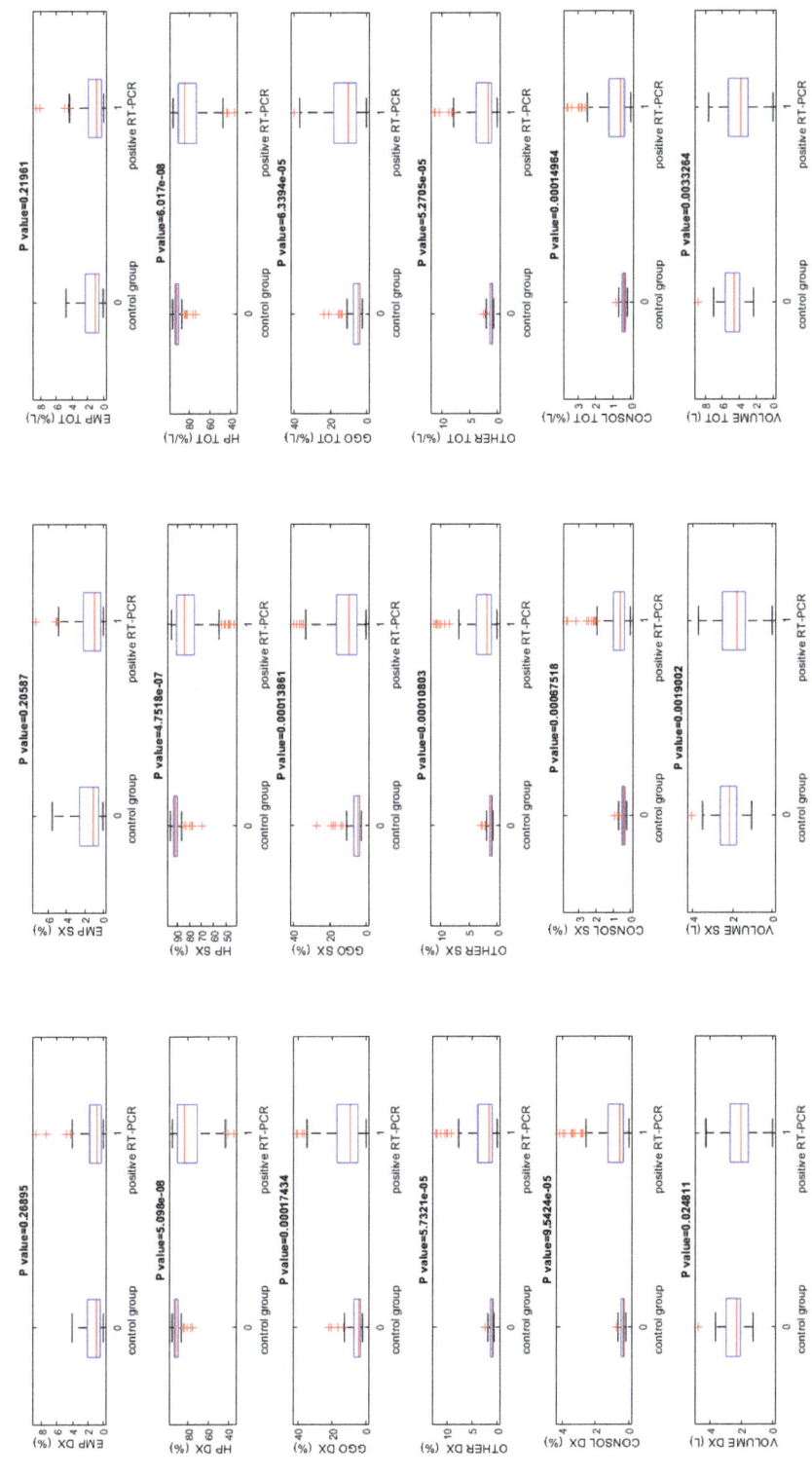

Figure 3. Boxplot of lung volumes quantified using the thoracic VCAR obtained on baseline CT scans. Note. EMP = emphysema; HP = health parenchyma; GGO = ground-glass opacity; CONSOL = consolidations.

Table 6. Lung volumes quantified using the ANKE ASG-340 CT workstation pneumonia tool in terms of median, minimum, and maximum values obtained on baseline CT scans.

		EMP DX (%)	EMP SX (%)	EMP TOT (%/L)	HP DX (%)	HP SX (%)	HP TOT (%/L)	GGO DX (%)	GGO SX (%)	GGO TOT (%/L)	OTHER DX (%)	OTHER SX (%)	OTHER TOT (%/L)	CONSOL DX (%)	CONSOL SX (%)	CONSOL TOT (%/L)	VOLUME DX (L)	VOLUME SX (L)	VOLUME TOT (L)
All Patients	Median	11.81	11.07	11.12	66.48	67.94	67.43	13.77	13.38	13.65	3.38	2.95	3.18	0.50	0.49	0.53	1.97	2.26	4.22
	Minimum	0.33	0.31	0.31	17.08	37.69	3.83	4.70	3.79	4.63	1.39	1.18	1.36	0.18	0.11	0.20	0.00	0.00	0.00
	Maximum	29.30	39.41	34.39	88.56	89.41	89.00	45.54	42.74	43.99	24.05	16.72	18.16	14.31	5.90	8.78	4.11	4.78	8.89
RT-PCR positive	Median	12.04	11.61	11.81	65.66	66.05	66.02	15.20	14.60	14.84	3.72	3.41	3.57	0.60	0.64	0.62	1.87	2.11	4.05
	Minimum	0.33	0.31	0.31	17.08	37.69	3.83	4.70	3.79	4.63	1.39	1.18	1.36	0.18	0.19	0.20	0.00	0.00	0.00
	Maximum	29.30	39.41	34.39	82.18	82.01	81.75	43.62	42.74	41.99	24.05	16.72	18.16	14.31	5.90	8.78	3.76	4.34	7.77
Control group	Median	11.27	9.75	10.77	69.46	71.52	70.79	9.78	10.24	10.02	2.49	2.40	2.44	0.34	0.34	0.35	2.13	2.37	4.61
	Minimum	1.29	1.08	1.24	43.62	45.18	43.35	5.04	5.89	5.80	1.56	1.53	1.56	0.23	0.11	0.22	1.06	1.29	2.35
	Maximum	25.29	24.04	24.54	88.56	89.41	89.00	45.54	42.67	43.99	8.15	8.03	8.08	1.39	1.32	1.34	4.11	4.78	8.89
p Value at Kruskal Wallis test		0.102	0.058	0.083	0.315	0.199	0.220	0.011	0.009	0.009	0.001	0.000	0.000	0.000	0.000	0.000	0.579	0.720	0.777

Note. EMP = emphysema; HP = health parenchyma; GGO = ground-glass opacity; CONSOL = consolidations.

Table 7. Percentage change of quantified volumes by two tools between baseline and follow-up in patients with positive RT-PCR in terms of median, minimum, and maximum values.

		EMP DX (%)	EMP SX (%)	EMP TOT (%/L)	HP DX (%)	HP SX (%)	HP TOT (%/L)	GGO DX (%)	GGO SX (%)	GGO TOT (%/L)	OTHER DX (%)	OTHER SX (%)	OTHER TOT (%/L)	CONSOL DX (%)	CONSOL SX (%)	CONSOL TOT (%/L)	VOLUME DX (L)	VOLUME SX (L)	VOLUME TOT (L)
Thoracic VCAR tool	Median	13.25	19.46	12.90	−6.57	−6.25	−6.44	53.24	48.48	50.39	42.11	44.58	43.84	28.21	33.33	30.93	−19.91	−12.96	−16.99
	Minimum	−28.00	−7.56	−15.86	−13.70	−9.77	−14.88	−5.46	−7.53	−27.66	−31.67	−37.86	−38.82	−49.38	−31.08	−33.78	−30.47	−23.03	−27.59
	Maximum	100.00	100.00	100.00	39.07	98.73	44.02	95.03	92.19	92.05	94.37	94.95	94.66	94.16	94.10	93.48	67.67	73.08	65.45
ANKE ASG-340 CT workstation pneumonia tool	Median	−4.51	0.49	−1.02	−11.20	−10.69	−7.52	31.03	33.87	31.99	35.60	36.03	35.63	37.50	39.55	39.66	−11.13	−11.56	−11.17
	Minimum	−19.24	−20.39	−20.61	−13.95	−9.52	−18.0	−12.41	−11.05	−11.20	−7.78	−40.61	−56.60	−112.86	−14.00	−14.00	−15.77	−12.39	−16.71
	Maximum	97.86	98.91	98.39	26.78	18.84	36.30	96.79	87.18	86.09	91.14	87.46	89.21	97.55	93.59	96.13	34.31	32.64	33.47

Note. EMP = emphysema; HP = health parenchyma; GGO = ground-glass opacity; CONSOL = consolidations.

Table 8. Lung volumes quantified by two tools in terms of median, minimum, and maximum values obtained on follow-up CT scans.

		EMP DX (%)	EMP SX (%)	EMP TOT (%/L)	HP DX (%)	HP SX (%)	HP TOT (%/L)	GGO DX (%)	GGO SX (%)	GGO TOT (%/L)	OTHER DX (%)	OTHER SX (%)	OTHER TOT (%/L)	CONSOL DX (%)	CONSOL SX (%)	CONSOL TOT (%/L)	VOLUME DX (L)	VOLUME SX (L)	VOLUME TOT (L)
Thoracic VCAR tool	Median	0.86	1.14	1.06	92.27	91.65	92.01	4.31	4.68	4.52	0.98	1.05	1.00	0.39	0.41	0.39	2.61	2.32	4.89
	Minimum	0.00	0.00	0.00	54.70	1.04	50.39	0.67	2.66	2.47	0.60	0.67	0.64	0.21	0.22	0.22	0.88	0.70	1.21
	Maximum	28.59	14.05	22.11	96.27	95.78	96.04	37.82	47.13	42.35	5.66	5.24	5.46	1.80	1.78	1.79	4.22	9.96	7.73
ANKE ASG-340 CT workstation pneumonia tool	Median	12.85	12.73	12.85	72.77	73.63	70.95	8.26	8.30	8.20	2.13	2.01	2.09	0.35	0.39	0.37	2.31	2.61	4.83
	Minimum	0.25	0.13	0.19	45.85	52.44	41.75	0.33	4.08	4.13	0.64	1.20	1.25	0.18	0.18	0.18	0.00	0.00	0.00
	Maximum	28.62	36.91	33.20	91.08	91.74	91.43	43.36	36.36	39.74	8.20	8.69	8.45	39.00	1.69	1.68	3.79	4.29	7.80

Note. EMP = emphysema; HP = health parenchyma; GGO = ground-glass opacity; CONSOL = consolidations.

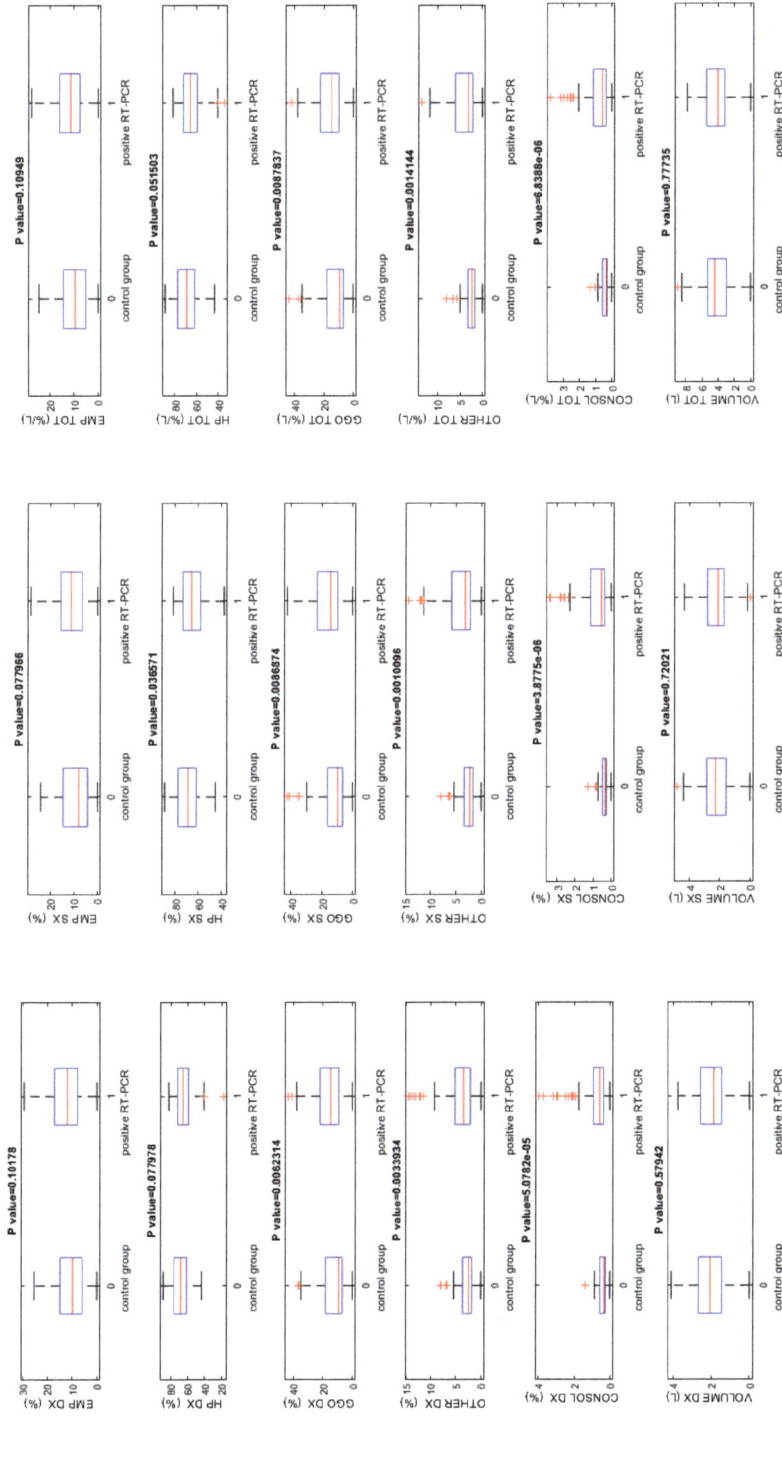

Figure 4. Boxplot of lung volumes quantified using the ANKE ASG-340 CT workstation pneumonia tool obtained on baseline CT scans. Note. EMP = emphysema; HP = health parenchyma; GGO = ground-glass opacity; CONSOL = consolidations.

Table 9. ROC analysis results for volumes measurements obtained on baseline CT scans for both software.

	ThoracicVCAR								ANKE ASG-340 CT Workstation Pneumonia					
	AUC	Sensitivity	Specificity	Positive Predictive Value	Negative Predictive Value	Accuracy	Cut-off	AUC	Sensitivity	Specificity	Positive Predictive Value	Negative Predictive Value	Accuracy	Cut-off
EMP DX (%)	0.42	0.04	1.00	1.00	0.26	0.28	4.06	0.50	0.51	0.58	0.78	0.28	0.53	11.44
EMP SX (%)	0.44	0.07	0.98	0.89	0.26	0.29	4.31	0.51	0.70	0.43	0.79	0.32	0.63	7.61
EMP TOT %/L	0.44	0.07	0.98	0.89	0.26	0.29	4.01	0.50	0.49	0.60	0.79	0.28	0.52	11.12
HP DX (%)	0.21	0.00	1.00	–	0.25	0.25	95.68	0.35	0.00	1.00	–	0.25	0.25	88.56
HP SX (%)	0.22	0.03	0.98	0.75	0.25	0.26	94.29	0.33	0.00	1.00	–	0.25	0.25	89.41
HP TOT (%/L)	0.21	0.00	1.00	–	0.25	0.25	95.58	0.34	0.00	1.00	–	0.25	0.25	89.00
GGO DX (%)	0.71	0.71	0.73	0.89	0.45	0.71	5.77	0.55	0.68	0.55	0.82	0.36	0.64	10.17
GGO SX (%)	0.70	0.70	0.73	0.88	0.45	0.71	5.74	0.55	0.68	0.53	0.81	0.35	0.64	10.26
GGO TOT (%/L)	**0.71**	**0.76**	**0.73**	**0.89**	**0.50**	**0.75**	**5.51**	0.55	0.68	0.55	0.82	0.37	0.65	10.03
OTHER DX (%)	0.71	0.48	0.98	0.98	0.38	0.60	1.89	0.60	0.50	0.75	0.86	0.33	0.56	3.64
OTHER SX (%)	0.71	0.52	0.90	0.94	0.38	0.61	1.92	0.61	0.25	0.98	0.97	0.30	0.43	6.42
OTHER TOT(%/L)	0.72	0.48	0.95	0.97	0.38	0.60	2.04	0.61	0.57	0.65	0.83	0.33	0.59	2.99
CONSOL DX (%)	0.72	0.55	0.88	0.93	0.39	0.63	0.50	0.64	0.64	0.63	0.84	0.37	0.64	0.42
CONSOL SX (%)	0.70	0.56	0.88	0.93	0.40	0.64	0.56	**0.68**	**0.77**	**0.55**	**0.84**	**0.44**	**0.71**	**0.35**
CONSOL TOT(%/L)	0.71	0.47	0.98	0.98	0.38	0.59	0.66	0.67	0.74	0.55	0.83	0.42	0.69	0.35
VOLUME DX (L)	0.38	0.04	0.98	0.83	0.25	0.28	3.65	0.37	0.00	1.00	–	0.25	0.25	4110.00
VOLUME SX (L)	0.34	0.00	1.00	NaN	0.25	0.25	4.08	0.39	0.00	1.00	–	0.25	0.25	4784.00
VOLUME TOT (L)	0.34	0.04	0.98	0.83	0.25	0.28	7.02	0.39	0.00	1.00	–	0.25	0.25	8894.00

Note. EMP = emphysema; HP = health parenchyma; GGO = ground-glass opacity; CONSOL = consolidations.

4. Discussions and Conclusions

In this study, we evaluated the quantitative analysis efficacy of chest CT sequelae in patients affected by COVID-19 pneumonia, comparing the consistency of two computerized tools. The visual evaluation of longitudinal changes in CT scans by radiologists is often a tedious task. There is a need to have a simple and fast automated method that can provide the segmentation and quantification of infection regions in order to evaluate the progression of the infected patients using lung CT scans [29–35]. Additionally, an objective evaluation by means of AI systems allows a data quantification, and therefore, an accurate definition of the disease progression; this is an element that otherwise is not very robust if entrusted to a simple visual inspection [36–38]. Recently, several computer tools have been proposed for the recognition of lung lesions from COVID-19 on CT examination [39–41]. However, many of them are not approved as medical devices, nor do they have the CE marking. Furthermore, the variability reported in the results obtained by these tools makes it difficult to choose the most accurate system [8].

To the best of our knowledge, this manuscript is the first with the aim to compare different computer tools for chest CT sequelae in patients affected by COVID-19 pneumonia. We demonstrated that there was a great variability among the quantitative measurements of the emphysema, residual healthy lung parenchyma volume, GGO, and consolidations volumes obtained by different computer tools when calculated on baseline CT scans. Instead, a good ICC was obtained for the quantitative measurements of the GGO and consolidations volumes obtained by two different computer tools when calculated on baseline CT scans, while considering the control group. Moreover, an excellent ICC was obtained for the quantitative measurements of the residual healthy lung parenchyma volume, GGO, and consolidations volumes obtained by two different computer tools when calculated on follow-up CT scans, and for the residual healthy lung parenchyma volume and GGO quantifications when the percentage change of these volumes was calculated between the baseline and follow-up scan. The lowest variability in the quantification was obtained for the GGO volume.

The Pearson correlation analyses showed a low correlation between the quantitative volume measurements determined by the thoracic VCAR tool and ANKE ASG-340 CT workstation pneumonia tool; exclusively, the measurement of the GGO showed a moderate correlation.

We think that the greater variability found at the baseline is linked to the complexity of the cases analyzed in this phase, which could affect the accuracy of lesion segmentation. As demonstrated by Herrmann et al. [42], in ARDS, image segmentation is especially difficult, since in some cases, it is almost impossible to discriminate the edge of the lung parenchyma from a pleural effusion, particularly in the most dependent lung regions and most severe ARDS forms. Also, at different airway pressures, they observed differences in lung weights. These variations may result either from the segmentation procedure and/or from actual changes in lung weight, primarily due to a possible airway pressure-dependent blood shift. It is unfortunately impossible to determine how much of the weight variation is due to an intrathoracic blood shift or to inaccuracies of the segmentation process. The decrease in intrathoracic blood volume we estimated in a previous work with increasing airway pressures was about 100 mL, leading to a small decrease in lung weight [43].

So, we believe that at follow-up, with a smaller extension of pulmonary involvement, the variability between the two systems is partially reduced, since the segmentation process is simpler in the absence of variables related to the presence of pleural effusion, and increase in pressures in the pulmonary vessels; the resolution of these variables favor the definition of the different pixels [44].

There were main critical points of the thoracic VCAR tool: automatic segmentation does not include areas of abundant consolidations of the lung parenchyma or pleural effusions, if conspicuous, requiring the manual segmentation modality; there was difficulty in the manual lung segmentation mode; its correction, performed on a single slice, takes time.

There were main critical points of the ANKE ASG-340 CT workstation pneumonia tool: it is slow in the analysis (120 s of median value compared to 10 s); it overestimates emphysema quantification; it is not able to segment complex cases with conspicuous effusion and/or areas of extensive consolidations.

Both tools, moreover, do not recognize several CT findings typical of the evolution of the disease, such as: (a) interlobular septal thickening, (b) fibrotic-like changes (reticular pattern and/or honeycombing), (c) bronchiectasis, (d) air bronchogram, (e) bronchial wall thickening, (f) pulmonary nodules surrounded by GGOs, (g) pleural and (h) pericardial effusion, and (i) lymphadenopathy, including these feature in others and reducing the accuracy of the assessment of the fibrotic-like changes.

According to Johns Hopkins University, case-fatality rates of COVID-19 patients ranges between 1% and 7% based on days since first confirmed case, testing efficacy, local pandemic response policies, and the population age [45–49]. Multi-organ manifestations of COVID-19 are now well-documented [50–57], but the potential long-term implications of these manifestations remain to be uncovered. Several studies have reported impaired exercise capacity and diffusing capacity for carbon monoxide (DL_{CO}) in SARS-CoV-1 survivors extending from 6 months to 15 years of follow-up [58–64], suggesting impairment of the intra-alveolar diffusion pathway. In this scenario, it is clear that it is important to have tools that objectively allow a stratification of patients based on the risk of developing chronic diseases that can impact their quality of life, and economically impact health care [65,66]. We believe that the computed assessment of CT findings could identify pulmonary abnormalities and lung recruitment, and we believe that knowledge of the percentage of potentially recruitable lung evolution may be important to establish the therapeutic management in chest sequelae in patients affected by COVID-19 pneumonia.

The present study has advantages: first, the homogeneity of the sample under examination and the follow-up at three months; second, the CT was performed at the same center, reducing the variability linked to different equipment; third, the high level of expertise of the group of radiologists who analyzed the images.

The major technical limitations for both tools is the lack of correlation of radiological data with clinical/functional data. It would be useful to evaluate how CT findings relate to functional investigations such as spirometry and/or lung scintigraphy. However, these data are present only for a small part of the population under examination.

In summary, computer-aided quantification could be an easy and feasible way to assess chest CT sequelae due to COVID-19 pneumonia; however, a great variability among the measurements provided by different tools should be considered.

Author Contributions: Conceptualization, R.G. (Roberto Grassi); Data curation, V.G., F.U. and R.G. (Roberto Grassi); Formal analysis, V.G., S.I., R.F., D.P., S.M., F.A. and R.G. (Roberta Grassi); Investigation, M.C., F.D.S., N.F., A.V. and F.G.; Methodology, S.I., R.F., F.A., P.C., A.P. and V.S.; Writing—original draft, V.G.; Writing—review & editing, V.G. All authors have read and agreed to the published version of the manuscript.

Funding: This research received no external funding.

Institutional Review Board Statement: This retrospective study included patients enrolled by the National Institute of Infec-tious Diseases Lazzaro Spallanzani Hospital, Rome, Italy.

Informed Consent Statement: Considering the emergency period, the local institutional review board waived in-formed consent for included patients in this retrospective study.

Data Availability Statement: All data are reported in the manuscript.

Acknowledgments: The authors are grateful to Alessandra Trocino, librarian at the National Cancer Institute of Naples, Italy.

Conflicts of Interest: The authors have no conflict of interest to be disclosed. The authors confirm that the article is not under consideration for publication elsewhere. Each author has participated sufficiently to take public responsibility for the content of the manuscript.

References

1. Stramare, R.; Carretta, G.; Capizzi, A.; Boemo, D.G.; Contessa, C.; Motta, R.; De Conti, G.; Causin, F.; Giraudo, C.; Donato, D. Radiological management of COVID-19: Structure your diagnostic path to guarantee a safe path. *Radiol. Med.* **2020**, *125*, 691–694. [CrossRef]
2. Granata, V.; Fusco, R.; Izzo, F.; Venanzio Setola, S.; Coppola, M.; Grassi, R.; Reginelli, A.; Cappabianca, S.; Grassi, R.; Petrillo, A. COVID-19 infection in cancer patients: The management in a diagnostic unit. *Radiol. Oncol.* **2021**, *55*, 121–129. [CrossRef]
3. Gaia, C.; Maria Chiara, C.; Silvia, L.; Chiara, A.; Maria Luisa, C.; Giulia, B.; Silvia, P.; Lucia, C.; Alessandra, T.; Annarita, S.; et al. Chest CT for early detection and management of coronavirus disease (COVID-19): A report of 314 patients admitted to Emergency Department with suspected pneumonia. *Radiol. Med.* **2020**, *125*, 931–942. [CrossRef]
4. Reginelli, A.; Grassi, R.; Feragalli, B.; Belfiore, M.P.; Montanelli, A.; Patelli, G.; La Porta, M.; Urraro, F.; Fusco, R.; Granata, V.; et al. Coronavirus Disease 2019 (COVID-19) in Italy: Double Reading of Chest CT Examination. *Biology* **2021**, *10*, 89. [CrossRef]
5. Giovagnoni, A. Facing the COVID-19 emergency: We can and we do. *Radiol. Med.* **2020**, *125*, 337–338. [CrossRef]
6. Montesi, G.; Di Biase, S.; Chierchini, S.; Pavanato, G.; Virdis, G.E.; Contato, E.; Mandoliti, G. Radiotherapy during COVID-19 pandemic. How to create a No fly zone: A Northern Italy experience. *Radiol. Med.* **2020**, *125*, 600–603. [CrossRef]
7. Ierardi, A.M.; Wood, B.J.; Arrichiello, A.; Bottino, N.; Bracchi, L.; Forzenigo, L.; Andrisani, M.C.; Vespro, V.; Bonelli, C.; Amalou, A.; et al. Preparation of a radiology department in an Italian hospital dedicated to COVID-19 patients. *Radiol. Med.* **2020**, *125*, 894–901. [CrossRef]
8. Grassi, R.; Cappabianca, S.; Urraro, F.; Feragalli, B.; Montanelli, A.; Patelli, G.; Granata, V.; Giacobbe, G.; Russo, G.M.; Grillo, A.; et al. Chest CT Computerized Aided Quantification of PNEUMONIA Lesions in COVID-19 Infection: A Comparison among Three Commercial Software. *Int. J. Environ. Res. Public Health* **2020**, *17*, 6914. [CrossRef] [PubMed]
9. Pediconi, F.; Galati, F.; Bernardi, D.; Belli, P.; Brancato, B.; Calabrese, M.; Camera, L.; Carbonaro, L.A.; Caumo, F.; Clauser, P.; et al. Breast imaging and cancer diagnosis during the COVID-19 pandemic: Recommendations from the Italian College of Breast Radiologists by SIRM. *Radiol. Med.* **2020**, *10*, 926–930. [CrossRef] [PubMed]
10. Available online: https://www.who.int (accessed on 6 March 2021).
11. Grassi, R.; Cappabianca, S.; Urraro, F.; Granata, V.; Giacobbe, G.; Magliocchetti, S.; Cozzi, D.; Fusco, R.; Galdiero, R.; Picone, C.; et al. Evolution of CT Findings and Lung Residue in Patients with COVID-19 Pneumonia: Quantitative Analysis of the Disease with a Computer Automatic Tool. *J. Pers. Med.* **2021**, *11*, 641. [CrossRef] [PubMed]
12. Koc, A.; Sezgin, O.S.; Kayipmaz, S. Comparing different planimetric methods on volumetric estimations by using cone beam computed tomography. *Radiol. Med.* **2020**, *125*, 398–405. [CrossRef]
13. Xu, G.X.; Liu, C.; Liu, J.; Ding, Z.; Shi, F.; Guo, M.; Zhao, W.; Li, X.; Wei, Y.; Gao, Y.; et al. Cross-Site Severity Assessment of COVID-19 from CT Images via Domain Adaptation. *IEEE Trans. Med. Imaging* **2021**. [CrossRef]
14. Agostini, A.; Floridi, C.; Borgheresi, A.; Badaloni, M.; Esposto Pirani, P.; Terilli, F.; Ottaviani, L.; Giovagnoni, A. Proposal of a low-dose, long-pitch, dual-source chest CT protocol on third-generation dual-source CT using a tin filter for spectral shaping at 100 kVp for CoronaVirus Disease 2019 (COVID-19) patients: A feasibility study. *Radiol. Med.* **2020**, *125*, 365–373. [CrossRef] [PubMed]
15. Borghesi, A.; Maroldi, R. COVID-19 outbreak in Italy: Experimental chest X-ray scoring system for quantifying and monitoring disease progression. *Radiol. Med.* **2020**, *125*, 509–513. [CrossRef]
16. Fiorini, F.; Granata, A.; Battaglia, Y.; Karaboue, M.A.A. Talking about medicine through mass media. *G. Ital. Nefrol.* **2019**, *36*, 2019-vol1. [PubMed]
17. Suri, J.S.; Agarwal, S.; Gupta, S.K.; Puvvula, A.; Biswa, M.; Saba, L.; Bit, A.; Tandel, G.S.; Agarwal, M.; Patrick, A.; et al. A narrative review on characterization of acute respiratory distress syndrome in COVID-19-infected lungs using artificial intelligence. *Comput. Biol. Med.* **2021**, *130*, 104210. [CrossRef]
18. Neri, E.; Miele, V.; Coppola, F.; Grassi, R. Use of CT and artificial intelligence in suspected or COVID-19 positive patients: Statement of the Italian Society of Medical and Interventional Radiology. *Radiol. Med.* **2020**, *125*, 505–508. [CrossRef] [PubMed]
19. Verschelden, G.; Noeparast, M.; Noparast, M.; Goossens, M.C.; Lauwers, M.; Cotton, F.; Michel, C.; Goyvaerts, C.; Hites, M. Plasma zinc status and hyperinflammatory syndrome in hospitalized COVID-19 patients: An observational study. *Int. Immunopharmacol.* **2021**, *100*, 108163. [CrossRef]
20. Merz, L.E.; Mistry, K.; Neuberg, D.; Freedman, R.; Menard, G.; Dorfman, D.M.; Park, H.S.; Jolley, K.; Achebe, M.O. Impact of sickle cell trait on morbidity and mortality from SARS-CoV-2 infection. *Blood Adv.* **2021**, *5*, 3690–3693. [CrossRef] [PubMed]
21. Carotti, M.; Salaffi, F.; Sarzi-Puttini, P.; Agostini, A.; Borgheresi, A.; Minorati, D.; Galli, M.; Marotto, D.; Giovagnoni, A. Chest CT features of coronavirus disease 2019 (COVID-19) pneumonia: Key points for radiologists. *Radiol. Med.* **2020**, *125*, 636–646. [CrossRef]
22. Zhou, S.; Wang, Y.; Zhu, T.; Xia, L. CT Features of Coronavirus Disease 2019 (COVID-19) Pneumonia in 62 Patients in Wuhan, China. *AJR Am. J. Roentgenol.* **2020**, *214*, 1287–1294. [CrossRef] [PubMed]
23. Xiong, Y.; Sun, D.; Liu, Y.; Fan, Y.; Zhao, L.; Li, X.; Zhu, W. Clinical and High-Resolution CT Features of the COVID-19 Infection: Comparison of the Initial and Follow-up Changes. *Investig. Radiol.* **2020**, *6*, 332–339. [CrossRef]
24. Belfiore, M.P.; Urraro, F.; Grassi, R.; Giacobbe, G.; Patelli, G.; Cappabianca, S.; Reginelli, A. Artificial intelligence to codify lung CT in COVID-19 patients. *Radiol. Med.* **2020**, *125*, 500–504. [CrossRef]

25. Grassi, R.; Belfiore, M.P.; Montanelli, A.; Patelli, G.; Urraro, F.; Giacobbe, G.; Fusco, R.; Granata, V.; Petrillo, A.; Sacco, P.; et al. COVID-19 pneumonia: Computer-aided quantification of healthy lung parenchyma, emphysema, ground glass and consolidation on chest computed tomography (CT). *Radiol. Med.* **2021**, *126*, 553–560. [CrossRef] [PubMed]
26. Kim, H.; Hong, H.; Yoon, S.H. Diagnostic performance of CT and reverse tran- scriptase-polymerase chain reaction for coronavirus disease 2019: A meta-analysis. *Radiology* **2020**, 201343. [CrossRef]
27. Caruso, D.; Guido, G.; Zerunian, M.; Polidori, T.; Lucertini, E.; Pucciarelli, F.; Polici, M.; Rucci, C.; Bracci, B.; Nicolai, M.; et al. Postacute Sequelae of COVID-19 Pneumonia: 6-month Chest CT Follow-up. *Radiology* **2021**, 210834. [CrossRef]
28. Hansell, D.M.; Bankier, A.A.; MacMahon, H.; McLoud, T.C.; Muller, N.L.; Remy, J. Fleischner Society: Glossary of terms for thoracic imaging. *Radiology* **2008**, *246*, 697–722. [CrossRef]
29. Lizzi, F.; Agosti, A.; Brero, F.; Cabini, R.F.; Fantacci, M.E.; Figini, S.; Lascialfari, A.; Laruina, F.; Oliva, P.; Piffer, S.; et al. Quantification of pulmonary involvement in COVID-19 pneumonia by means of a cascade of two U-nets: Training and assessment on multiple datasets using different annotation criteria. *Int. J. Comput. Assist. Radiol. Surg.* **2021**. [CrossRef]
30. Naudé, W. Artificial intelligence vs. COVID-19: Limitations, constraints and pitfalls. *AI Soc.* **2020**, *35*, 761–765. [CrossRef] [PubMed]
31. Wu, J.; Wang, J.; Nicholas, S.; Maitland, E.; Fan, Q. Application of big data technology for COVID-19 prevention and control in China: Lessons and recommendations. *J. Med. Internet Res.* **2020**, *22*, e21980. [CrossRef]
32. Alballa, N.; Al-Turaiki, I. Machine learning approaches in COVID-19 diagnosis, mortality, and severity risk prediction: A review. *Inform. Med. Unlocked* **2021**, *24*, 100564. [CrossRef] [PubMed]
33. Grassi, R.; Fusco, R.; Belfiore, M.P.; Montanelli, A.; Patelli, G.; Urraro, F.; Petrillo, A.; Granata, V.; Sacco, P.; Mazzei, M.; et al. Coronavirus disease 2019 (COVID-19) in Italy: Features on chest computed tomography using a structured report system. *Sci. Rep.* **2020**, *10*, 17236. [CrossRef] [PubMed]
34. Di Serafino, M.; Notaro, M.; Rea, G.; Iacobellis, F.; Paoli, V.D.; Acampora, C.; Ianniello, S.; Brunese, L.; Romano, L.; Vallone, G. The lung ultrasound: Facts or artifacts? In the era of COVID-19 outbreak. *Radiol. Med.* **2020**, *8*, 738–753. [CrossRef]
35. Agbehadji, I.E.; Awuzie, B.O.; Ngowi, A.B.; Millham, R.C. Review of big data analytics, artificial intelligence and nature-inspired computing models towards accurate detection of COVID-19 pandemic cases and contact tracing. *Int. J. Environ. Res. Public Health* **2020**, *17*, 5330. [CrossRef]
36. van Assen, M.; Muscogiuri, G.; Caruso, D.; Lee, S.J.; Laghi, A.; De Cecco, C.N. Artificial intelligence in cardiac radiology. *Radiol. Med.* **2020**, *125*, 1186–1199. [CrossRef]
37. Zhang, L.; Kang, L.; Li, G.; Zhang, X.; Ren, J.; Shi, Z.; Li, J.; Yu, S. Computed tomography-based radiomics model for discriminating the risk stratification of gastrointestinal stromal tumors. *Radiol. Med.* **2020**, *125*, 465–473. [CrossRef] [PubMed]
38. Hu, H.T.; Shan, Q.Y.; Chen, S.L.; Li, B.; Feng, S.T.; Xu, E.J.; Li, X.; Long, J.Y.; Xie, X.Y.; Lu, M.D.; et al. CT-based radiomics for preoperative prediction of early recurrent hepatocellular carcinoma: Technical reproducibility of acquisition and scanners. *Radiol. Med.* **2020**, *125*, 697–705. [CrossRef]
39. Li, L.; Qin, L.; Xu, Z.; Yin, Y.; Wang, X.; Kong, B.; Bai, J.; Lu, Y.; Fang, Z.; Song, Q.; et al. Artificial Intelligence Distinguishes COVID-19 from Community Acquired Pneumonia on Chest CT. *Radiology* **2020**, *19*, 200905. [CrossRef]
40. Tárnok, A. Machine Learning, COVID-19 (2019-nCoV), and multi-OMICS. *Cytometry* **2020**, *97*, 215–216. [CrossRef]
41. Gozes, O.; Frid-Adar, M.; Greenspan, H.; Browning, P.; Zhang, H.; Ji, W.; Bernheim, A.; Siegel, E. Rapid AI Development Cycle for the Coronavirus (COVID-19) Pandemic: Initial Results for Automated Detection & Patient Monitoring using Deep Learning CT Image Analysis. *arXiv* **2020**, arXiv:2003.05037.
42. Herrmann, P.; Busana, M.; Cressoni, M.; Lotz, J.; Moerer, O.; Saager, L.; Meissner, K.; Quintel, M.; Gattinoni, L. Using Artificial Intelligence for Automatic Segmentation of CT Lung Images in Acute Respiratory Distress Syndrome. *Front. Physiol.* **2021**, *12*, 676118. [CrossRef]
43. Chiumello, D.; Carlesso, E.; Aliverti, A.; Dellaca, R.L.; Pedotti, A.; Pelosi, P.P.; Gattinoni, L. Effects of volume shift on the pressure-volume curve of the respiratory system in ALI/ARDS patients. *Minerva Anestesiol.* **2007**, *73*, 109–118. [PubMed]
44. Oulefki, A.; Agaian, S.; Trongtirakul, T.; Kassah Laouar, A. Automatic COVID-19 lung infected region segmentation and measurement using CT-scans images. *Pattern Recognit.* **2021**, *114*, 107747. [CrossRef]
45. Johns Hopkins University. Coronavirus Resource Center: Mortality Analyses. Available online: https://coronavirus.jhu.edu/data/mortality (accessed on 24 November 2020).
46. D'Agostino, V.; Caranci, F.; Negro, A.; Piscitelli, V.; Tuccillo, B.; Fasano, F.; Sirabella, G.; Marano, I.; Granata, V.; Grassi, R.; et al. A Rare Case of Cerebral Venous Thrombosis and Disseminated Intravascular Coagulation Temporally Associated to the COVID-19 Vaccine Administration. *J. Pers. Med.* **2021**, *11*, 285. [CrossRef]
47. Ghayda, R.A.; Lee, K.H.; Han, Y.J.; Ryu, S.; Hong, S.H.; Yoon, S.; Jeong, G.H.; Lee, J.; Lee, J.Y.; Yang, J.W.; et al. Estimation of global case fatality rate of coronavirus disease 2019 (COVID-19) using meta-analyses: Comparison between calendar date and days since the outbreak of the first confirmed case. *Int. J. Infect Dis.* **2020**, *100*, 302–308. [CrossRef] [PubMed]
48. La Seta, F.; Buccellato, A.; Tesè, L.; Biscaldi, E.; Rollandi, G.A.; Barbiera, F.; Cappabianca, S.; Di Mizio, R.; Grassi, R. Multidetector-row CT enteroclysis: Indications and clinical applications. *Radiol. Med.* **2006**, *111*, 141–158. [CrossRef]
49. Cantisani, V.; Iannetti, G.; Miele, V.; Grassi, R.; Karaboue, M.; Cesarano, E.; Vimercati, F.; Calliada, F. Addendum to the sonographic medical act. *J. Ultrasound* **2021**, *24*, 229–230. [CrossRef] [PubMed]

50. Granata, V.; Fusco, R.; Costa, M.; Picone, C.; Cozzi, D.; Moroni, C.; La Casella, G.V.; Montanino, A.; Monti, R.; Mazzoni, F.; et al. Preliminary Report on Computed Tomography Radiomics Features as Biomarkers to Immunotherapy Selection in Lung Adenocarcinoma Patients. *Cancers* **2021**, *13*, 3992. [CrossRef]
51. Nardone, V.; Boldrini, L.; Grassi, R.; Franceschini, D.; Morelli, I.; Becherini, C.; Loi, M.; Greto, D.; Desideri, I. Radiomics in the Setting of Neoadjuvant Radiotherapy: A New Approach for Tailored Treatment. *Cancers* **2021**, *13*, 3590. [CrossRef]
52. Fichera, G.; Stramare, R.; De Conti, G.; Motta, R.; Giraudo, C. It's not over until it's over: The chameleonic behavior of COVID-19 over a six-day period. *Radiol. Med.* **2020**, *5*, 514–516. [CrossRef]
53. Granata, V.; Grassi, R.; Miele, V.; Larici, A.R.; Sverzellati, N.; Cappabianca, S.; Brunese, L.; Maggialetti, N.; Borghesi, A.; Fusco, R.; et al. Structured Reporting of Lung Cancer Staging: A Consensus Proposal. *Diagnostics* **2021**, *11*, 1569. [CrossRef] [PubMed]
54. Borghesi, A.; Zigliani, A.; Masciullo, R.; Golemi, S.; Maculotti, P.; Farina, D.; Maroldi, R. Radiographic severity index in COVID-19 pneumonia: Relationship to age and sex in 783 Italian patients. *Radiol. Med.* **2020**, *125*, 461–464. [CrossRef]
55. Maio, F.; Tari, D.U.; Granata, V.; Fusco, R.; Grassi, R.; Petrillo, A.; Pinto, F. Breast Cancer Screening during COVID-19 Emergency: Patients and Department Management in a Local Experience. *J. Pers. Med.* **2021**, *11*, 380. [CrossRef] [PubMed]
56. Nardone, V.; Reginelli, A.; Vinciguerra, C.; Correale, P.; Calvanese, M.G.; Falivene, S.; Sangiovanni, A.; Grassi, R.; Di Biase, A.; Polifrone, M.A.; et al. Mood Disorder in Cancer Patients Undergoing Radiotherapy During the COVID-19 Outbreak. *Front. Psychol.* **2021**, *12*, 568839. [CrossRef]
57. Granata, V.; Fusco, R.; Setola, S.V.; Galdiero, R.; Picone, C.; Izzo, F.; D'Aniello, R.; Miele, V.; Grassi, R.; Grassi, R.; et al. Lymphadenopathy after BNT162b2Covid-19 Vaccine: Preliminary Ultrasound Findings. *Biology* **2021**, *10*, 214. [CrossRef] [PubMed]
58. Ngai, J.C.; Ko, F.W.S.; Ng, S.; To, K.-W.; Tong, M.; Hui, D. The long-term impact of severe acute respiratory syndrome on pulmonary function, exercise capacity and health status. *Respirology* **2010**, *15*, 543–550. [CrossRef] [PubMed]
59. Su, M.-C.; Hsieh, Y.-T.; Wang, Y.-H.; Lin, A.-S.; Chung, Y.-H.; Lin, M.-C. Exercise capacity and pulmonary function in hospital workers recovered from severe acute respiratory syndrome. *Respiration* **2007**, *74*, 511–516. [CrossRef]
60. Liu, Y.-X.; Ye, Y.-P.; Zhang, P.; Chen, J.; Ye, H.; He, Y.-H.; Li, N. Changes in pulmonary function in SARS patients during the three-year convalescent period. *Zhongguo Wei Zhong Bing Ji Jiu Yi Xue.* **2007**, *19*, 536–538.
61. Hui, D.S.; Joynt, G.; Wong, K.T.; Gomersall, C.; Li, T.S.; Antonio, G.; Ko, F.W.S.; Chan, M.C.; Chan, D.P.; Tong, M.W.; et al. Impact of severe acute respiratory syndrome (SARS) on pulmonary function, functional capacity and quality of life in a cohort of survivors. *Thorax* **2005**, *60*, 401–409. [CrossRef]
62. Cozzi, D.; Albanesi, M.; Cavigli, E.; Moroni, C.; Bindi, A.; Luvara, S.; Lucarini, S.; Busoni, S.; Mazzoni, L.N.; Miele, V. Chest X-ray in new Coronavirus Disease 2019 (COVID-19) infection: Findings and correlation with clinical outcome. *Radiol. Med.* **2020**, *125*, 730–737. [CrossRef]
63. Gatti, M.; Calandri, M.; Barba, M.; Biondo, A.; Geninatti, C.; Gentile, S.; Greco, M.; Morrone, V.; Piatti, C.; Santonocito, A.; et al. Baseline chest X-ray in coronavirus disease 19 (COVID-19) patients: Association with clinical and laboratory data. *Radiol. Med.* **2020**, *125*, 1271–1279. [CrossRef] [PubMed]
64. Giannitto, C.; Sposta, F.M.; Repici, A.; Vatteroni, G.; Casiraghi, E.; Casari, E.; Ferraroli, G.M.; Fugazza, A.; Sandri, M.T.; Chiti, A.; et al. Chest CT in patients with a moderate or high pretest probability of COVID-19 and negative swab. *Radiol. Med.* **2020**, *125*, 1260–1270. [CrossRef]
65. Fusco, R.; Grassi, R.; Granata, V.; Setola, S.V.; Grassi, F.; Cozzi, D.; Pecori, B.; Izzo, F.; Petrillo, A. Artificial Intelligence and COVID-19 Using Chest CT Scan and Chest X-ray Images: Machine Learning and Deep Learning Approaches for Diagnosis and Treatment. *J. Pers. Med.* **2021**, *11*, 993. [CrossRef] [PubMed]
66. Scoccianti, S.; Perna, M.; Olmetto, E.; Delli Paoli, C.; Terziani, F.; Ciccone, L.P.; Detti, B.; Greto, D.; Simontacchi, G.; Grassi, R.; et al. Local treatment for relapsing glioblastoma: A decision-making tree for choosing between reirradiation and second surgery. *Crit. Rev. Oncol. Hematol.* **2021**, *157*, 103184. [CrossRef] [PubMed]

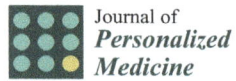

Systematic Review

Artificial Intelligence and COVID-19 Using Chest CT Scan and Chest X-ray Images: Machine Learning and Deep Learning Approaches for Diagnosis and Treatment

Roberta Fusco [1], Roberta Grassi [2,3], Vincenza Granata [4,*], Sergio Venanzio Setola [4], Francesca Grassi [2], Diletta Cozzi [5], Biagio Pecori [6], Francesco Izzo [7] and Antonella Petrillo [4]

1. IGEA SpA Medical Division—Oncology, Via Casarea 65, Casalnuovo di Napoli, 80013 Naples, Italy; r.fusco@igeamedical.com
2. Division of Radiology, Università Degli Studi Della Campania Luigi Vanvitelli, 80138 Naples, Italy; grassi.roberta89@gmail.com (R.G.); francescagrassi1996@gmail.com (F.G.)
3. Italian Society of Medical and Interventional Radiology (SIRM), SIRM Foundation, 20122 Milan, Italy
4. Division of Radiology, Istituto Nazionale Tumori IRCCS Fondazione Pascale—IRCCS di Napoli, 80131 Naples, Italy; s.setola@istitutotumori.na.it (S.V.S.); a.petrillo@istitutotumori.na.it (A.P.)
5. Division of Radiology, Azienda Ospedaliera Universitaria Careggi, 50134 Florence, Italy; cozzid@aou-careggi.toscana.it
6. Division of Radiotherapy and Innovative Technologies, Istituto Nazionale Tumori IRCCS Fondazione Pascale—IRCCS di Napoli, 80131 Naples, Italy; b.pecori@istitutotumori.na.it
7. Division of Hepatobiliary Surgery, Istituto Nazionale Tumori IRCCS Fondazione Pascale—IRCCS di Napoli, 80131 Naples, Italy; f.izzo@istitutotumori.na.it
* Correspondence: v.granata@istitutotumori.na.it

Citation: Fusco, R.; Grassi, R.; Granata, V.; Setola, S.V.; Grassi, F.; Cozzi, D.; Pecori, B.; Izzo, F.; Petrillo, A. Artificial Intelligence and COVID-19 Using Chest CT Scan and Chest X-ray Images: Machine Learning and Deep Learning Approaches for Diagnosis and Treatment. *J. Pers. Med.* **2021**, *11*, 993. https://doi.org/10.3390/jpm11100993

Academic Editors: Sabina Tangaro and Moon-Soo Lee

Received: 15 August 2021
Accepted: 28 September 2021
Published: 30 September 2021

Publisher's Note: MDPI stays neutral with regard to jurisdictional claims in published maps and institutional affiliations.

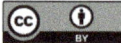

Copyright: © 2021 by the authors. Licensee MDPI, Basel, Switzerland. This article is an open access article distributed under the terms and conditions of the Creative Commons Attribution (CC BY) license (https://creativecommons.org/licenses/by/4.0/).

Abstract: Objective: To report an overview and update on Artificial Intelligence (AI) and COVID-19 using chest Computed Tomography (CT) scan and chest X-ray images (CXR). Machine Learning and Deep Learning Approaches for Diagnosis and Treatment were identified. Methods: Several electronic datasets were analyzed. The search covered the years from January 2019 to June 2021. The inclusion criteria were studied evaluating the use of AI methods in COVID-19 disease reporting performance results in terms of accuracy or precision or area under Receiver Operating Characteristic (ROC) curve (AUC). Results: Twenty-two studies met the inclusion criteria: 13 papers were based on AI in CXR and 10 based on AI in CT. The summarized mean value of the accuracy and precision of CXR in COVID-19 disease were 93.7% ± 10.0% of standard deviation (range 68.4–99.9%) and 95.7% ± 7.1% of standard deviation (range 83.0–100.0%), respectively. The summarized mean value of the accuracy and specificity of CT in COVID-19 disease were 89.1% ± 7.3% of standard deviation (range 78.0–99.9%) and 94.5 ± 6.4% of standard deviation (range 86.0–100.0%), respectively. No statistically significant difference in summarized accuracy mean value between CXR and CT was observed using the Chi square test (p value > 0.05). Conclusions: Summarized accuracy of the selected papers is high but there was an important variability; however, less in CT studies compared to CXR studies. Nonetheless, AI approaches could be used in the identification of disease clusters, monitoring of cases, prediction of the future outbreaks, mortality risk, COVID-19 diagnosis, and disease management.

Keywords: COVID-19; computed tomography; X-ray; artificial intelligence; machine learning; deep learning

1. Introduction

In December 2019, a large outbreak of a novel coronavirus infection occurred in Wuhan, Hubei Province, China. The novel coronavirus was named severe acute respiratory syndrome coronavirus 2 (SARS-CoV-2) by the International Committee on Taxonomy of Viruses and led to a dramatic pneumonia outbreak in China [1–3]. The disease caused by the virus, named coronavirus disease (COVID-19) by the World Health Organization (WHO), can be spread through human-to-human contact. On January 30, 2020, the WHO declared a global public health emergency against the outbreak of COVID-19 [4–6].

The COVID-19 diagnosis is confirmed by the positive results of the nucleic acid amplification test of the respiratory tract or blood specimens using reverse transcription real-time fluorescence polymerase chain reaction (RT-PCR) [7,8]. However, methods like chest X-ray (CXR) and chest Computed Tomography (CT) scan are medical imaging techniques, which are widely used to assess the pneumonia due to COVID-19 [9–19]. The reported sensitivity of CXR for COVID-19 pneumonia is relatively low in the early phase of the disease and in mild cases (69%). Conversely, CT shows greater sensitivity for early pneumonic change, disease progression, and alternative diagnosis; the administration of the intravenous contrast medium, is essential for the diagnosis of pulmonary thromboembolism [20–37]. Despite recent advances in diagnostic tools, radiologic imaging alone is not sufficient for the COVID-19 pneumonia diagnosis. Imaging should be associated to clinical and laboratory testing. In addition, the American College of Radiology, so as the Italian Society of Radiology (SIRM) does not recommend chest CT as a screening tool, suggesting this method only for symptomatic patients with specific clinical indications. Bilateral distribution of ground glass opacities (GGO) with or without consolidation in posterior and peripheral lungs was the cardinal hallmark of COVID-19 disease [6,22]. Among COVID-19 patients, it is reasonable to assume that those with a very severe disease could exhibit high risk of venous thromboembolism, including deep vein thrombosis and/or pulmonary embolism. In this scenario, it is opened the question on the use of contrast medium during CT studies [20–22].

The mathematical models for COVID-19 pandemic, confirmed by practical evidence in China, in Italy, and in the rest of the world, have shown that the rapid substantial increase in the number of critically ill patients exceeds in the total capacity of Intensive care units (ICUs), even excluding routine critical admissions for trauma, stroke, and other emergencies.

In the context of the COVID-19 outbreak, there is a painstaking need for ready-to-use resources for data acquisition and artificial intelligence (AI) algorithms to accelerate the search for effective and safe treatments. The progressive integration of radiomics approaches and AI-based solutions in healthcare is already changing established paradigms in the entire healthcare ecosystem, leveraging the progressive digitalization of medical data [38–53]. Specifically, diagnostic and decision support systems developed for medical imaging are the first successful examples of innovation for health. AI-based methods have led to diagnostic applications that accelerate image acquisition, preprocessing, annotation and interpretation, offering an "augmentation" of the radiologists, rather than their unrealistic substitution. In particular, the application of AI in medical imaging has improved the assessment, diagnosis and early detection of neurodegenerative diseases, heart diseases, with a specifically high impact on breast and lung cancer [38–53].

Deep learning (DL) and machine learning (ML) are branches of AI that focus on producing systems that can learn from examples and improve without being explicitly programmed. ML is the study of computer algorithms that can improve automatically through experience and using data. Machine learning algorithms build a model based on sample data, known as "training data", to make predictions or decisions without being explicitly programmed to do so. Machine learning algorithms are used in a wide variety of applications, such as in medicine, email filtering, speech recognition, and computer vision, where it is difficult or unfeasible to develop conventional algorithms to perform the needed tasks. A subset of machine learning is closely related to computational statistics, which focus on making predictions using computers; but not all machine learning is statistical learning. The study of mathematical optimization delivers methods, theory and application domains to the field of machine learning. Data mining is a related field of study, focusing on exploratory data analysis through unsupervised learning.

Deep learning is a class of machine learning algorithms that uses multiple layers to progressively extract higher-level features from the raw input. For example, in image processing, lower layers may identify edges, while higher layers may identify the concepts relevant to a human such as digits or letters or faces. Deep-learning architectures such as deep neural networks, deep belief networks, deep reinforcement learning, recurrent neural networks and convolutional neural networks have been applied to fields including computer vision, speech recognition, natural language processing, machine translation, bioinformatics, drug design, medical image analysis, material inspection and board game programs, where they have produced results comparable to and in some cases surpassing human expert performance.

DL and ML have been applied successfully in many fields, including health care and medical informatics. One important research direction leverages DL and ML to understand and fight COVID-19. Numerous lines of research have been initiated for the application and development of COVID-19-related DL and ML algorithms.

Several review articles have been published on the use of artificial intelligence approaches in COVID-19 research. Agbehadji et al. [54], summarized how big data and AI models can be used for case detection and contact tracing of COVID-19. Bullock et al. [55], discussed how AI is used to evaluate the challenges of COVID-19 at different scales, including molecular, medical, and epidemiological applications. Naudé [56] highlighted the actual and potential applications of AI in fighting COVID-19. Wu et al. [57], surveyed the application of big data technology for preventing and managing COVID-19 in China.

Alballa et al. [58], review the recent ML algorithms in this field and focus on their potential in two main applications: diagnosis of COVID-19 and prediction of mortality risk and severity, using simple clinical and laboratory data; they analyze the main features that were found to be the most relevant to these applications.

Our aim is to report an overview and update on AI-based methods application in COVID-19 disease using radiological images including CXR and CT focus on their potential in two main applications: diagnosis of COVID-19 and prediction of mortality risk and severity.

This narrative review is the result of an autonomous study without protocol and a registration number.

2. Methods

2.1. Search Criterion

Several electronic datasets were searched: PubMed (US National Library of Medicine, http://www.ncbi.nlm.nih.gov/pubmed accessed on 24 June 2021), Scopus (Elsevier, http://www.scopus.com/ accessed on 24 June 2021), Web of Science (Thomson Reuters, http://apps.webof knowledge.com/ accessed on 24 June 2021) and Google Scholar (https://scholar.google.it/ accessed on 24 June 2021). The following search criteria have been used: "COVID-19" and "X-ray" and "ARTIFICIAL INTELLIGENCE"; "COVID-19" and "CT" and "ARTIFICIAL INTELLIGENCE"; "COVID-19" and "X-ray" and "DEEP LEARNING"; "COVID-19" and "CT" and "DEEP LEARNING"; "COVID-19" and "X-ray" and "MACHINE LEARNING"; "COVID-19" and "CT" and "MACHINE LEARNING".

The search covered the years from January 2019 to June 2021. The reference lists of the found papers were analyzed for papers not indexed in the electronic databases. All titles and abstracts were analyzed. The inclusion criteria were studied evaluating the use of AI methods in COVID-19 disease reporting performance results in terms of accuracy or precision or area under Receiver Operating Characteristic (ROC) curve (AUC). Articles published in the English language were included. Exclusion criteria were different topics, unavailability of full text, and not sufficient data.

2.2. Statistical Analysis

The summarized accuracy, precision or specificity were calculated in terms of mean, standard deviation value and range. The Chi square test was used to assess differences statistically significant between CXR and CT results. p value < 0.05 was considered significant for all tests.

All analyses were performed using IBM SPSS Statistics 24 (IBM, Armonk, NY, USA).

3. Results

We identified 84 potentially relevant references through electronic searches. We identified 15 references through scanning reference lists of the identified paper that we added to the 84 references previously selected (total number of articles was 99). We then excluded 51 clearly irrelevant articles through screening titles and reading abstracts. We excluded 25 articles for the reasons listed in the exclusion criteria. A total of 23 article met the inclusion criteria. A diagram of included and excluded studies was summarized in the study flow diagram (Figure 1).

Table 1 reports the classification problem, the classification approach and the performance results of the selected papers.

Thirteen papers using CXR and AI approaches in the COVID-19 disease were identified. The summarized mean value of the accuracy and precision of CRX in COVID-19 disease were 93.7% $\pm$ 10.0% of standard deviation (range 68.4–99.9%) and 95.7% $\pm$ 7.1% of standard deviation (range 83.0–100.0%), respectively.

Ten papers using chest CT and AI approaches in the COVID-19 disease were found. The summarized mean value of the accuracy and specificity of CT in COVID-19 disease were 89.1% $\pm$ 7.3% of standard deviation (range 78.0–99.9%) and 94.5% $\pm$ 6.4% of standard deviation (range 86.0–100.0%), respectively.

No statistically significant difference in summarized accuracy mean value between CXR and CT was observed using the Chi square test (p value > 0.05).

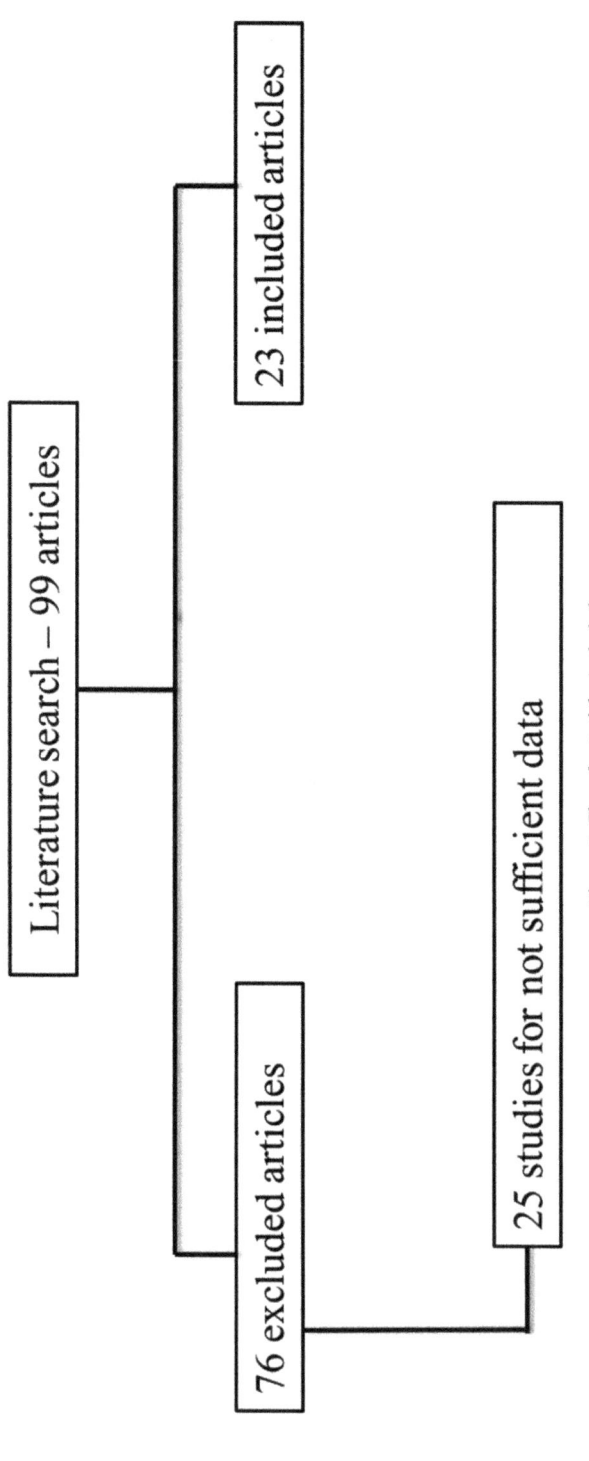

Figure 1. Flowchart of the included papers.

Table 1. Imaging Modality, Dataset, classification problem, classification approach and performance results of the selected papers.

Authors	Methodology	Imaging Modality	Dataset	Limits	Classification Problem	Classification Model	Accuracy [%]	Specificity [%]	Precision [%]	Area Under ROC Curve
Sethy et al.	deep learning	CXR	Firt dataset: 25 number of COVID-19+ and 25 number of COVID-19- X-ray images. Second dataset: 133 X-ray images of COVID-19+, including MERS, SARS, and ARDS and 133 chest X-ray images as COVID-19-	Number of patients. Moreover, the limitation of this methodology is that if the patient is in a critical situation and unable to attend for CXR scanning. The model is limited to classify the input chest X-ray image into only two classes either normal or COVID-19	COVID-19 detection	resnet50 plus Support Vector Machine	95.38			

Table 1. Cont.

Authors	Methodology	Imaging Modality	Dataset	Limits	Classification Problem	Classification Model	Accuracy [%]	Specificity [%]	Precision [%]	Area Under ROC Curve
Jiao et al.	deep learning	CXR	1834 patients were identified and assigned to the model training (n = 1285), validation (n = 183), or testing (n = 366) sets. The number of patients that were identified for external testing of the model were 475.	The artificial intelligence model showed decreased performance on the external testing set relative to the internal testing set, indicating that generalization might not be possible. This finding could have been due to several factors, including heterogeneous data and image acquisition between the different hospital systems. The model is limited to classifying the input chest X-ray image into only two classes either normal or COVID-19	predict the binary outcome of COVID-19 disease severity (critical or non-critical)	EfficientNet deep neural network and clinical data				0.85 on internal testing and 0.80 on external testing
Al-Waisy et al.	deep learning	CXR	200 X-ray images with confirmed COVID-19 infection come by Cohen's GitHub database [58]; 200 COVID-19 CXR gathered from three different repository: Radiopaedia dataset [59], Italian Society of Medical and Interventional Radiology (SIRM) [60], and Radiological Society of North America (RSNA) [61]; 400 normal CXR by Kaggle's CXR dataset [62]	Cases used in this study come from different databases. The model is limited to classifying the input chest X-ray image into only two classes, either normal or COVID-19	COVID-19 detection	COVID-CheXNet system made by combining the results generated from two different deep learning models	99.99	100	100	
Ozcan et al.	deep learning	CXR	127 X-ray images diagnosed with COVID-19, 500 no-findings and 500 pneumonia class	No external testing of the model and the patient number is low for multi class classification	COVID-19 versus no findings classification/multi-class classification COVID-19 versus no findings versus pneumonia	single layer-based (SLB) and a feature fusion based (FFB) composite systems using deep features	99.52/87.64		98.03/99.7	
Ozturk et al.	deep learning	CXR	127 X-ray images diagnosed with COVID-19, 500 no-findings and 500 pneumonia class	No external testing of the model and the patient number is low for multi class classification	COVID-19 versus no findings classification/multi-class classification COVID-19 versus no findings versus pneumonia	DarkNet model implementing 17 convolutional layers and introducing different filtering on each layer	98.08/87.02		98.03/89.96	

Table 1. Cont.

Authors	Methodology	Imaging Modality	Dataset	Limits	Classification Problem	Classification Model	Accuracy [%]	Specificity [%]	Precision [%]	Area Under ROC Curve
Du et al.	machine learning	CXR	447 cases with COVID-19; 405 with other viral PNA, 1515 with bacterial PNA, 1862 with Clinical PNA, 256 with other infections and 663 with other diseases	The model has a moderate specificity	COVID-19 detection		68.4			
Dey et al.	classifier ensemble technique	CXR	A total of 506 viral lung infection cases including 468 cases with COVID-19,46 bacterial lung infection and 26 fungal lung infection by https://github.com/ieee8023/covid-chestxray-dataset; 1583 normal CXR and 4273 COVID-19+ CXR by https://www.kaggle.com/paultimothymooney/chest-xray-pneumonia/version/2.	No external testing of the model and patient number.	classification of Normal, COVID-19, and Pneumonia cases	Choquet fuzzy integral using two dense layers and one softmax layer	99.02		99	
Alruwaili et al.	deep learning	CXR	2905 CXR images, which are distributed into 219 COVID-19 images, 1345 viral pneumonia images, and 1341 for normal category	No external testing of the model and patient number.	COVID-19 vs. normal vs. viral pneumonia classification	Inception-ResNetV2 deep learning model	99.83		98.11	
Bukhari et al.	deep learning	CXR	93 CXR which have no radiological abnormality; 96 CXR with the radiological features of pneumonia different from COVID-19 infection; 89 digital images of chest X-rays of patients diagnosed with COVID-19 infection	The model takes a roughly higher training and testing run time compared to other models due to the complex structure of the inside modules.	healthy normal, bacterial pneumonia, viral pneumonia, and COVID-19 classification	resnet50	98.18		98.14	
Khan et al.	deep learning	CXR	1203 normal, 660 bacterial Pneumonia and 931 viral Pneumonia cases	Small prepared dataset which indicates that given more data, the proposed model can achieve better results with minimum pre-processing of data	viral pneumonia, COVID-19, bacterial pneumonia, and normal classification/normal, COVID-19, and pneumonia classification	CoroNet: pretrained Xception convolution network	89.6/95.0			

Table 1. *Cont.*

Authors	Methodology	Imaging Modality	Dataset	Limits	Classification Problem	Classification Model	Accuracy [%]	Specificity [%]	Precision [%]	Area Under ROC Curve
Hemdan et al.	deep learning	CXR	25 normal cases and 25 positive COVID-19 images	The model is limited to classifying the input chest X-ray image into only two classes, either normal or COVID-19. Another limit is the number of patients	COVID-19 detection	InceptionV3, MobileNetV2, VGG19, DenseNet201, Inception-ResNetV2, ResNetV2, and Xception model	90		83	
Sethy and Behera	deep learning and machine learning	CXR	25 normal cases and 25 positive COVID-19 images	The model is limited to classifying the input chest X-ray image into only two classes, either normal or COVID-19	detecting COVID-19 (ignoring SARS, MERS and ARDS)	deep learning for feature extraction and support vector machine (SVM) for classification	95.38			
Ouchicha et al.	deep learning	CXR	219 COVID-19, 1341 normal and 1345 viral pneumonia	The model has been trained on a small dataset of few images of various COVID-19, viral pneumonia and normal cases from publically available database	classification of Normal, COVID-19, and Pneumonia cases	local and global features of CXR using two parallel layers with reaching various kernel sizes	97.2			
Gozes et al.	deep learning	CT	106 COVID-19 chest CT scans and 99 normal ones	Patient number is low	COVID-19 versus no COVID-19	robust 2D and 3D deep learning models				0.948
Wang et al. [63]	deep learning	CT	740 for COVID-19 negative and 325 for COVID-19 positive	Sample size was relatively small	COVID-19 versus no COVID-19	GoogleNet Inception v3 convolution neural network	89.5	88		
Li et al.	deep learning	CT	1292 with COVID-19, 1735 for community-acquired pneumonia, and 1325 for non-pneumonia abnormalities	The model is limited to classifying the input chest X-ray image into only two classes, either normal or COVID-19	COVID-19 versus no COVID-19	resnet50		90		0.96
Ko et al.	deep learning	CT	1194 chest CT COVID-19 images and 1357 chest CT images with non-COVID-19 pneumonia	The model is limited to classifying the input chest X-ray image into only two classes, either normal or COVID-19	Classification of COVID-19 patients	FCONet developed by transfer learning using one of four state-of-the-art pretrained deep learning models (VGG16, ResNet-50, Inception-v3, or Xception)	99.87	100		

Table 1. Cont.

Authors	Methodology	Imaging Modality	Dataset	Limits	Classification Problem	Classification Model	Accuracy [%]	Specificity [%]	Precision [%]	Area Under ROC Curve
Nguyen et al.	deep learning	CT	101 with COVID-19, 118 with common Pneumonia and 118 for non-pneumonia abnormalities	Patient number is low for three classes classification	normal, COVID-19, and pneumonia classification	convolutional neural network	87			0.83
			1544 with COVID-19, 1556 with common Pneumonia and 118 for non-pneumonia abnormalities				97			0.99
			281 with COVID-19 and 1068 for non-pneumonia abnormalities				86			0.87
Zhang et al. [64]	CT	CT	There were 406 clearer COVID-19-positive lung CT images. The marked areas in the mask images are 0-"ground glass opacity," 1-"consolidations," 2-"lungs other," 3-"background.	The complexity of the model and the number of patients	segment ground glass opaque lesions in COVID-19 lung CT images	COVSeg-NET model is based on the fully convolutional neural network model structure, which mainly includes convolutional layer, nonlinear unit activation function, maximum pooling layer, batch normalization layer, merge layer, flattening layer, sigmoid layer, and so forth		100		
Song et al.	deep learning	CT	A total of 88 patients diagnosed with the COVID-19, 101 patients infected with bacteria pneumonia, and 86 healthy persons	Patient number is low for a three classes classification	normal verus COVID-19 classification/discriminating COVID-19 patients from others	resnet50	78	96/86		0.99/0.95
Wang et al. [65]	machine learning	CT	A total of 1051 patients with RT-PCR confirmed COVID-19 and chest CT was included in this study	Patient selection bias, retrospective and multi-institutional nature of the study.	for prediction of COVID-19 progression using CT imaging and clinical data				80	

Table 1. Cont.

Authors	Methodology	Imaging Modality	Dataset	Limits	Classification Problem	Classification Model	Accuracy [%]	Specificity [%]	Precision [%]	Area Under ROC Curve
Xu et al.	deep learning	CT	A total of 618 CT samples were collected: 219 samples from 110 patients with COVID-19 and 224 samples from 224 patients with influenza-A viral pneumonia (IAVP)	Patient selection bias, patient number is low	early screening model to distinguish COVID-19 from IAVP and healthy cases through pulmonary CT images	3D deep learning network that consists of four basic stages, which are pre-processing, candidate region segmentation, classification	86.7			

4. Discussions

Artificial intelligence approaches have been used to predict the outbreak, to diagnose the disease, to analyze CXR and CT scan images, and more recently to predict mortality or progression risk to severe respiratory failure. This evidence clearly indicates the need for the most rapid and accurate diagnostic and stratification of patients with COVID-19, with technologies and expertise easily accessible from all nodes of the healthcare system with responsibility of diagnosis of COVID-19 and management of patients (either in the health structures or at home) [59].

Chest radiographs are first-line investigations in many countries. Researchers could examine not only the initial imaging findings and extent of respiratory involvement, but also how radiographic progression in serial studies correlates with patients' clinical outcome [60–62,66]. CT examination has been used extensively worldwide to evaluate the grade and the extension of the viral pneumonia by COVID-19 and in the follow-up, which are also based on AI algorithms [67–70]. Several radiological organizations do not recommend CT as primary diagnostic/screening tool for COVID-19 [71–74] or have excluded CT findings from its diagnostic criteria [75]. Radiologists focus on main CT findings (GGO, consolidation, reticulation/thickened interlobular septa, nodules), and lesion distribution (left, right or bilateral lungs) [76–80].

AI methods seek to exploit mainly for characterizing COVID-19 pneumonia CT patterns, for monitoring patients in clinical settings and for estimating efficacy of treatment. Based on the data derived from clinical parameters, AI may provide critical data for resource allocation and decision-making by prioritizing the need of ventilators and respiratory supports in the Intensive Care Unit [81–83]. AI was used for the COVID-19 disease detection and quantification from CXR and CT images [63,81–88]. AI can also be used for predicting the chances of recovery or mortality in COVID-19 and to provide daily updates, storage and trend analysis and charting the course of treatment.

CT scan-based and CXR-based identification and detection of COVID-19 have been implemented using pretrained networks such as InceptionV3, VGGNet, InceptionResNetV2, ResNet, etc., and achieved benchmark accuracies as high as 99% [84].

At the same time, radiomics approaches can be usefully implemented, focusing on segmentation techniques of the lung parenchyma based on region growing techniques and on other radiomics COVID-19 specific features and their use with machine learning such as Support Vector Machines (SVMs) or Random Forests [86–88].

4.1. Application on Chest X-Ray Images

In the study of Sethy et al. [83], the deep learning methodology is reported for detection of a coronavirus infected patient by CXR. The suggested classification model, Resnet50 plus Support Vector Machine (SVM), achieved accuracy and false positive rate of 95.38% and 95.52% respectively for detecting COVID-19.

Jiao et al. [89], using the CXR as input to an EfficientNet deep neural network combined with clinical data, assessed the ability to predict COVID-19 disease severity (critical or non-critical). They reported that when CXR was added to clinical data for severity prediction, the area under the receiver operating characteristic curve (ROC-AUC) increased from 0.821 to 0.846 on internal testing and from 0.731 to 0.792 on external testing; when deep-learning features were added to clinical data for progression prediction, the concordance index (C-index) increased from 0.769 to 0.805 on internal testing and from 0.707 to 0.752 on external testing; when image and clinical data were combined C-index increase from 0.805 to 0.781 on internal testing and from 0.752 to 0.715 on and internal testing.

Al-Waisy et al. [90], proposed COVID-CheXNet system that is made by combining the results generated from two different deep learning models (e.g., ResNet34 and HRNet) on CXR: two predicted probability scores are computed, and the highest probability score is used to assign the input image to one of two classes for detecting COVID-19. The proposed COVID-CheXNet system reached to diagnose the COVID-19 patients with a detection accuracy rate of 99.99%, a sensitivity of 99.98%, a specificity of 100% and a precision of

100%. Cases used in this study come from different databases: 200 X-ray images with confirmed COVID-19 infections come by Cohen's GitHub database [91]; 200 COVID-19 CXRs gathered from three different repositories: Radiopaedia dataset [92], Italian Society of Medical and Interventional Radiology (SIRM) [93] and Radiological Society of North America (RSNA) [94]; 400 normal CXR by Kaggle's CXR dataset [95].

Ozcan et al. [96], proposed single layer-based (SLB) and feature fusion based (FFB) composite systems to detect COVID-19 in X-ray images using deep features. Four types of SLB (including AlexNet-fc6 (SLB1), ResNet18-pool5 (SLB2), ResNet18-fc1000 (SLB3), and ResNet50-fc1000 (SLB4)) and six types of FFB (including fc6-pool5 (FFB1), fc6-fc1000 (FFB2), fc6-fc1000 (FFB3), pool5-fc1000 (FFB4), pool5-fc1000 (FFB5), fc1000-fc1000 (FFB6)) were used in the study. The proposed FFB3 model reached the best average recognition rate of 87.64% in COVID-19, no-finding, and pneumonia classifications while reached as the best average recognition rate of 99.52% in COVID-19 and no-finding classifications.

Ozturc at al. [97] proposed a model for automatic COVID-19 detection using raw CXR images in order to perform the binary classification COVID-19 versus no findings and multi-class classification COVID-19 versus no findings. Their model produced a classification accuracy of 98.08% for binary classes and 87.02% for multi-class cases. The DarkNet model was used in the study as a classifier implementing 17 convolutional layers and introducing different filtering on each layer.

Du et al. [98], applied machine learning (ML) to the task of detection of SARS-CoV-2 infection using basic laboratory markers. Moreover, they tested ML accuracy adding at laboratory markers the radiologist interpretations of chest radiographs. When they used the combination of laboratory markers and radiologist interpretations, the sensitivity of ML was over 90% while keeping moderate specificity.

Dey et al. [99], proposed a classifier ensemble technique, utilizing Choquet fuzzy integral. It classifies CXR images in common pneumonia, confirmed COVID-19, and healthy lungs. They utilized the pre-trained convolutional neural network models to extract features and classify the CXR images using two dense layers and one softmax layer. The proposed method provides 99.00%, 99.00%, 99.00%, and 99.02% average recall, precision, F-score, and accuracy, respectively.

Alruwaili et al. [100], proposed an enhanced Inception-ResNetV2 deep learning model that can diagnose chest X-ray scans with high accuracy of 99.83%. Besides, a Grad-CAM algorithm is used to enhance the visualization of the infected regions of the lungs in CXR images.

Bukhari et al. [101], employed ResNet50 for COVID-19 detection using CXR images. They tried to differentiate four types of classes, which are healthy normal, bacterial pneumonia, viral pneumonia, and COVID-19 cases. They achieved an average accuracy of 98.18% and a F1-score of 98.19%.

Khan et al. [102], proposed a model named CoroNet to identify COVID-19 in x-ray and CT scans utilizing a pretrained Xception convolution network. For the four classes (viral pneumonia, COVID-19, bacterial pneumonia, and normal), the first experiment attained an accuracy of 89.6%, while for three classes (normal, COVID-19, and pneumonia) obtained a total accuracy of 95.0%.

A COVIDX-Net model to help radiologists in identifying and diagnosing COVID-19 in CXR images was developed by Hemdan et al. [103]. They compared seven performances of seven pretrained deep learning networks; they are the InceptionV3, MobileNetV2, VGG19, DenseNet201, Inception-ResNetV2, ResNetV2, and Xception model. Based on their experiments, the VGG19 model achieved the highest accuracy of 90%.

Sethy and Behera [83], introduced a hybrid approach that utilizes deep learning for feature extraction and support vector machine (SVM) for detecting patients contaminated with COVID-19 by using CXR images. Using the pretrained 13 distinct Convolutional Neural Network models, the SVM provided the best results on the deep features of the ResNet50 model achieving accuracy of 95.38% for detecting COVID-19 (ignoring SARS, MERS and ARDS).

Ouchicha et al. [104], proposed a model named CVDNet to diagnose the COVID-19 cases. This model employed local and global features of CXR by using two parallel layers with various kernel sizes reaching an average accuracy of 97.20% for detecting COVID-19 cases.

4.2. Application on Chest CT images

Gozes et al. [81], used deep learning models to explore AI CT image analysis tools in the detection, quantification, and tracking of coronavirus. A total of 106 COVID-19 chest CT scans (50 labeled by a radiologist, and other 56 by RT-PCR test) and 99 normal ones were used to find potential COVID-19 thoracic CT features and to evaluate disease progression over time, generating a quantitative score. Utilizing the deep-learning image analysis system developed, they achieved classification results for COVID-19 versus no COVID-19 by chest CT of 0.948 of AUC (95%CI: 0.912–0.985).

Proof of principle of diagnostic capability of deep learning methods using CT images to detect COVID-19 disease have been demonstrated by Wang et al. [63] on 1119 CT images of pathogen-confirmed COVID-19 cases versus typical viral pneumonia. Their internal validation achieved a total accuracy of 89.5% with a specificity of 0.88 and sensitivity of 0.87. The external testing dataset showed a total accuracy of 79.3% with a specificity of 0.83 and sensitivity of 0.67.

Li et al. [85], investigated a deep learning model, COVID-19 detection neural network (COVNet), by extraction of visual features from volumetric chest CT images to detect COVID-19. The datasets were collected from six hospitals between August 2016 and February 2020. The sensitivity and specificity for detecting COVID-19 was 114 of 127 (90% [95% CI: 83%, 94%]) and 294 of 307 (96% [95% CI: 93%, 98%]), respectively, with an AUC of 0.96 (p-value < 0.001).

Ko et al. [105], investigated a simple 2D deep learning framework, and named the fast-track COVID-19 classification network (FCONet), in order to diagnose COVID-19 pneumonia based on a single chest CT image. FCONet was developed by transfer learning using one of four state-of-the-art pretrained deep learning models (VGG16, ResNet-50, Inception-v3, or Xception) as a backbone. Among the four pretrained models of FCONet, ResNet-50 showed excellent diagnostic performance (sensitivity 99.58%, specificity 100.00%, and accuracy 99.87%) and outperformed the other three pretrained models in the testing data set. In the additional external testing data set using low-quality CT images, the detection accuracy of the ResNet-50 model was the highest (96.97%).

Nguyen et al. [106], examined deep learning models in order to identify COVID-19-positive patients on 3D CT datasets from different countries. The models achieved accuracy/AUC values of 0.87/0.826 (dataset at UT Southwestern), 0.97/0.988 (dataset at China), and 0.86/0.873 (dataset at Iran).

Zhang et al. [64], used artificial intelligence technology proposing a COVSeg-NET model that can segment GGO lesions in COVID-19 chest CT images. The COVSeg-NET model is based on the fully convolutional neural network model structure, which mainly includes convolutional layer, nonlinear unit activation function, maximum pooling layer, batch normalization layer, merge layer, flattening layer, sigmoid layer, and so forth. The results showed a sensitivity and specificity of the COVSeg-NET model of 0.447 and 0.996 respectively.

Song et al. [107], developed a deep learning network, which is called DeepPneumonia, to diagnose COVID-19 cases analyzing CT scans. Their proposed system was built on the ResNet50 using transfer learning technology. It could localize the essential lesion characteristics, especially GGO. Their system achieved an average AUC of 0.99 and sensitivity score of 93%. Besides, it reached an average AUC of 0.95 and sensitivity of 96% for bacterial pneumonia-infected cases.

Wang et al. [65], developed an artificial intelligence system in a time-to-event analysis framework to integrate chest CT and clinical data for risk prediction of future deterioration to critical illness in patients with COVID-19. The artificial intelligence system achieved a C-index of 0.80 for predicting individual COVID-19 patients as having critical illness, and successfully stratified the patients into high-risk and low-risk groups with distinct progression risks ($p < 0.0001$).

Xu et al. [108], proposed a fully automated COVID-19 diagnosis based on a 3D deep learning network-using chest CT scans. Their proposed system consists of four basic stages, which are pre-processing, candidate region segmentation, classification for each candidate region, and overall infection probability. The experimental results of this study showed that the summarized accuracy rate was 86.7%.

4.3. Critical Considerations and Conclusions

In addition, if the summarized accuracy of the selected papers is high, there was an important variability. The accuracy and applicability of AI approaches in COVID-19 from CXR or chest CTs have questioned, based on concerns of the radiologists' association, and given the impact of selection bias reported in first published results. Moreover, the limitation of this methodology is that if the patient is in a critical situation and unable to attend for CXR or CT scanning.

The analyzed papers showed the great potential of AI in COVID-19 pandemic by helping complex decision-making. However, most of the analyzed papers were experimental, and the produced models have not been deployed in real-world clinical setting. Those reported are impeded by several limitations. The available data sets may suffer from selection bias. The prognosis studies mostly encompass inpatients, who are usually sicker, whereas the diagnosis studies typically involve patients who already exhibit symptoms fitting with COVID-19. More data are needed on asymptomatic individuals and those with mild symptoms, who might not visit the hospital. Moreover, most of the studies reviewed employed imbalanced data sets, that is, those where many records in the training data set represent the negative class, and the positive class is under-represented. Thus, the reported performance of various AI algorithms applied in this context may have been affected by polarization of the context: a pandemic scenario. A high accuracy value in such cases could be attributed to the ability of the model to accurately identify negative samples and erroneously exclude all the positive COVID-19 cases. More effort is required to handle imbalanced data sets prior to the application of AI to COVID-19. The predictive performance of the models might also differ when using representative data that incorporates the targeted population, which merits further investigation.

Moreover, although AI is a promising tool in precision medicine, many factors such as low signal-to-noise ratio and complex data integration have challenged its efficacy. Both CXR and CT showed a high accuracy to detect pneumonia by COVID-19 and to predict the disease evolution, but which CXR is the first examination in this context and thus more data is available, CT is more capable to investigate extension and critical issues of the disease. However, CT images represent a difficult classification task due to the relatively large number of variable objects, specifically the imaged areas outside the lungs that are irrelevant to the diagnosis of pneumonia. Notably, the assessed features of the CT images were from patients with severe lung lesions at later stages of disease development. A larger number of databases to associate this with the disease progress and all pathologic stages of COVID-19 are necessary to optimize the diagnostic system.

In conclusion, AI approaches could be used in the identification of disease clusters, monitoring of cases, prediction of the future outbreaks, mortality risk, diagnosis of COVID-19, disease management by resource allocation, facilitating training, record maintenance and pattern recognition for studying the disease trend.

Author Contributions: Conceptualization, R.F. and V.G.; methodology and investigation, R.F., R.G., V.G., S.V.S., F.G., D.C., B.P., F.I., A.P. Writing—original draft preparation, writing—review and editing, R.F. and V.G. All authors have read and agreed to the published version of the manuscript.

Funding: This research received no external funding.

Institutional Review Board Statement: Not applicable.

Informed Consent Statement: Not applicable.

Data Availability Statement: All data are reported in the manuscript.

Acknowledgments: The authors are grateful to Alessandra Trocino, librarian at the National Cancer Institute of Naples, Italy. Moreover, for their collaboration, authors are grateful to Andrea Esposito, Paola Gargiulo, Giuditta Giannotti, Paolo Pariante, Martina Totaro (research support) of Radiology Division, "Istituto Nazionale Tumori IRCCS Fondazione Pascale—IRCCS di Napoli", Naples, I-80131, Italy.

Conflicts of Interest: The authors declare no conflict of interest.

References

1. WHO. Summary of Probable SARS Cases with onset of Illness from 1 November 2002 to 31 July 2003 (based on data as of 31 December 2003). Available online: https://www.who.int/home/search?indexCatalogue=genericsearchindex1 (accessed on 24 June 2021).
2. WHO. Middle East Respiratory Syndrome Coronavirus (MERS-CoV). Available online: https://www.who.int/health-topics/middle-east-respiratory-syndrome-coronavirus-mers#tab=tab_1 (accessed on 24 June 2021).
3. WHO. Naming the Coronavirus Disease (COVID-2019) and the Virus That Causes It. Available online: https://www.who.int/emergencies/diseases/novel-coronavirus-2019/technical-guidance/naming-the-coronavirus-disease-(covid-2019)-and-the-virus-that-causes-it (accessed on 24 June 2021).
4. Giovanetti, M.; Angeletti, S.; Benvenuto, D.; Ciccozzi, M. A doubt of multiple introduction of SARS-CoV-2 in Italy: A preliminary overview. *J. Med. Virol.* **2020**, *92*, 1634–1636. [CrossRef]
5. Center for Systems Science and Engineering (CSSE) at Johns Hopkins University (JHU). COVID-19 Dashboard. Available online: https://gisanddata.maps.arcgis.com/apps/opsdashboard/index.html#/bda7594740fd40299423467b48e9ecf6 (accessed on 5 August 2020).
6. Kinross, P.; Suetens, C.; Dias, J.G.; Alexakis, L.; Wijermans, A.; Colzani, E.; Monnet, D.L. European Centre for Disease Prevention and Control (ECDC) Public Health Emergency Team Rapidly increasing cumulative incidence of coronavirus disease (COVID-19) in the European Union/European Economic Area and the United Kingdom, 1 January to 15 March 2020. *Eurosurveillance* **2020**, *25*, 2000285. [CrossRef]
7. Kostoulas, P.; Eusebi, P.; Hartnack, S. Diagnostic Accuracy Estimates for COVID-19 Real-Time Polymerase Chain Reaction and Lateral Flow Immunoassay Tests with Bayesian Latent-Class Models. *Am. J. Epidemiol.* **2021**, *190*, 1689–1695. [CrossRef]
8. Deeks, J.J.; Dinnes, J.; Takwoingi, Y.; Davenport, C.; Spijker, R.; Taylor-Phillips, S.; Adriano, A.; Beese, S.; Dretzke, J.; di Ruffano, L.F.; et al. Antibody tests for identification of current and past infection with SARS-CoV-2. *Cochrane Database Syst. Rev.* **2020**, *2020*, CD013652. [CrossRef]
9. Beigmohammadi, M.T.; Bitarafan, S.; Abdollahi, A.; Amoozadeh, L.; Salahshour, F.; Abadi, M.M.A.; Soltani, D.; Motallebnejad, Z.A. The association between serum levels of micronutrients and the severity of disease in patients with COVID-19. *Nutrition* **2021**, *91–92*, 111400. [CrossRef] [PubMed]
10. Stramare, R.; Carretta, G.; Capizzi, A.; Boemo, D.G.; Contessa, C.; Motta, R.; De Conti, G.; Causin, F.; Giraudo, C.; Donato, D. Radiological management of COVID-19: Structure your diagnostic path to guarantee a safe path. *Radiol. Med.* **2020**, *125*, 691–694. [CrossRef] [PubMed]
11. Ierardi, A.M.; Wood, B.J.; Arrichiello, A.; Bottino, N.; Bracchi, L.; Forzenigo, L.; Andrisani, M.C.; Vespro, V.; Bonelli, C.; Amalou, A.; et al. Preparation of a radiology department in an Italian hospital dedicated to COVID-19 patients. *Radiol. Med.* **2020**, *125*, 894–901. [CrossRef] [PubMed]
12. Cappabianca, S.; Fusco, R.; de Lisio, A.; Paura, C.; Clemente, A.; Gagliardi, G.; Lombardi, G.; Giacobbe, G.; Russo, G.M.; Belfiore, M.P.; et al. Correction to: Clinical and laboratory data, radiological structured report findings and quantitative evaluation of lung involvement on baseline chest CT in COVID-19 patients to predict prognosis. *Radiol. Med.* **2021**, *126*, 643. [CrossRef]
13. Carvalho, E.D.; Silva, R.R.; Araújo, F.H.; Rabelo, R.D.A.; Filho, A.O.D.C. An approach to the classification of COVID-19 based on CT scans using convolutional features and genetic algorithms. *Comput. Biol. Med.* **2021**, *136*, 104744. [CrossRef]
14. Nakazono, T.; Yamaguchi, K.; Egashira, R.; Mizuguchi, M.; Irie, H. Anterior mediastinal lesions: CT and MRI features and differential diagnosis. *JPN J. Radiol.* **2021**, *39*, 101–117. [CrossRef]
15. Koç, A.; Sezgin, S.; Kayıpmaz, S. Comparing different planimetric methods on volumetric estimations by using cone beam computed tomography. *Radiol. Med.* **2020**, *125*, 398–405. [CrossRef] [PubMed]
16. Xu, G.-X.; Liu, C.; Liu, J.; Ding, Z.; Shi, F.; Guo, M.; Zhao, W.; Li, X.; Wei, Y.; Gao, Y.; et al. Cross-Site Severity Assessment of COVID-19 from CT Images via Domain Adaptation. *IEEE Trans. Med Imaging* **2021**, *1*. [CrossRef]
17. Gaia, C.; Chiara, C.M.; Silvia, L.; Chiara, C.; Luisa, D.C.M.; Giulia, B.; Silvia, P.; Lucia, C.; Alessandra, T.; Annarita, S.; et al. Chest CT for early detection and management of coronavirus disease (COVID-19): A report of 314 patients admitted to Emergency Department with suspected pneumonia. *Radiol. Med.* **2020**, *125*, 931–942. [CrossRef] [PubMed]
18. Giannitto, C.; Sposta, F.M.; Repici, A.; Vatteroni, G.; Casiraghi, E.; Casari, E.; Ferraroli, G.M.; Fugazza, A.; Sandri, M.T.; Chiti, A.; et al. Chest CT in patients with a moderate or high pretest probability of COVID-19 and negative swab. *Radiol. Med.* **2020**, *125*, 1260–1270. [CrossRef] [PubMed]
19. Crimì, F.; Cabrelle, G.; Zanon, C.; Quaia, E. Chest computed tomography in COVID-19 infection. *Clin. Transl. Imaging* **2021**, *8*, 1–2. [CrossRef]

20. Giovagnoni, A. Facing the COVID-19 emergency: We can and we do. *Radiol. Med.* **2020**, *125*, 337–338. [CrossRef] [PubMed]
21. Montesi, G.; Di Biase, S.; Chierchini, S.; Pavanato, G.; Virdis, G.E.; Contato, E.; Mandoliti, G. Radiotherapy during COVID-19 pandemic. How to create a No fly zone: A Northern Italy experience. *Radiol. Med.* **2020**, *125*, 600–603. [CrossRef]
22. Agostini, A.; Floridi, C.; Borgheresi, A.; Badaloni, M.; Pirani, P.E.; Terilli, F.; Ottaviani, L.; Giovagnoni, A. Proposal of a low-dose, long-pitch, dual-source chest CT protocol on third-generation dual-source CT using a tin filter for spectral shaping at 100 kVp for CoronaVirus Disease 2019 (COVID-19) patients: A feasibility study. *Radiol. Med.* **2020**, *125*, 365–373. [CrossRef] [PubMed]
23. Borghesi, A.; Maroldi, R. COVID-19 outbreak in Italy: Experimental chest X-ray scoring system for quantifying and monitoring disease progression. *Radiol. Med.* **2020**, *125*, 509–513. [CrossRef]
24. Fichera, G.; Stramare, R.; De Conti, G.; Motta, R.; Giraudo, C. It's not over until it's over: The chameleonic behavior of COVID-19 over a six-day period. *Radiol. Med.* **2020**, *125*, 514–516. [CrossRef]
25. Granata, V.; Fusco, R.; Setola, S.; Galdiero, R.; Picone, C.; Izzo, F.; D'Aniello, R.; Miele, V.; Grassi, R.; Grassi, R.; et al. Lymphadenopathy after *BNT162b2* Covid-19 Vaccine: Preliminary Ultrasound Findings. *Biology* **2021**, *10*, 214. [CrossRef] [PubMed]
26. Belfiore, M.P.; Urraro, F.; Grassi, R.; Giacobbe, G.; Patelli, G.; Cappabianca, S.; Reginelli, A. Artificial intelligence to codify lung CT in Covid-19 patients. *Radiol. Med.* **2020**, *125*, 500–504. [CrossRef] [PubMed]
27. Neri, E.; Miele, V.; Coppola, F.; Grassi, R. Use of CT and artificial intelligence in suspected or COVID-19 positive patients: Statement of the Italian Society of Medical and Interventional Radiology. *Radiol. Med.* **2020**, *125*, 505–508. [CrossRef] [PubMed]
28. Carotti, M.; Salaffi, F.; Sarzi-Puttini, P.; Agostini, A.; Borgheresi, A.; Minorati, D.; Galli, M.; Marotto, D.; Giovagnoni, A. Chest CT features of coronavirus disease 2019 (COVID-19) pneumonia: Key points for radiologists. *Radiol. Med.* **2020**, *125*, 636–646. [CrossRef] [PubMed]
29. Shaw, B.; Daskareh, M.; Gholamrezanezhad, A. The lingering manifestations of COVID-19 during and after convalescence: Update on long-term pulmonary consequences of coronavirus disease 2019 (COVID-19). *Radiol. Med.* **2020**, *126*, 40–46. [CrossRef] [PubMed]
30. Di Serafino, M.; Notaro, M.; Rea, G.; Iacobellis, F.; Delli Paoli, V.; Acampora, C.; Ianniello, S.; Brunese, L.; Romano, L.; Vallone, G. The lung ultrasound: Facts or artifacts? In the era of COVID-19 outbreak. *Radiol Med.* **2020**, *125*, 738–753. [CrossRef] [PubMed]
31. Cozzi, D.; Albanesi, M.; Cavigli, E.; Moroni, C.; Bindi, A.; Luvarà, S.; Lucarini, S.; Busoni, S.; Mazzoni, L.N.; Miele, V. Chest X-ray in new Coronavirus Disease 2019 (COVID-19) infection: Findings and correlation with clinical outcome. *Radiol. Med.* **2020**, *125*, 730–737. [CrossRef]
32. Pediconi, F.; Galati, F.; Bernardi, D.; Belli, P.; Brancato, B.; Calabrese, M.; Camera, L.; Carbonaro, L.A.; Caumo, F.; Clauser, P.; et al. Breast imaging and cancer diagnosis during the COVID-19 pandemic: Recommendations from the Italian College of Breast Radiologists by SIRM. *Radiol. Med.* **2020**, *125*, 926–930. [CrossRef]
33. Borghesi, A.; Zigliani, A.; Masciullo, R.; Golemi, S.; Maculotti, P.; Farina, D.; Maroldi, R. Radiographic severity index in COVID-19 pneumonia: Relationship to age and sex in 783 Italian patients. *Radiol. Med.* **2020**, *125*, 461–464. [CrossRef]
34. Gatti, M.; Calandri, M.; Barba, M.; Biondo, A.; Geninatti, C.; Gentile, S.; Greco, M.; Morrone, V.; Piatti, C.; Santonocito, A.; et al. Baseline chest X-ray in coronavirus disease 19 (COVID-19) patients: Association with clinical and laboratory data. *Radiol. Med.* **2020**, *125*, 1271–1279. [CrossRef] [PubMed]
35. Caruso, D.; Polici, M.; Zerunian, M.; Pucciarelli, F.; Polidori, T.; Guido, G.; Rucci, C.; Bracci, B.; Muscogiuri, E.; De Dominicis, C.; et al. Quantitative Chest CT analysis in discriminating COVID-19 from non-COVID-19 patients. *Radiol. Med.* **2020**, *126*, 243–249. [CrossRef] [PubMed]
36. Grassi, R.; Belfiore, M.P.; Montanelli, A.; Patelli, G.; Urraro, F.; Giacobbe, G.; Fusco, R.; Granata, V.; Petrillo, A.; Sacco, P.; et al. COVID-19 pneumonia: Computer-aided quantification of healthy lung parenchyma, emphysema, ground glass and consolidation on chest computed tomography (CT). *Radiol. Med.* **2020**, *126*, 553–560. [CrossRef] [PubMed]
37. Grassi, R.; Cappabianca, S.; Urraro, F.; Granata, V.; Giacobbe, G.; Magliocchetti, S.; Cozzi, D.; Fusco, R.; Galdiero, R.; Picone, C.; et al. Evolution of CT Findings and Lung Residue in Patients with COVID-19 Pneumonia: Quantitative Analysis of the Disease with a Computer Automatic Tool. *J. Pers. Med.* **2021**, *11*, 641. [CrossRef] [PubMed]
38. Grassi, R.; Miele, V.; Giovagnoni, A. Artificial intelligence: A challenge for third millennium radiologist. *Radiol. Med.* **2019**, *124*, 241–242. [CrossRef]
39. Neri, E.; Coppola, F.; Miele, V.; Bibbolino, C.; Grassi, R. Artificial intelligence: Who is responsible for the diagnosis? *Radiol. Med.* **2020**, *125*, 517–521. [CrossRef]
40. Van Assen, M.; Muscogiuri, G.; Caruso, D.; Lee, S.J.; Laghi, A.; De Cecco, C.N. Artificial intelligence in cardiac radiology. *Radiol. Med.* **2020**, *125*, 1186–1199. [CrossRef]
41. Chen, T.; Ning, Z.; Xu, L.; Feng, X.; Han, S.; Roth, H.R.; Xiong, W.; Zhao, X.; Hu, Y.; Liu, H.; et al. Radiomics nomogram for predicting the malignant potential of gastrointestinal stromal tumours preoperatively. *Eur. Radiol.* **2019**, *29*, 1074–1082. [CrossRef] [PubMed]
42. Hu, H.-T.; Shan, Q.-Y.; Chen, S.-L.; Li, B.; Feng, S.-T.; Xu, E.-J.; Li, X.; Long, J.-Y.; Xie, X.-Y.; Lu, M.-D.; et al. CT-based radiomics for preoperative prediction of early recurrent hepatocellular carcinoma: Technical reproducibility of acquisition and scanners. *Radiol. Med.* **2020**, *125*, 697–705. [CrossRef] [PubMed]
43. Choi, H.; Chang, W.; Kim, J.H.; Ahn, C.; Lee, H.; Kim, H.Y.; Cho, J.; Lee, Y.J.; Kim, Y.H. Dose reduction potential of vendor-agnostic deep learning model in comparison with deep learning–based image reconstruction algorithm on CT: A phantom study. *Eur. Radiol.* **2021**, *8*, 1–9. [CrossRef]

44. Ma, J.; He, N.; Yoon, J.H.; Ha, R.; Li, J.; Ma, W.; Meng, T.; Lu, L.; Schwartz, L.H.; Wu, Y.; et al. Distinguishing benign and malignant lesions on contrast-enhanced breast cone-beam CT with deep learning neural architecture search. *Eur. J. Radiol.* **2021**, *142*, 109878. [CrossRef] [PubMed]
45. Liu, Z.; Ni, S.; Yang, C.; Sun, W.; Huang, D.; Su, H.; Shu, J.; Qin, N. Axillary lymph node metastasis prediction by contrast-enhanced computed tomography images for breast cancer patients based on deep learning. *Comput. Biol. Med.* **2021**, *136*, 104715. [CrossRef] [PubMed]
46. Cozzi, D.; Bicci, E.; Bindi, A.; Cavigli, E.; Danti, G.; Galluzzo, M.; Granata, V.; Pradella, S.; Trinci, M.; Miele, V. Role of Chest Imaging in Viral Lung Diseases. *Int. J. Environ. Res. Public Health* **2021**, *18*, 6434. [CrossRef] [PubMed]
47. Kirienko, M.; Ninatti, G.; Cozzi, L.; Voulaz, E.; Gennaro, N.; Barajon, I.; Ricci, F.; Carlo-Stella, C.; Zucali, P.; Sollini, M.; et al. Computed tomography (CT)-derived radiomic features differentiate prevascular mediastinum masses as thymic neoplasms versus lymphomas. *Radiol. Med.* **2020**, *125*, 951–960. [CrossRef] [PubMed]
48. Nazari, M.; Shiri, I.; Hajianfar, G.; Oveisi, N.; Abdollahi, H.; Deevband, M.R.; Oveisi, M.; Zaidi, H. Noninvasive Fuhrman grading of clear cell renal cell carcinoma using computed tomography radiomic features and machine learning. *Radiol. Med.* **2020**, *125*, 754–762. [CrossRef] [PubMed]
49. Palumbo, P.; Cannizzaro, E.; Bruno, F.; Schicchi, N.; Fogante, M.; Agostini, A.; De Donato, M.C.; De Cataldo, C.; Giovagnoni, A.; Barile, A.; et al. Coronary artery disease (CAD) extension-derived risk stratification for asymptomatic diabetic patients: Usefulness of low-dose coronary computed tomography angiography (CCTA) in detecting high-risk profile patients. *Radiol. Med.* **2020**, *125*, 1249–1259. [CrossRef]
50. Zhang, L.; Kang, L.; Li, G.; Zhang, X.; Ren, J.; Shi, Z.; Li, J.; Yu, S. Computed tomography-based radiomics model for discriminating the risk stratification of gastrointestinal stromal tumors. *Radiol. Med.* **2020**, *125*, 465–473. [CrossRef] [PubMed]
51. Abdollahi, H.; Mofid, B.; Shiri, I.; Razzaghdoust, A.; Saadipoor, A.; Mahdavi, A.; Galandooz, H.M.; Mahdavi, S.R. Machine learning-based radiomic models to predict intensity-modulated radiation therapy response, Gleason score and stage in prostate cancer. *Radiol. Med.* **2019**, *124*, 555–567. [CrossRef] [PubMed]
52. Grassi, R.; Fusco, R.; Belfiore, M.P.; Montanelli, A.; Patelli, G.; Urraro, F.; Petrillo, A.; Granata, V.; Sacco, P.; Mazzei, M.A.; et al. Coronavirus disease 2019 (COVID-19) in Italy: Features on chest computed tomography using a structured report system. *Sci. Rep.* **2020**, *10*, 17236. [CrossRef]
53. Reginelli, A.; Grassi, R.; Feragalli, B.; Belfiore, M.; Montanelli, A.; Patelli, G.; La Porta, M.; Urraro, F.; Fusco, R.; Granata, V.; et al. Coronavirus Disease 2019 (COVID-19) in Italy: Double Reading of Chest CT Examination. *Biology* **2021**, *10*, 89. [CrossRef]
54. Agbehadji, I.E.; Awuzie, B.O.; Ngowi, A.B.; Millham, R.C. Review of Big Data Analytics, Artificial Intelligence and Nature-Inspired Computing Models towards Accurate Detection of COVID-19 Pandemic Cases and Contact Tracing. *Int. J. Environ. Res. Public Health* **2020**, *17*, 5330. [CrossRef]
55. Bullock, J.; Luccioni, A.; Pham, K.H.; Lam, C.S.N.; Luengo-Oroz, M. Mapping the landscape of Artificial Intelligence applications against COVID-19. *J. Artif. Intell. Res.* **2020**, *69*, 807–845. [CrossRef]
56. Naudé, W. Artificial intelligence vs. covid-19: Limitations, constraints and pitfalls. *AI Soc.* **2020**, *35*, 761–765. [CrossRef] [PubMed]
57. Wu, J.; Wang, J.; Nicholas, S.; Maitland, E.; Fan, Q. Application of Big Data Technology for COVID-19 Prevention and Control in China: Lessons and Recommendations. *J. Med. Internet Res.* **2020**, *22*, e21980. [CrossRef] [PubMed]
58. Alballa, N.; Al-Turaiki, I. Machine Learning Approaches in COVID-19 Diagnosis, Mortality, and Severity Risk Prediction: A Review. *Inform. Med. Unlocked* **2021**, *24*, 100564. [CrossRef]
59. Raiano, N.; Raiano, C.; Mazio, F.; Rossi, I.; Bordino, U.; De Simone, G.; Fusco, R.; Granata, V.; Cerciello, V.; Setola, S.V.; et al. Home mobile radiography service in the COVID-19 era. *Eur. Rev. Med. Pharmacol. Sci.* **2021**, *25*, 3338–3341. [CrossRef]
60. Granata, V.; Fusco, R.; Izzo, F.; Setola, S.V.; Coppola, M.; Grassi, R.; Reginelli, A.; Cappabianca, S.; Petrillo, A. Covid-19 infection in cancer patients: The management in a diagnostic unit. *Radiol. Oncol.* **2021**, *55*, 121–129. [CrossRef]
61. Bandirali, M.; Sconfienza, L.M.; Serra, R.; Brembilla, R.; Albano, D.; Pregliasco, F.E.; Messina, C. Chest Radiograph Findings in Asymptomatic and Minimally Symptomatic Quarantined Patients in Codogno, Italy during COVID-19 Pandemic. *Radiology* **2020**, *295*, E7. [CrossRef] [PubMed]
62. Zhang, G.; Yang, Z.; Gong, L.; Jiang, S.; Wang, L.; Zhang, H. Classification of lung nodules based on CT images using squeeze-and-excitation network and aggregated residual transformations. *Radiol. Med.* **2020**, *125*, 374–383. [CrossRef]
63. Wang, S.; Kang, B.; Ma, J.; Zeng, X.; Xiao, M.; Guo, J.; Cai, M.; Yang, J.; Li, Y.; Meng, X.; et al. A deep learning algorithm using CT images to screen for Corona virus disease (COVID-19). *Eur. Radiol.* **2021**, *31*, 6096–6104. [CrossRef]
64. Zhang, X.; Wang, G.; Zhao, S. COVSeg-NET: A deep convolution neural network for COVID -19 lung CT image segmentation. *Int. J. Imaging Syst. Technol.* **2021**, *31*, 1071–1086. [CrossRef]
65. Wang, R.; Jiao, Z.; Yang, L.; Choi, J.W.; Xiong, Z.; Halsey, K.; Tran, T.M.L.; Pan, I.; Collins, S.A.; Feng, X.; et al. Artificial intelligence for prediction of COVID-19 progression using CT imaging and clinical data. *Eur. Radiol.* **2021**, *7*, 1–8. [CrossRef]
66. Peng, Q.-Y.; Chinese Critical Care Ultrasound Study Group (CCUSG); Wang, X.-T.; Zhang, L.-N. Findings of lung ultrasonography of novel corona virus pneumonia during the 2019–2020 epidemic. *Intensiv. Care Med.* **2020**, *46*, 849–850. [CrossRef] [PubMed]
67. Li, Y.; Xia, L. Coronavirus Disease 2019 (COVID-19): Role of Chest CT in Diagnosis and Management. *Am. J. Roentgenol.* **2020**, *214*, 1280–1286. [CrossRef] [PubMed]
68. Huang, C.; Wang, Y.; Li, X.; Ren, L.; Zhao, J.; Hu, Y.; Zhang, L.; Fan, G.; Xu, J.; Gu, X.; et al. Clinical features of patients infected with 2019 novel coronavirus in Wuhan, China. *Lancet* **2020**, *395*, 497–506. [CrossRef]

69. Lei, J.; Li, J.; Li, X.; Qi, X. CT Imaging of the 2019 Novel Coronavirus (2019-nCoV) Pneumonia. *Radiology* **2020**, *295*, 18. [CrossRef]
70. Novel Coronavirus Pneumonia Emergency Response Epidemiology Team. The epidemiological characteristics of an outbreak of 2019 novel coronavirus diseases (COVID-19) in China. *Zhonghua Liu Xing Bing Xue Za Zhi* **2020**, *41*, 145–151.
71. American College of Radiology. ACR Recommendations for the Use of Chest Radiography and Computed Tomography (CT) for Suspected COVID-19 Infection. Available online: https://www.acr.org/Advocacy-and-Economics/ACR-Position-Statements/Recommendations-for-Chest-Radiography-and-CT-for-Suspected-COVID19-Infection (accessed on 24 June 2021).
72. The Royal Australian and New Zealand College of Radiologist. COVID-19 Updates. Available online: https://www.ranzcr.com/our-work/coronavirus (accessed on 24 June 2021).
73. The Royal College of Radiologists. RCR position on the role of CT in patients suspected with COVID-19 infection. Available online: https://www.rcr.ac.uk/search-v2?search=the%20role%20of%20CT%20in%20patients%20suspected%20with%20COVID-19%20infection%20 (accessed on 24 June 2021).
74. Canadian Association of Radiologists. Canadian Society of Thoracic Radiology and Canadian Association of Radiologists' Statement on COVID-19. Available online: https://car.ca/news/canadian-society-of-thoracic-radiology-and-canadian-association-of-radiologists-statement-on-covid-19/ (accessed on 24 June 2021).
75. Mossa-Basha, M.; Meltzer, C.C.; Kim, D.C.; Tuite, M.J.; Kolli, K.P.; Tan, B.S. Radiology Department Preparedness for COVID-19: Radiology Scientific Expert Review Panel. *Radiology* **2020**, *296*, E106–E112. [CrossRef]
76. Zu, Z.Y.; Di Jiang, M.; Xu, P.P.; Chen, W.; Ni, Q.Q.; Lu, G.M.; Zhang, L.J. Coronavirus Disease 2019 (COVID-19): A Perspective from China. *Radiology* **2020**, *296*, E15–E25. [CrossRef]
77. Chung, M.; Bernheim, A.; Mei, X.; Zhang, N.; Huang, M.; Zeng, X.; Cui, J.; Xu, W.; Yang, Y.; Fayad, Z.A.; et al. CT Imaging Features of 2019 Novel Coronavirus (2019-nCoV). *Radiology* **2020**, *295*, 202–207. [CrossRef]
78. Wang, D.; Hu, B.; Hu, C.; Zhu, F.; Liu, X.; Zhang, J.; Wang, B.; Xiang, H.; Cheng, Z.; Xiong, Y.; et al. Clinical Characteristics of 138 Hospitalized Patients With 2019 Novel Coronavirus–Infected Pneumonia in Wuhan, China. *JAMA* **2020**, *323*, 1061. [CrossRef]
79. Fang, Y.; Zhang, H.; Xu, Y.; Xie, J.; Pang, P.; Ji, W. CT Manifestations of Two Cases of 2019 Novel Coronavirus (2019-nCoV) Pneumonia. *Radiology* **2020**, *295*, 208–209. [CrossRef] [PubMed]
80. Qian, L.; Yu, J.; Shi, H. Severe Acute Respiratory Disease in a Huanan Seafood Market Worker: Images of an Early Casualty. *Radiol. Cardiothorac. Imaging* **2020**, *2*, e200033. [CrossRef] [PubMed]
81. Gozes, O.; Frid-Adar, M.; Greenspan, H.; Browning, P.D.; Zhang, H.; Ji, W.; Bernheim, A.; Siegel, E. Rapid AI Development Cycle for the Coronavirus (COVID-19) Pandemic: Initial Results for Automated Detection & Patient Monitoring using Deep Learning CT Image Analysis. *arXiv* **2020**, arXiv:2003.05037.
82. Rahmatizadeh, S.; Valizadeh-Haghi, S.; Dabbagh, A. The role of artificial intelligence in management of critical COVID-19 patients. *J. Cell. Mol. Anes.* **2020**, *5*, 16–22.
83. Sethy, P.K.; Behera, S.K.; Ratha, P.K.; Biswas, P. Detection of coronavirus Disease (COVID-19) based on Deep Features and Support Vector Machine. *Int. J. Math. Eng. Manag. Sci.* **2020**, *5*, 643–651. [CrossRef]
84. Kassani, S.H.; Kassasni, P.H.; Wesolowski, M.J.; Schneider, K.A.; Deters, R. Automatic detection of coronavirus disease (COVID-19) in X-ray and CT images. A machine learning-based approach. *arXiv* **2020**, arXiv:2004.10641.
85. Li, L.; Qin, L.; Xu, Z.; Yin, Y.; Wang, X.; Kong, B.; Bai, J.; Lu, Y.; Fang, Z.; Song, Q.; et al. Using Artificial Intelligence to Detect COVID-19 and Community-acquired Pneumonia Based on Pulmonary CT: Evaluation of the Diagnostic Accuracy. *Radiology* **2020**, *296*, E65–E71. [CrossRef]
86. Ginneken, B.; Armato, S.J., III; Hoop, B.; van de Vorst, S.A.; Duindam, T.; Murphy, N.; Schilham, A.; Retico, A.; Fantacci, M.E.; Fujita, H.; et al. Comparing and combining algorithms for computer-aided detection of pulmonary nodules in computed tomography scans: The ANODE09 study. *Med. Image Anal.* **2010**, *14*, 707–722. [CrossRef]
87. Bellotti, R.; De Carlo, F.; Gargano, G.; Tangaro, S.; Cascio, D.; Catanzariti, E.; Cerello, P.; Cheran, S.C.; Delogu, P.; De Mitri, I.; et al. A CAD system for nodule detection in low-dose lung CTs based on region growing and a new active contour model. *Med. Phys.* **2007**, *34*, 4901–4910. [CrossRef] [PubMed]
88. Shi, L.; Campbell, G.; Jones, W.D.; Campagne, F.; Wen, Z.; Walker, S.J.; Su, Z.; Chu, T.M.; Goodsaid, F.M.; Pusztai, L.; et al. The MicroArray Quality Control (MAQC)-II study of common practices for the development and validation of microarray-based predictive models. *Nat. Biotechnol.* **2010**, *28*, 827–838. [PubMed]
89. Jiao, Z.; Choi, J.W.; Halsey, K.; Tran, T.M.L.; Hsieh, B.; Wang, D.; Eweje, F.; Wang, R.; Chang, K.; Wu, J.; et al. Prognostication of patients with COVID-19 using artificial intelligence based on chest X-rays and clinical data: A retrospective study. *Lancet Digit. Health* **2021**, *3*, e286–e294. [CrossRef]
90. Al-Waisy, A.S.; Al-Fahdawi, S.; Mohammed, M.A.; Abdulkareem, K.H.; Mostafa, S.A.; Maashi, M.S.; Arif, M.; Garcia-Zapirain, B. COVID-CheXNet: Hybrid deep learning framework for identifying COVID-19 virus in chest X-rays images. *Soft Comput.* **2020**, *11*, 1–16. [CrossRef]
91. Cohen, J.P.; Morrison, P.; Dao, L. COVID-19 Image Data Collection. 2020. Available online: https://github.com/ieee8023/covid-chestxray-dataset (accessed on 24 June 2021).
92. Cornacchia, S.; Errico, R.; La Tegola, L.; Maldera, A.; Simeone, G.; Fusco, V.; Niccoli-Asabella, A.; Rubini, G.; Guglielmi, G. The new lens dose limit: Implication for occupational radiation protection. *Radiol. Med.* **2019**, *124*, 728–735. [CrossRef] [PubMed]
93. Italian Society of Medical and Interventional Radiology (SIRM). 2020. Available online: https://www.sirm.org/en/italian-society-of-medical-and-interventional-radiology/ (accessed on 11 May 2020).

94. Radiological Society of North America (RSNA). 2020. Available online: https://www.kaggle.com/c/rsna-pneumonia-detection-challenge/data (accessed on 11 May 2020).
95. Kaggle's Chest X-ray Images (Pneumonia) Dataset. 2020. Available online: https://www.kaggle.com/paultimothymooney/chest-xray-pneumonia (accessed on 11 May 2020).
96. Ozcan, T. A new composite approach for COVID-19 detection in X-ray images using deep features. *Appl. Soft Comput.* **2021**, *111*, 107669. [CrossRef]
97. Ozturk, T.; Talo, M.; Yildirim, E.A.; Baloglu, U.B.; Yildirim, O.; Acharya, U.R. Automated detection of COVID-19 cases using deep neural networks with X-ray images. *Comput. Biol. Med.* **2020**, *121*, 103792. [CrossRef] [PubMed]
98. Du, R.; Tsougenis, E.D.; Ho, J.W.K.; Chan, J.K.Y.; Chiu, K.W.H.; Fang, B.X.H.; Ng, M.Y.; Leung, S.-T.; Lo, C.S.Y.; Wong, H.-Y.F.; et al. Machine learning application for the prediction of SARS-CoV-2 infection using blood tests and chest radiograph. *Sci. Rep.* **2021**, *11*, 1–13. [CrossRef] [PubMed]
99. Dey, S.; Bhattacharya, R.; Malakar, S.; Mirjalili, S.; Sarkar, R. Choquet fuzzy integral-based classifier ensemble technique for COVID-19 detection. *Comput. Biol. Med.* **2021**, *135*, 104585. [CrossRef] [PubMed]
100. Alruwaili, M.; Shehab, A.; El-Ghany, S.A. COVID-19 Diagnosis Using an Enhanced Inception-ResNetV2 Deep Learning Model in CXR Images. *J. Health Eng.* **2021**, *2021*, 1–16. [CrossRef] [PubMed]
101. Bukhari, S.U.; Bukhari, S.S.; Syed, A.; Shah, S.S. *The Diagnostic Evaluation of Convolutional Neural Network (CNN) for the Assessment of Chest X-ray of Patients Infected with COVID-19*; medRxiv: Long Island, NY, USA, 2020.
102. Khan, A.I.; Shah, J.L.; Bhat, M.M. CoroNet: A deep neural network for detection and diagnosis of COVID-19 from chest x-ray images. *Comput. Methods Programs Biomed.* **2020**, *196*, 105581. [CrossRef] [PubMed]
103. Hemdan, E.E.-D.; Shouman, M.A.; Karar, M.E. COVIDx-Net: A Framework of Deep Learning Classifiers to Diagnose COVID-19 in X-ray Images. 2020. Available online: http://arxiv.org/abs/2003.11055 (accessed on 24 June 2021).
104. Ouchicha, C.; Ammor, O.; Meknassi, M. CVDNet: A novel deep learning architecture for detection of coronavirus (Covid-19) from chest x-ray images. *Chaos Solitons Fractals* **2020**, *140*, 110245. [CrossRef]
105. Ko, H.; Chung, H.; Kang, W.S.; Kim, K.W.; Shin, Y.; Kang, S.J.; Lee, J.H.; Kim, Y.J.; Kim, N.Y.; Jung, H.; et al. COVID-19 Pneumonia Diagnosis Using a Simple 2D Deep Learning Framework With a Single Chest CT Image: Model Development and Validation. *J. Med. Internet Res.* **2020**, *22*, e19569. [CrossRef] [PubMed]
106. Nguyen, D.; Kay, F.; Tan, J.; Yan, Y.; Ng, Y.S.; Iyengar, P.; Peshock, R.; Jiang, S. Deep Learning–Based COVID-19 Pneumonia Classification Using Chest CT Images: Model Generalizability. *Front. Artif. Intell.* **2021**, *4*, 694875. [CrossRef] [PubMed]
107. Song, Y.; Zheng, S.; Li, L.; Zhang, X.; Zhang, X.; Huang, Z.; Chen, J.; Wang, R.; Zhao, H.; Zha, Y.; et al. Deep learning Enables Accurate Diagnosis of Novel Coronavirus (COVID-19) with CT images. *IEEE/ACM Trans. Comput. Biol. Bioinform.* **2021**, *3*, PP. [CrossRef]
108. Xu, X.; Jiang, X.; Ma, C.; Du, P.; Li, X.; Lv, S.; Yu, L.; Ni, Q.; Chen, Y.; Su, J.; et al. A Deep Learning System to Screen Novel Coronavirus Disease 2019 Pneumonia. *Engineering* **2020**, *6*, 1122–1129. [CrossRef] [PubMed]

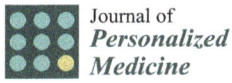

Article

Evolution of CT Findings and Lung Residue in Patients with COVID-19 Pneumonia: Quantitative Analysis of the Disease with a Computer Automatic Tool

Roberto Grassi [1,2], Salvatore Cappabianca [1], Fabrizio Urraro [1], Vincenza Granata [3,*], Giuliana Giacobbe [1], Simona Magliocchetti [1], Diletta Cozzi [4], Roberta Fusco [5], Roberta Galdiero [3], Carmine Picone [3], Maria Paola Belfiore [1], Alfonso Reginelli [1], Umberto Atripaldi [1], Ornella Picascia [1], Michele Coppola [6], Elio Bignardi [6], Roberta Grassi [1,2] and Vittorio Miele [4]

1. Division of Radiodiagnostic, Università degli Studi della Campania Luigi Vanvitelli, 80138 Naples, Italy; roberto.grassi@unicampania.it (R.G.); salvatore.cappabianca@unicampania.it (S.C.); fabrizio.urraro@unicampania.it (F.U.); giuliana.giacobbe@unicampania.it (G.G.); simona.magliocchetti@unicampania.it (S.M.); mariapaola.belfiore@unicampania.it (M.P.B.); alfonso.reginelli@unicampania.it (A.R.); umberto.atripaldi@studenti.unicampania.it (U.A.); ornella.picascia@studenti.unicampania.it (O.P.); robertagrassi89@gmail.com (R.G.)
2. Italian Society of Medical and Interventional Radiology (SIRM), SIRM Foundation, 20122 Milan, Italy
3. Radiology Division, Istituto Nazionale Tumori IRCCS Fondazione Pascale—IRCCS di Napoli, 80131 Naples, Italy; r.galdiero@istitutotumori.na.it (R.G.); c.picone@istitutotumori.na.it (C.P.)
4. Division of Radiodiagnostic, Azienda Ospedaliero—Universitaria Careggi, 50139 Florence, Italy; dilettacozzi@gmail.com (D.C.); vmiele@sirm.org (V.M.)
5. Medical Oncology Division, Igea SpA, 80013 Naples, Italy; r.fusco@igeamedical.com
6. Diagnostic Imaging Unit, "Azienda Ospedaliera dei Colli"—Ospedale Monaldi, 80131 Naples, Italy; michele.coppola@ospedalideicolli.it (M.C.); elio.bignardi@ospedalideicolli.it (E.B.)
* Correspondence: v.granata@istitutotumori.na.it; Tel.: +39-081-590-3714

Abstract: Purpose: the purpose of this study was to assess the evolution of computed tomography (CT) findings and lung residue in patients with COVID-19 pneumonia, via quantified evaluation of the disease, using a computer aided tool. Materials and methods: we retrospectively evaluated 341 CT examinations of 140 patients (68 years of median age) infected with COVID-19 (confirmed by real-time reverse transcriptase polymerase chain reaction (RT-PCR)), who were hospitalized, and who received clinical and CT examinations. All CTs were evaluated by two expert radiologists, in consensus, at the same reading session, using a computer-aided tool for quantification of the pulmonary disease. The parameters obtained using the computer tool included the healthy residual parenchyma, ground glass opacity, consolidation, and total lung volume. Results: statistically significant differences (p value ≤ 0.05) were found among quantified volumes of healthy residual parenchyma, ground glass opacity (GGO), consolidation, and total lung volume, considering different clinical conditions (stable, improved, and worsened). Statistically significant differences were found among quantified volumes for healthy residual parenchyma, GGO, and consolidation (p value ≤ 0.05) between dead patients and discharged patients. CT was not performed on cadavers; the death was an outcome, which was retrospectively included to differentiate findings of patients who survived vs. patients who died during hospitalization. Among discharged patients, complete disease resolutions on CT scans were observed in 62/129 patients with lung disease involvement $\leq 5\%$; lung disease involvement from 5% to 15% was found in 40/129 patients, while 27/129 patients had lung disease involvement between 16 and 30%. Moreover, 8–21 days (after hospital admission) was an "advanced period" with the most severe lung disease involvement. After the extent of involvement started to decrease—particularly after 21 days—the absorption was more obvious. Conclusions: a complete disease resolution on chest CT scans was observed in 48.1% of discharged patients using a computer-aided tool to quantify the GGO and consolidation volumes; after 16 days of hospital admission, the abnormalities identified by chest CT began to improve; in particular, the absorption was more obvious after 21 days.

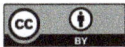

Keywords: COVID-19; computed tomography; computer aided quantification

1. Introduction

The spread of severe acute respiratory syndrome coronavirus 2 (SARS-CoV-2) has already assumed pandemic proportions, affecting over 100 countries in few weeks [1,2].

Currently, the "gold standard" for diagnosis of COVID-19 infection is a real-time reverse transcriptase polymerase chain reaction (RT-PCR) amplification of the viral DNA. However, radiological imaging is of great significance in the surveillance of COVID-19 infection [3–5]. Recent studies have demonstrated that CT findings of COVID-19 pneumonia show ground glass opacity (GGO) with surrounding consolidation, with bilateral involvement, peripheral distribution, and multi-lobar distribution [3–7].

However, the consolidation, or GGO with consolidation, increased, and reticular was observed in the later stages (scan > 1 week after symptom onset), this represents the conversion of findings from GGO to consolidation, and an increase in the reticulation pattern in affected lung parenchyma. CT features had rapid sever changes, from focal unilateral pulmonary parenchyma to diffuse bilateral GGO, or GGO with consolidation, within 1–3 weeks [6,7]. Although several studies have described the CT imaging features of COVID-19 pneumonia, so far, there is a lack of large-sample CT imaging studies and follow-up observations [8–20].

CT investigation in patients with suspected COVID-19 pneumonia involves the use of high-resolution techniques. Artificial intelligence (AI) software for quantification of pneumonia lesions has been employed to integrate CT diagnosis [15,16]. Computer software could be useful to categorize the disease into different severities, with quantitative, objective assessments of the extent of the lesions [17–20]. Computer tools have recently been proposed for the recognition of lung lesions (from COVID-19) on CT examinations [21–23]. However, many of them are not recognized as medical devices nor do they have the CE marking.

To the best of our knowledge, no study in the literature reports on the temporal changes of CT findings, using an automatic tool to quantify the abnormality in lung parenchyma, due to COVID-19 pneumonia, in a large dataset of patients.

We investigate the use of a computer-aided tool in order to quantify the abnormalities visible on chest CT images in patients with COVID-19 pneumonia.

The aim of this study was to assess the evolution of CT findings and lung residue in patients with COVID-19 pneumonia, performing quantitative analysis of the disease with the commercially available system.

2. Methods

2.1. Patient Characteristics

This retrospective study included patients enrolled by "Hospital of Colli (Monaldi-Cotugno-CTO)" in Naples. In relation to the ongoing epidemic emergency, the institutional local review boards gave up written informed consent for this retrospective study that evaluated anonymized data and involved no potential risk to patients. The population included 140 patients (50 women and 90 men; 68 years of median age—range, 25–92 years) subjected to the nucleic acid amplification test of the respiratory tract or blood specimens, using a reverse transcription real-time fluorescence polymerase chain reaction test, for suspicion of COVID-19, between 2 March 2020 and 5 May 2020. The virus investigation for etiological diagnosis was executed by the current gold standard test. All patients with a positive RT-PCR test at hospital admission and with respiratory distress were hospitalized and followed-up. The clinical evolution of the disease was subdivided in stable, improved, and worsened. The parameters considered took into account the fever (≤ 37.3, 37.4–38.0, >38.0) and the breathing with SpO2 value in ambient air, and the ratio PaO2/FiO2 (mild >200 up to 300 mm Hg; moderate >100 and ≤ 200 mm Hg, severe ≤ 100 mm Hg). The following laboratory parameters were assessed: white blood cells (Lymphopenia, leukopenia), PCR, VES, procalcitonin (PCT), D-dimer. The worsened picture was evaluated, considering organ dysfunction with the delta sequential organ failure assessment score (SOFA), in ranges from 0 to 24, and included points related to six organ systems: respiratory (hypoxemia), coagulatory (thrombocytopenia), liver (hyperbilirubinemia), cardiovascular system (hypotension), neurologic (low-level consciousness), and renal (oliguria or elevated creatinine).

2.2. CT Technique

Chest CT scans were performed at the time of hospital admission and during the hospital stay, with a 64-slice scanner (Toshiba Aquilion 64-Slice CT, Tokyo, Japan) dedicated to COVID-19 patients. CT examinations were performed with the patient in the supine position using a standard dose protocol, without contrast intravenous injection. The scanning range was from the apex to the base of the lungs. The tube voltage and the current tube were 120 kV and 100–200 mA, respectively. All images were obtained with a standard dose scanning protocol, reconstructed at 1.0 mm slice thickness, with 1 mm increment, 512 × 512 mm. Images were reconstructed with a sharp reconstruction kernel for parenchyma (FC13 on Toshiba). The lung window setting was at a window level of −600 Hounsfield units (HU) and window width of 1600 HU.

2.3. CT Post Processing

DICOM data were transferred into a PACS workstation and CT images were evaluated by two expert radiologists, in consensus, at the same reading session, using the clinically available computer tool Thoracic VCAR software (GE Healthcare, Chicago, IL, USA). The software provides automatic segmentation of the lungs and automatic segmentation and tracking of the airway tree. It provides the classification of voxels based on Hounsfield units and a color-coded display of the thresholds within a segmented region. Thoracic VCAR provided automatic segmentation of the lungs, and was performed using adaptive density based morphology. The lungs were extracted by using an optimal thresholding to identify low-density fields in the scans, region growing (automating seed generation method to segment an image into regions, with respect to a set of seeds) and void filling. The three-dimensional hole filling was used to fill the lung cavities created by the elimination of normal blood vessels during the thresholding process, while airways were automatically segmented and exempted by iterative application of increasingly restrictive constraints, to a thresholding and 3D region growing process. The software complies with the regulatory requirements of Council Directive 93/42/EEC concerning medical devices (CE 0459) and FDA regulations. Lung parenchyma was divided by Hounsfield unit (HU) intervals from −1024 to less than −977 HU, representing emphysematous changes [24]; values higher than −977 to −703 HU, representing normal parenchyma [25,26]; values from −703 to −368 HU, representing ground glass opacity (GGO); and values higher than −100 to 5 HU, representing consolidations [17,25,27,28]; the remaining lung parenchyma is classified as other. Thoracic VCAR software, representing the percentages of ground-glass opacity volume, consolidation volume, and emphysema volume in both lungs. Total lesion calculation was also performed, which made a total of ground-glass opacity and consolidation volumes [17]. The Thoracic VCAR is already in clinical practice in Chest CT affected by COVID-19 infections [17,29,30].

2.4. Statistical Analysis

Continuous data were expressed in terms of median value and range.

The Mann–Whitney test and Kruskal–Wallis test were used to assess statistically significant differences among groups. p value < 0.05 was considered significant for all tests.

All analyses were performed using Statistics Toolbox of MATLAB R2007a (The MathWorks Inc., Natick, MA, USA).

3. Results

A total of 341 CT examinations, including baseline and follow-up CTs, were analyzed. Thoracic VCAR software was unable to perform the quantification in 16/341 (4.7%) cases, both automatically and manually; therefore, the findings of 325 CTs were reported in the results. Among 140 enrolled patients, 11 patients died, while 129 patients were discharged after a median hospitalization period of 14 days (range, 4–50 days).

No statistically significant difference was found in the quantified volume distribution in the right and left lungs (p value > 0.23 at Mann–Whitney test).

Table 1 reports the percentage changes on quantified volumes between baseline CT and follow-up CTs, grouping the patients based on their clinical conditions (stable condition, improved, and worsened condition). Statistically significant differences were found (p value $\leq$ 0.05 at Kruskal–Wallis test) among quantified volumes of healthy residual parenchyma, GGO, consolidation and total pulmonary volume, considering different clinical conditions (stable, worsened, improved) (see Figure 1).

Table 2 reports the quantified volumes at the last CT follow-up as percentage values of the total lung volumes, grouping the patients based on outcome in those dead and those discharged. CT was not performed on cadavers; the death was an outcome, which was retrospectively included, to differentiate findings of patients who survived vs. patients who died during the hospitalization.

Statistically significant differences were also found (p value $\leq$ 0.05 at Kruskal–Wallis test), based on patients outcomes between dead patients and discharged patients, for quantified volumes of healthy residual parenchyma (42.9% versus 87.5%, retrospectively), of GGO (33.5% versus 9.0%, retrospectively), and of consolidation (3.2% versus 0.7%, retrospectively) (Figure 2). GGO and consolidation at the last follow-up, considering the discharged patients, had, as a median value, 0.37 and 0.03 L, respectively. Among discharged patients, a complete disease resolution of the CT scan was observed in 62/129 (48.1%) patients with a lung disease involvement $\leq$5%; a lung disease involvement from 5% to 15% was found in 40/129 (31.0%) patients, while 27/129 (20.9%) patients had lung disease involvement included, between 16 and 30%.

In Figure 3, we reported the evolution of the quantified GGO and consolidation volumes calculated on chest CT. Figure 3a,c shows the boxplots of GGO volume and consolidation volume, grouping the temporal course in 0–7 days, 8–14 days, 15–21 days, and $\geq$22 days after hospital admission. Exclusively GGO volume presented statistically significant differences among these groups. Considering Figure 3b,d, we can observe that GGO volume increased until the 16 days and consolidation volume until the 12 days, 8–21 days is the advanced period with the most severe lung involvement; after the extent of involvement started to decrease, particularly, after 21 days, the absorption was more obvious.

Figure 4 showed two representative cases: a patient with a CT panel improved and then discharged Figure 4a,b and a case of a patient with a CT panel worsened and then died Figure 4c,d.

Table 1. Percentage change of quantified volume between baseline CT and follow-up CTs.

		H. PAR. R (%)	H. PAR. L (%)	TOTAL H. PAR. (%)	GGO R (%)	GGO L (%)	TOTAL GGO (%)	OTHER R (%)	OTHER L (%)	TOTAL OTHER (%)	CONSOL. R (%)	CONSOL. L (%)	TOTAL CON-SOLID. (%)	TOTAL LUNG VOL. R (%)	TOTAL LUNG VOL. L (%)	TOTAL LUNG VOL. (%)
Worsened (N. 10)	Median value	−23.32	−11.87	−18.32	21.19	50.23	42.29	32.42	12.59	22.90	45.88	54.41	37.61	−6.70	−5.56	−3.50
	Minimum value	−76.59	−83.42	−79.78	−67.78	−68.76	−68.21	−71.78	−74.55	−71.02	−86.73	−83.40	−82.67	−49.03	−60.31	−54.36
	Maximum value	101.71	81.72	85.30	139.50	207.06	168.57	200.23	628.14	242.41	694.60	507.97	543.48	43.43	41.13	41.64
Stable (N. 11)	Median value	−15.10	−11.11	−12.87	5.92	−2.52	2.20	−12.24	−5.45	−7.25	−9.78	−0.94	3.34	−5.34	−5.85	−8.06
	Minimum value	−85.69	−85.58	−82.97	−66.78	−56.24	−62.03	−74.14	−76.63	−71.11	−93.67	−93.98	−93.84	−47.81	−46.60	−47.26
	Maximum value	115.23	185.07	95.99	203.05	517.48	289.99	334.34	412.35	365.69	1030.43	900.34	971.51	69.84	397.22	142.59
Improved (N. 119)	Median value	23.99	22.26	23.17	−19.21	−17.66	−17.78	−32.71	−29.74	−31.09	−20.80	−18.31	−21.63	10.00	13.20	13.32
	Minimum value	−45.43	−72.40	−52.02	−77.15	−77.58	−75.48	−83.24	−89.89	−87.02	−96.29	−96.07	−96.22	−33.14	−66.22	−38.05
	Maximum value	329.90	488.56	389.44	240.24	180.80	192.19	516.14	592.85	388.46	872.45	1756.37	500.33	147.37	192.86	165.33
Total (N. 140)	Median value	15.21	18.93	17.01	−10.11	−15.02	−13.97	−26.81	−23.56	−26.12	−18.99	−11.82	−14.10	7.25	10.81	8.56
	Minimum value	−85.69	−85.58	−82.97	−77.15	−77.58	−75.48	−83.24	−89.89	−87.02	−96.29	−96.07	−96.22	−49.03	−66.22	−54.36
	Maximum value	329.90	488.56	389.44	240.24	517.48	289.99	516.14	628.14	388.46	1030.43	1756.37	971.51	147.37	397.22	165.33

Note: H. PAR. = healthy parenchyma, GGO = ground glass opacity; CONSOL = consolidation; TOTAL LUN VOL. = total lung volume; R= right; L = left; Lung parenchyma was divided by Hounsfield unit (HU) intervals from −1024 HU to less than −977 HU representing emphysematous changes, values higher than −977 HU to −703 HU representing normal parenchyma, values from −703 HU to −368 HU representing ground glass opacity (GGO) and values higher than −100 HU to 5 HU representing consolidations; the remaining lung parenchyma is classified as other.

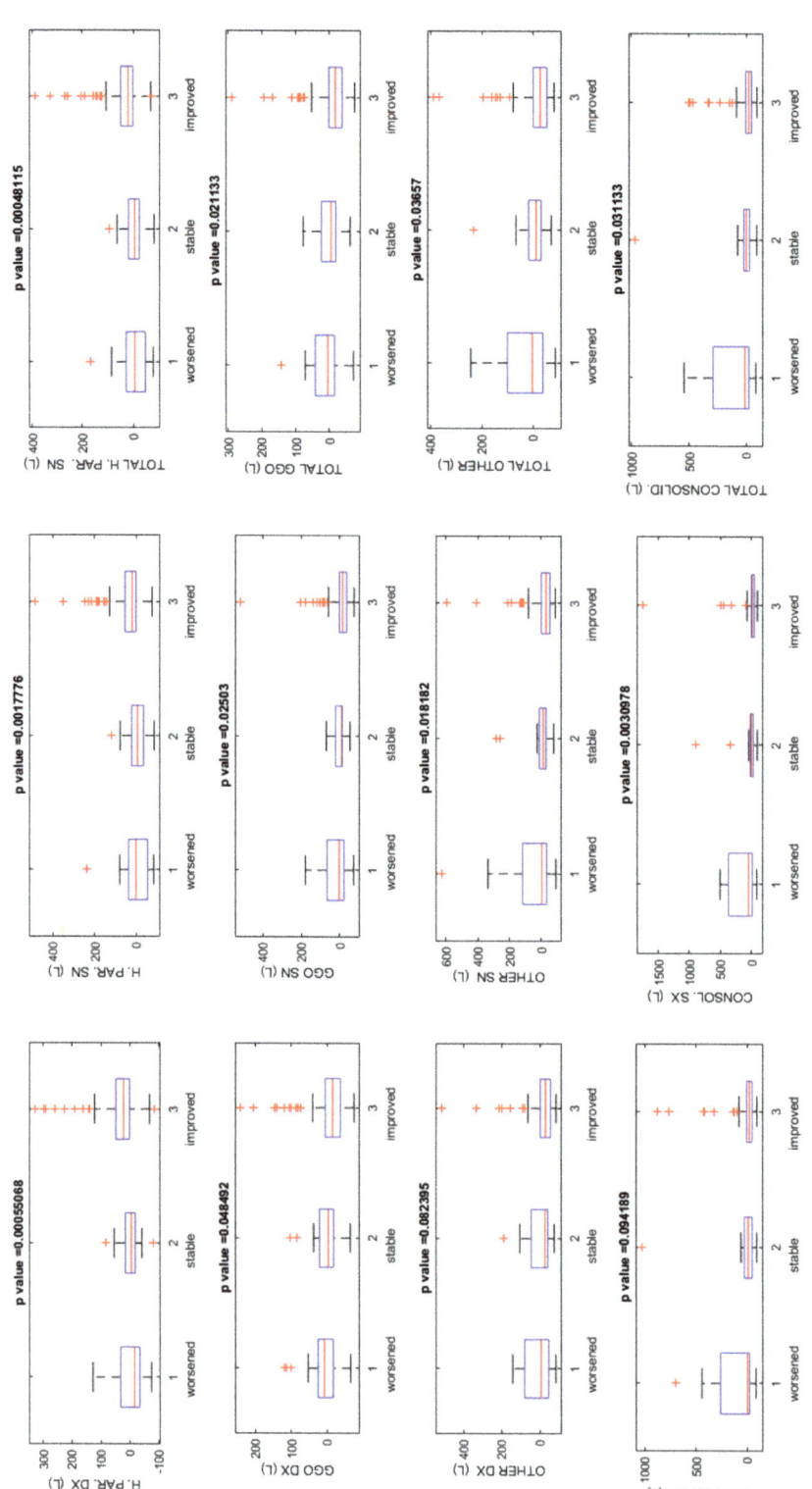

Figure 1. Boxplots of quantified volumes on CT using the computer tool based on the clinical condition (stable, improved, and worsened). Note: H. PAR. = healthy parenchyma, GGO = ground glass opacity; CONSOL = consolidation; R = right; L = left.

Table 2. Quantified volumes on CT at the last follow-up.

		H. PAR. R (%)	H. PAR. L (%)	TOTAL H. PAR. L (%)	GGO R (%)	GGO L (%)	TOTAL GGO (%)	OTHER R (%)	OTHER L (%)	TOTAL OTHER (%)	CONSOL. R (%)	CONSOL. L (%)	TOTAL CONSOLID. (%)
Dead (N. 11)	Median value	44.46	44.06	42.89	34.01	33.12	33.58	8.09	9.30	8.55	2.34	3.55	3.21
	Minimum value	18.34	15.94	23.36	7.03	7.30	7.15	1.31	1.20	1.26	0.32	0.33	0.32
	Maximum value	90.72	90.40	90.58	63.00	53.70	58.55	24.08	34.00	28.12	11.05	17.92	13.78
Discharged (N. 129)	Median value	87.36	87.71	87.48	8.67	9.19	9.02	1.57	1.51	1.56	0.69	0.61	0.65
	Minimum value	4.55	8.64	6.41	2.73	2.71	2.72	0.51	0.56	0.54	0.27	0.30	0.29
	Maximum value	95.76	95.14	95.45	75.17	79.12	76.99	25.65	23.37	24.61	21.28	23.94	21.95
Total (N. 140)	Median value	86.67	87.10	86.31	9.77	9.96	9.96	1.61	1.61	1.69	0.72	0.65	0.69
	Minimum value	4.55	8.64	6.41	2.73	2.71	2.72	0.51	0.56	0.54	0.27	0.30	0.29
	Maximum value	95.76	95.14	95.45	75.17	79.12	76.99	25.65	34.00	28.12	21.28	23.94	21.95

Note: H. PAR. = healthy parenchyma, GGO = ground glass opacity; CONSOL = consolidation; TOTAL LUN VOL. = total lung volume; R= right; L = left; Lung parenchyma was divided by Hounsfield unit (HU) intervals from −1024 HU to less than −977 HU representing emphysematous changes, values higher than −977 HU to −703 HU representing normal parenchyma, values from −703 HU to −368 HU representing ground glass opacity (GGO) and values higher than −100 HU to 5 HU representing consolidations; the remaining lung parenchyma is classified as other.

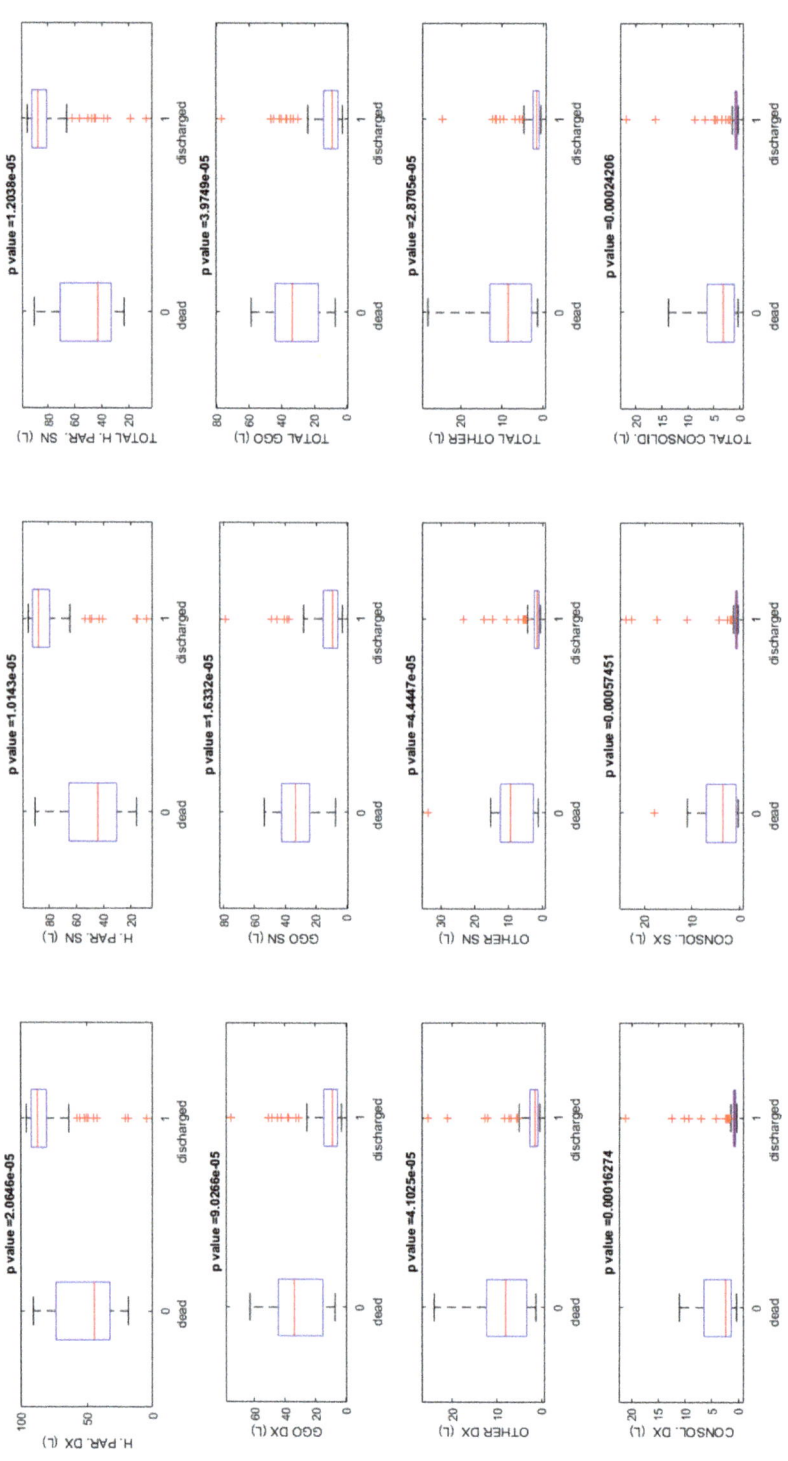

Figure 2. Boxplots of the quantified volume considering dead patients and discharged patients. Note: H. PAR. = healthy parenchyma, GGO = ground glass opacity; CONSOL = consolidation; R = right; L = left.

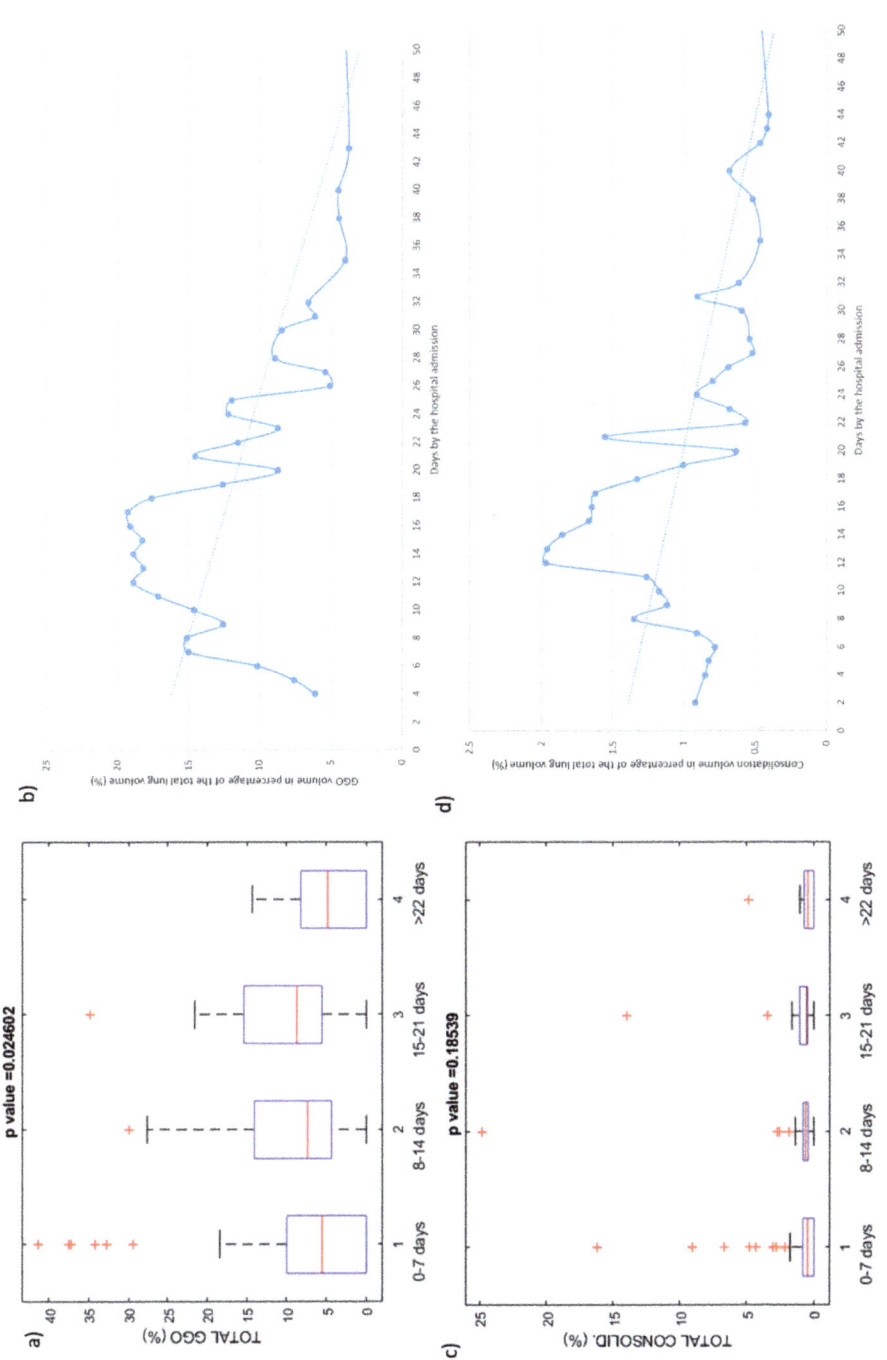

Figure 3. Temporal course of quantified volume on chest CT: in (**a**) and (**c**) boxplots of GGO volume and consolidation volume grouping the temporal course in 0–7 days (N. 25), 8–14 days (N. 50), 15–21 days (N. 37), and >22 days (N. 28); in (**b**) and (**d**) the temporal course of GGO and consolidation volume as a percentage value of total lung volume.

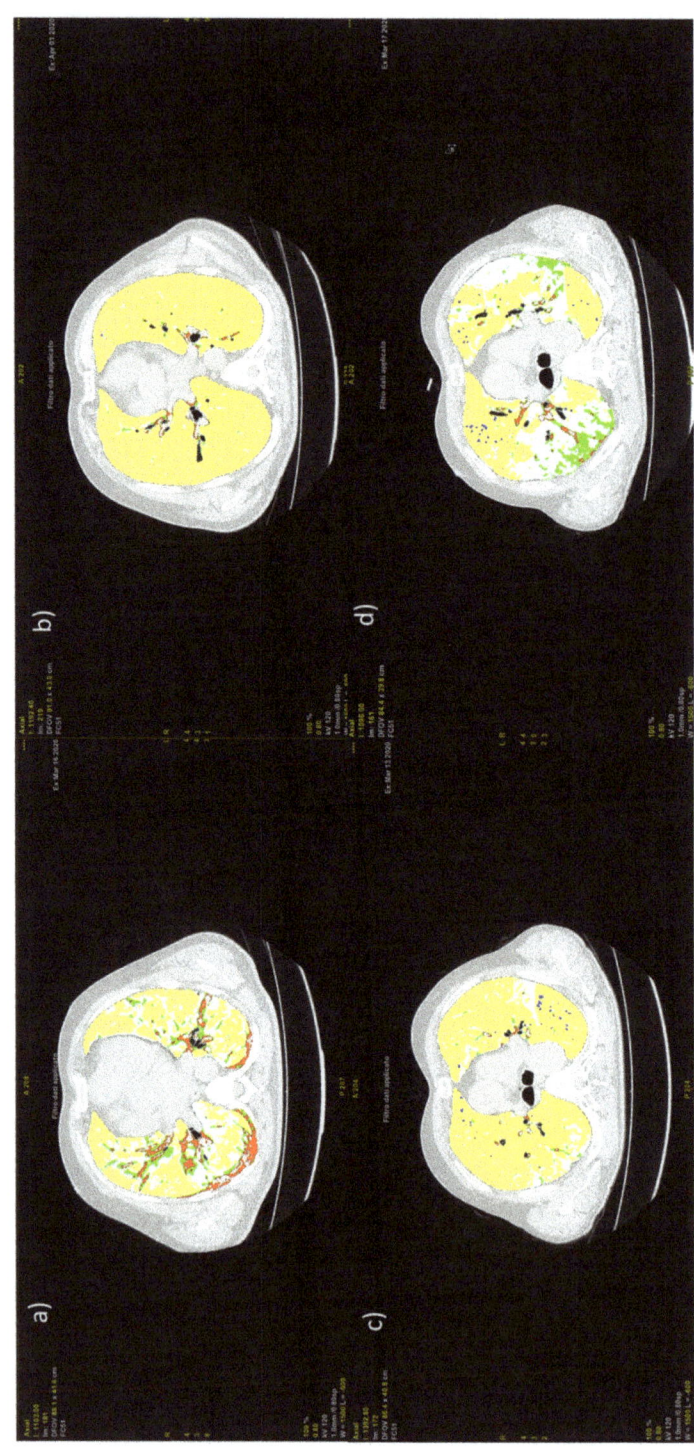

Figure 4. Representative cases of a patient with a CT panel improved and then discharged (**a**) and (**b**) (at baseline and follow-up CT), and of a case of a patient with a CT panel worsened and then died (**c**) and (**d**) (at baseline and follow -up CT).

4. Discussion

Several previous studies [6–16] have described the main CT signs of COVID-19, summarized as GGO, crazy-paving pattern, and consolidation. Several methods of disease extent quantification at chest CT using machine learning and AI tools have been proposed, including the extent of emphysema, GGO, and consolidation [31–51]. Few studies have investigated the changes in CT findings associated with COVID-19 pneumonia in the follow-up, quantifying the evolution and the absorption of the abnormalities visible on CT using a computer automatic aided tool.

Zhou et al. [36] investigated CT images of 100 confirmed COVID-19 pneumonia patients, to describe the lesion distribution, CT signs, and evolution during different courses. They reported that the course of COVID-19 pneumonia consists of three stages: 1–7 days is the early rapid progressive stage, 8–14 days is the advanced stage, and after 14 days, the abnormalities start to decrease. In the early rapid progressive stage, GGO plus a reticular pattern, GGO plus consolidation, and GGO, were all common signs; in the advanced stage, signs of progression and absorption coexisted; lung abnormalities showed an asynchronous process, with parts with absorption and parts progressing. Lung abnormalities predominantly showed peripheral, middle, and lower distribution.

Pan et al. [5] assessed the chest CT to determine the changes in the findings associated with COVID-19 from initial diagnosis until patient recovery. They reported that lung abnormalities on chest CT scans showed the greatest severity approximately 10 days after the initial onset of symptoms.

Wang at al [50] reported the analysis on 366 CT scans to assess the temporal changes of CT findings in 90 patients with COVID-19 pneumonia. Their results showed that CT findings progressed rapidly, and peaked during illness days 6–11. The predominant pattern of abnormalities after symptom onset was ground-glass opacity. The percentage of mixed patterns peaked on illness days 12–17, and became the second most predominant pattern thereafter. Pure ground-glass opacity was the most prevalent subtype of ground-glass opacity after symptom onset. The percentage of ground-glass opacity with irregular linear opacity peaked on illness days 6–11 and became the second most prevalent subtype thereafter. The distribution of lesions was predominantly bilateral and subpleural. Sixty-six of the 70 patients discharged (94%) had residual disease on final CT scans.

However, to the best of our knowledge, there is no study in the literature reporting on the temporal changes of CT findings, using an automatic tool to quantify the abnormality in lung parenchyma (due to COVID-19 pneumonia).

According to the recent literature, we reported that GGO is the most representative sign of COVID-19 disease on chest CT, and that statistically significant differences were found among quantified volumes of healthy residual parenchyma, GGO, consolidation and total pulmonary volume, considering different clinical conditions (stable, improved, and worsened). Statistically significant differences were also found, based on patient outcomes between dead patients and discharged patients, for quantified volumes of healthy residual parenchyma (42.9% versus 87.5%, retrospectively), of GGO (33.5% versus 9.0%, retrospectively), and of consolidation (3.2% versus 0.7%, retrospectively). We reported that, among discharged patients, a complete disease resolution on CT scans was observed in 62/129 patients with lung disease involvement ≤5; lung disease involvement ranging from 5% to 15% was found in 40/129 patients, while 27/129 (20.9%) patients had lung disease involvement, between 16 and 30%. The discharged patients at the last follow-up had a percentage change of lung disease involvement of 12.5% while the dead patients of 57.1%.

Moreover, we demonstrated that GGO and consolidation at the last follow-up were almost completely absorbed, and that 8–21 days of hospital admission was the advanced period with the most severe lung involvement. After 16 days of hospital admission, the abnormalities identified by chest CTs started to improve and, in particular, after 21 days, the absorption was more obvious.

In this study, we reported that no statistically significant difference was found in the quantified volume distribution in the right and left lung—in contrast to what was reported by Li et al. [52] and Nagra et al. [53]. Li et al. [52] noticed a side-preference of lung lesions in COVID-19. The lesions in the right lungs were significantly larger and developed faster than those on the left. Moreover, the level of the right-over-left preference of lung injury was significantly correlated with the potential need for intensive care and inpatient mortality. Nagra et al. [53] concluded that in COVID-19 the right lung has a higher degree of opacification on a plain radiograph than the left lung.

We believe that analysis of CT findings, using a computer tool based on different thresholding Hounsfield unit settings, could identify pulmonary abnormalities and lung recruitment, and we believe that knowledge of the percentage of potentially recruitable lung evolution may be important to establish the therapeutic efficacy in COVID-19 disease.

There are still some limitations in this study. First, the time for CT re-examination of each patient is not standardized. Second, the retrospective and monocentric nature of the study. Third, the absence of laboratory findings to correlate with the CT results.

5. Conclusions

In conclusion, we reported that CT findings, using a computer automatic tool based on different thresholding Hounsfield Unit settings, could identify pulmonary abnormalities and lung recruitment. Moreover, we demonstrated that discharged patients had lung disease involvement of 12.5%, while for dead patients it was 57.1%; a complete disease resolution on chest CT scans was observed in 48.1% of patients using a computer aided tool to quantify the GGO and consolidation volumes. Moreover, 8–21 days of hospital admission is the advanced stage, with peak levels of abnormalities on CTs; after 16 days, the abnormalities started to improve. Therefore, CT has proven to be a useful tool in following the evolution of the disease, by clarifying the progression/regression timing of the disease.

Author Contributions: Data curation, R.G. (Roberto Grassi), V.G. and R.F.; Formal analysis, R.G. (Roberto Grassi), V.G. and R.F.; Investigation, A.R. and V.M.; Methodology, R.G. (Roberto Grassi), S.C., F.U., V.G., R.G. (Roberta Galdiero), C.P., G.G., S.M., D.C., R.F., M.P.B., U.A., O.P., M.C., E.B., R.G. (Roberta Grassi) and V.M.; Supervision, R.G. (Roberto Grassi) and S.C. All authors have read and agreed to the published version of the manuscript.

Funding: This research received no external funding.

Institutional Review Board Statement: This retrospective study included patients enrolled by "Hospital of Colli (Monaldi-Cotugno-CTO)" in Naples.

Informed Consent Statement: In relation to the ongoing epidemic emergency, the institutional local review boards gave up written informed consent for this retrospective study that evaluated anonymized data and involved no potential risk to patients.

Data Availability Statement: All data are reported in the manuscript.

Conflicts of Interest: The authors declare no conflict of interest.

References

1. World Health Organization. Naming the Coronavirus Disease (COVID-2019) and the Virus that Causes It. Available online: www.who.int/emergencies/diseases/ (accessed on 21 March 2020).
2. Wuhan Coronavirus (2019-nCoV) Global Cases (by Johns Hopkins CSSE). Case Dashboard. Available online: https://gisanddata.maps.arcgis.com/apps/opsdashboard/index.html#/bda7594740fd40299423467b48e9ecf6 (accessed on 21 March 2020).
3. Xu, Y.-H.; Dong, J.-H.; An, W.-M.; Lv, X.-Y.; Yin, X.-P.; Zhang, J.-Z.; Dong, L.; Ma, X.; Zhang, H.-J.; Gao, B.-L. Clinical and computed tomographic imaging features of novel coronavirus pneumonia caused by SARS-CoV-2. *J. Infect.* **2020**, *80*, 394–400. [CrossRef]
4. Yang, W.; Cao, Q.; Qin, L.; Wang, X.; Cheng, Z.; Pan, A.; Dai, J.; Sun, Q.; Zhao, F.; Qu, J.; et al. Clinical characteristics and imaging manifestations of the 2019 novel coronavirus disease (COVID-19): A multi-center study in Wenzhou city, Zhejiang, China. *J. Infect.* **2020**, *80*, 388–393. [CrossRef]
5. Pan, F.; Ye, T.; Sun, P.; Gui, S.; Liang, B.; Li, L.; Zheng, D.; Wang, J.; Hesketh, R.L.; Yang, L.; et al. Time course of lung changes on chest CT during recovery from 2019 novel coronavirus (COVID-19) pneumonia. *Radiology* **2020**, *295*, 715–721. [CrossRef]

6. Shi, H.; Han, X.; Jiang, N.; Cao, Y.; Alwalid, O.; Gu, J.; Fan, Y.; Zheng, C. Radiological findings from 81 patients with COVID-19 pneumonia in Wuhan, China: A descriptive study. *Lancet Infect. Dis.* **2020**, *20*, 425–434. [CrossRef]
7. Yoon, S.H.; Lee, K.H.; Kim, J.Y.; Lee, Y.K.; Ko, H.; Kim, K.H.; Park, K.M.; Kim, Y.-H. Chest radiographic and CT findings of the 2019 novel coronavirus disease (COVID-19): Analysis of nine patients treated in Korea. *Korean J. Radiol.* **2020**, *21*, 1144173. [CrossRef]
8. Agostini, A.; Floridi, C.; Borgheresi, A.; Badaloni, M.; Pirani, P.E.; Terilli, F.; Ottaviani, L.; Giovagnoni, A. Proposal of a low-dose, long-pitch, dual-source chest CT protocol on third-generation dual-source CT using a tin filter for spectral shaping at 100 kVp for CoronaVirus Disease 2019 (COVID-19) patients: A feasibility study. *Radiol. Med.* **2020**, *125*, 365–373. [CrossRef] [PubMed]
9. Borghesi, A.; Maroldi, R. COVID-19 outbreak in Italy: Experimental chest X-ray scoring system for quantifying and monitoring disease progression. *Radiol. Med.* **2020**, *125*, 509–513. [CrossRef] [PubMed]
10. Fichera, G.; Stramare, R.; De Conti, G.; Motta, R.; Giraudo, C. It's not over until it's over: The chame-leonic behavior of COVID-19 over a six-day period. *Radiol. Med.* **2020**, *125*, 514–516. [CrossRef] [PubMed]
11. Gaia, C.; Chiara, C.M.; Silvia, L.; Chiara, A.; Luisa, D.C.M.; Giulia, B.; Silvia, P.; Lucia, C.; Alessandra, T.; Annarita, S.; et al. Chest CT for early detection and management of coronavirus disease (COVID-19): A report of 314 patients admitted to Emergency Department with suspected pneumonia. *Radiol. Med.* **2020**, *125*, 931–942. [CrossRef] [PubMed]
12. Giannitto, C.; Sposta, F.M.; Repici, A.; Vatteroni, G.; Casiraghi, E.; Casari, E.; Ferraroli, G.M.; Fugazza, A.; Sandri, M.T.; Chiti, A.; et al. Chest CT in patients with a moderate or high pretest probability of COVID-19 and negative swab. *Radiol. Med.* **2020**, *125*, 1260–1270. [CrossRef]
13. Ierardi, A.M.; Wood, B.J.; Arrichiello, A.; Bottino, N.; Bracchi, L.; Forzenigo, L.; Andrisani, M.C.; Vespro, V.; Bonelli, C.; Amalou, A.; et al. Preparation of a radiology department in an Italian hospital dedicated to COVID-19 patients. *Radiol. Med.* **2020**, *125*, 894–901. [CrossRef] [PubMed]
14. Cappabianca, S.; Fusco, R.; de Lisio, A.; Paura, C.; Clemente, A.; Gagliardi, G.; Lombardi, G.; Giacobbe, G.; Russo, G.M.; Belfiore, M.P.; et al. Correction to: Clinical and laboratory data, radiological structured report findings and quantitative evaluation of lung involvement on baseline chest CT in COVID-19 patients to predict prognosis. *Radiol. Med.* **2021**, *126*, 643. [CrossRef]
15. Huang, C.; Wang, Y.; Li, X.; Ren, L.; Zhao, J.; Hu, Y.; Zhang, P.L.; Fan, G.; Xu, J.; Gu, X.; et al. Clinical features of patients infected with 2019 novel coronavirus in Wuhan, China. *Lancet* **2020**, *15*, 497–506. [CrossRef]
16. Lei, J.; Li, J.; Li, X.; Qi, X. CT Imaging of the 2019 Novel Coronavirus (2019-nCoV) Pneumonia. *Radiology* **2020**, *295*, 18. [CrossRef] [PubMed]
17. Belfiore, M.P.; Urraro, F.; Grassi, R.; Giacobbe, G.; Patelli, G.; Cappabianca, S.; Reginelli, A. Artificial intelligence to codify lung CT in Covid-19 patients. *Radiol. Med.* **2020**, *125*, 500–504. [CrossRef] [PubMed]
18. Neri, E.; Miele, V.; Coppola, F.; Grassi, R. Use of CT and artificial intelligence in suspected or COVID-19 positive patients: Statement of the Italian Society of Medical and Interventional Radiology. *Radiol. Med.* **2020**, *125*, 505–508. [CrossRef]
19. Laghi, A.; Grassi, R. Italian Radiology's Response to the COVID-19 Outbreak. *J. Am. Coll. Radiol.* **2020**, *17*, 699–700. [CrossRef] [PubMed]
20. Neri, E.; Coppola, F.; Miele, V.; Bibbolino, C.; Grassi, R. Artificial intelligence: Who is responsible for the diagnosis? *Radiol. Med.* **2020**, *31*. [CrossRef]
21. Li, L.; Qin, L.; Xu, Z.; Yin, Y.; Wang, X.; Kong, B.; Bai, J.; Lu, Y.; Fang, Z.; Song, Q.; et al. Artificial Intelligence Distinguishes COVID-19 from Community Acquired Pneumonia on Chest CT. *Radiology* **2020**, *19*, 200905. [CrossRef]
22. Tárnok, A. Machine Learning, COVID-19 (2019-nCoV), and multi-OMICS. *Cytometry A* **2020**, *97*, 215–216. [CrossRef] [PubMed]
23. Gozes, O.; Frid-Adar, M.; Greenspan, H.; Browning, P.; Zhang, H.; Ji, W.; Bernheim, A.; Siegel, E. Rapid AI Development Cycle for the Coronavirus (COVID-19) Pandemic: Initial Results for Automated Detection & Patient Monitoring using Deep Learning CT Image Analysis. *arXiv* **2020**, arXiv:2003.05037.
24. Wang, Z.; Gu, S.; Leader, J.K.; Kundu, S.; Tedrow, J.R.; Sciurba, F.; Gur, D.; Siegfried, J.M.; Pu, J. Optimal threshold in CT quantification of emphysema. *Eur. Radiol.* **2013**, *23*, 975–984. [CrossRef] [PubMed]
25. Gattinoni, L.; Caironi, P.; Cressoni, M.; Chiumello, D.; Ranieri, V.M.; Quiten, M.; Russo, S.; Patroniti, N.; Cornejo, R.; Bugedo, G. Lung recruitment in patients with the acute espiratory distress syndrome. *N. Engl. J. Med.* **2006**, *354*, 1775–1786. [CrossRef]
26. Ohkubom, H.; Kanemitsu, Y.; Uemura, T.; Takakuwa, O.; Takemura, M.; Maeno, K.; Ito, Y.; Ogury, T.; Kazawa, N.; Mikami, R.; et al. Normal Lung Quanti-fication in Usual Interstitial Pneumonia Pattern: The Impact of Threshold-based Volumetric CT Analysis for the Staging of Idiopathic Pulmonary Fibrosis. *PLoS ONE* **2016**, *11*, e0152505.
27. Çinkooğlu, A.; Bayraktaroğlu, S.; Savaş, R. Lung Changes on Chest CT During 2019 Novel Coronavirus (COVID-19) Pneumonia. *Eur. J. Breast Health* **2020**, *16*, 89–90. [CrossRef] [PubMed]
28. Albarello, F.; Pianura, E.; Di Stefano, F.; Cristofaro, M.; Petrone, A.; Marchioni, L.; Palazzolo, C.; Schinina, J.; Nicastri, E.; Petrosillo, N.; et al. COVID 19 INMI Study Group. 2019-novel Coronavirus severe adult respiratory distress syndrome in two cases in Italy: An un-common radiological presentation. *Int. J. Infect. Dis.* **2020**, *93*, 192–197. [CrossRef]
29. Rorat, M.; Jurek, T.; Simon, K.; Guziński, M. Value of quantitative analysis in lung computed tomography in patients severely ill with COVID-19. *PLoS ONE* **2021**, *16*, e0251946. [CrossRef] [PubMed]
30. Grassi, R.; Cappabianca, S.; Urraro, F.; Feragalli, B.; Montanelli, A.; Patelli, G.; Granata, V.; Giacobbe, G.; Russo, G.M.; Grillo, A.; et al. Chest CT Computerized Aided Quantification of PNEUMONIA Lesions in COVID-19 Infection: A Comparison among Three Commercial Software. *Int. J. Environ. Res. Public Health* **2020**, *17*, 6914. [CrossRef]

31. Allam, Z.; Jones, D.S. On the Coronavirus (COVID-19) Outbreak and the Smart City Network: Universal Data Sharing Standards Coupled with Artificial Intelligence (AI) to Benefit Urban Health Monitoring and Management. *Healthcare* **2020**, *8*, 46. [CrossRef] [PubMed]
32. Meng, Y.; Liu, C.L.; Cai, Q.; Shen, Y.Y.; Chen, S.Q. Contrast analysis of the relationship between the HRCT sign and new pathologic classification in small ground glass nodule-like lung adenocarcinoma. *Radiol. Med.* **2019**, *124*, 8–13. [CrossRef]
33. Hoesein, M.F.A.; de Hoop, B.; Zanen, P.; Gietema, H.; Kruitwagen, C.L.; van Ginneken, B.; Isgum, I.; Mol, C.; van Klaveren, R.J.; Dijkstra, A.E.; et al. CT-quantified emphysema in male heavy smokers: Association with lung function decline. *Thorax* **2011**, *66*, 782–787. [CrossRef]
34. Maldonado, F.; Moua, T.; Rajagopalan, S.; Karwoski, R.A.; Raghunath, S.; Decker, P.A.; Hartman, T.E.; Bartholmai, B.J.; Robb, R.A.; Ryu, J.H. Automated quantification of radiological patterns predicts survival in idiopathic pulmonary fibrosis. *Eur. Respir. J.* **2014**, *43*, 204–212. [CrossRef] [PubMed]
35. Yang, R.; Li, X.; Liu, H.; Zhen, Y.; Zhang, X.; Xiong, Q.; Luo, Y.; Gao, C.; Zeng, W. Chest CT Severity Score: An Imaging Tool for Assessing Severe COVID-19. *Radiol. Cardiothorac. Imaging* **2020**, *2*, e200047. [CrossRef]
36. Zhou, S.; Zhu, T.; Wang, Y.; Xia, L. Imaging features and evolution on CT in 100 COVID-19 pneumonia patients in Wuhan, China. *Eur. Radiol.* **2020**, *30*, 5446–5454. [CrossRef]
37. Carotti, M.; Salaffi, F.; Sarzi-Puttini, P.; Agostini, A.; Borgheresi, A.; Minorati, D.; Galli, M.; Marotto, D.; Giovagnoni, A. Chest CT features of coronavirus disease 2019 (COVID-19) pneumonia: Key points for radiologists. *Radiol. Med.* **2020**, *125*, 636–646. [CrossRef]
38. Shaw, B.; Daskareh, M.; Gholamrezanezhad, A. The lingering manifestations of COVID-19 during and after convalescence: Update on long-term pulmonary consequences of coronavirus disease 2019 (COVID-19). *Radiol. Med.* **2021**, *126*, 40–46. [CrossRef] [PubMed]
39. Di Serafino, M.; Notaro, M.; Rea, G.; Iacobellis, F.; Paoli, D.V.; Acampora, C.; Ianniello, S.; Brunese, L.; Romano, L.; Vallone, G. The lung ultrasound: Facts or artifacts? In the era of COVID-19 outbreak. *Radiol. Med.* **2020**, *125*, 738–753. [CrossRef] [PubMed]
40. Cozzi, D.; Albanesi, M.; Cavigli, E.; Moroni, C.; Bindi, A.; Luvarà, S.; Lucarini, S.; Busoni, S.; Mazzoni, L.N.; Miele, V. Chest X-ray in new Coronavirus Disease 2019 (COVID-19) infection: Findings and correlation with clinical outcome. *Radiol. Med.* **2020**, *125*, 730–737. [CrossRef]
41. Pediconi, F.; Galati, F.; Bernardi, D.; Belli, P.; Brancato, B.; Calabrese, M.; Camera, L.; Carbonaro, L.A.; Caumo, F.; Clauser, P.; et al. Breast imaging and cancer diagnosis during the COVID-19 pandemic: Recommendations from the Italian College of Breast Radiologists by SIRM. *Radiol. Med.* **2020**, *125*, 926–930. [CrossRef] [PubMed]
42. Borghesi, A.; Zigliani, A.; Masciullo, R.; Golemi, S.; Maculotti, P.; Farina, D.; Maroldi, R. Radiographic severity index in COVID-19 pneumonia: Relationship to age and sex in 783 Italian patients. *Radiol. Med.* **2020**, *125*, 461–464. [CrossRef]
43. Gatti, M.; Calandri, M.; Barba, M.; Biondo, A.; Geninatti, C.; Gentile, S.; Greco, M.; Morrone, V.; Piatti, C.; Santonocito, A.; et al. Baseline chest X-ray in coronavirus disease 19 (COVID-19) patients: Association with clinical and laboratory data. *Radiol. Med.* **2020**, *125*, 1271–1279. [CrossRef]
44. Caruso, D.; Polici, M.; Zerunian, M.; Pucciarelli, F.; Polidori, T.; Guido, G.; Rucci, C.; Bracci, B.; Muscogiuri, E.; De Dominicis, C.; et al. Quantitative Chest CT analysis in discriminating COVID-19 from non-COVID-19 patients. *Radiol. Med.* **2021**, *126*, 243–249. [CrossRef]
45. Grassi, R.; Belfiore, M.P.; Montanelli, A.; Patelli, G.; Urraro, F.; Giacobbe, G.; Fusco, R.; Granata, V.; Petrillo, A.; Sacco, P.; et al. COVID-19 pneumonia: Computer-aided quantification of healthy lung parenchyma, emphysema, ground glass and consolidation on chest computed tomography (CT). *Radiol. Med.* **2021**, *126*, 553–560. [CrossRef] [PubMed]
46. Grassi, R.; Fusco, R.; Belfiore, M.P.; Montanelli, A.; Patelli, G.; Urraro, F.; Petrillo, A.; Granata, V.; Sacco, P.; Mazzei, M.A.; et al. Coronavirus disease 2019 (COVID-19) in Italy: Features on chest computed tomography using a structured report system. *Sci. Rep.* **2020**, *10*, 17236. [CrossRef] [PubMed]
47. Reginelli, A.; Grassi, R.; Feragalli, B.; Belfiore, M.; Montanelli, A.; Patelli, G.; La Porta, M.; Urraro, F.; Fusco, R.; Granata, V.; et al. Coronavirus Disease 2019 (COVID-19) in Italy: Double Reading of Chest CT Examination. *Biology* **2021**, *10*, 89. [CrossRef]
48. Granata, V.; Fusco, R.; Izzo, F.; Setola, S.V.; Coppola, M.; Grassi, R.; Reginelli, A.; Cappabianca, S.; Petrillo, A. COVID-19 infection in cancer patients: The management in a diagnostic unit. *Radiol. Oncol.* **2021**, *55*, 121–129. [CrossRef]
49. Granata, V.; Fusco, R.; Setola, S.; Galdiero, R.; Picone, C.; Izzo, F.; D'Aniello, R.; Miele, V.; Grassi, R.; Grassi, R.; et al. Lymphadenopathy after *BNT162b2* COVID-19 Vaccine: Preliminary Ultrasound Findings. *Biology* **2021**, *10*, 214. [CrossRef]
50. Wang, Y.; Dong, C.; Hu, Y.; Li, C.; Ren, Q.; Zhang, X.; Shi, H.; Zhou, M. Temporal Changes of CT Findings in 90 Patients with COVID-19 Pneumonia: A Longitudinal Study. *Radiology* **2020**, *296*, E55–E64. [CrossRef] [PubMed]
51. Maio, F.; Tari, D.U.; Granata, V.; Fusco, R.; Grassi, R.; Petrillo, A.; Pinto, F. Breast Cancer Screening during COVID-19 Emergency: Patients and Department Management in a Local Experience. *J. Pers. Med.* **2021**, *11*, 380. [CrossRef] [PubMed]
52. Li, J.; Yu, X.; Hu, S.; Lin, Z.; Xiong, N.; Gao, Y. COVID-19 targets the right lung. *Crit. Care* **2020**, *24*, 339. [CrossRef] [PubMed]
53. Nagra, D.; Russell, M.; Yates, M.; Galloway, J.; Barker, R.; Desai, S.R.; Norton, S. COVID-19: Opacification score is higher in the right lung and right lung involvement is a better predictor of ICU admission. *Eur. Respir. J.* **2020**, *56*, 2002340. [CrossRef] [PubMed]

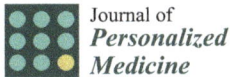

Article

Cerebral Vasoreactivity Evaluated by Transcranial Color Doppler and Breath-Holding Test in Patients after SARS-CoV-2 Infection

Marino Marcic [1,*], Ljiljana Marcic [2], Barbara Marcic [3], Vesna Capkun [4] and Katarina Vukojevic [3,4,*]

1. Department of Neurology, University Hospital Center Split, 21000 Split, Croatia
2. Department of Radiology, Polyclinic Medicol, 2100 Split, Croatia; lmarcic@mefst.hr
3. Department of Medical Genetics, University of Mostar School of Medicine, 88000 Mostar, Bosnia and Herzegovina; barbara.marcic@mef.sum.ba
4. Department of Anatomy, Histology and Embryology, University of Split School of Medicine, 21000 Split, Croatia; vesna.capkun@mefst.hr
* Correspondence: marino.marcic@yahoo.com (M.M.); katarina.vukojevic@mefst.hr (K.V.)

Abstract: From the beginning of the SARS-CoV-2 virus pandemic, it was clear that the virus is highly neurotrophic. Neurological manifestations can range from nonspecific symptoms such as dizziness, headaches and olfactory disturbances to severe forms of neurological dysfunction. Some neurological complication can occur even after mild forms of respiratory disease. This study's aims were to assess cerebrovascular reactivity in patients with nonspecific neurological symptoms after SARS-CoV-2 infection. A total of 25 patients, aged 33–62 years, who had nonspecific neurological symptoms after SARS-CoV-2 infection, as well as 25 healthy participants in the control group, were assessed for cerebrovascular reactivity according to transcranial color Doppler (TCCD) which we combined with a breath-holding test (BHT). In subjects after SARS-CoV-2 infection, there were statistically significantly lower flow velocities through the middle cerebral artery at rest period, lower maximum velocities at the end of the breath-holding period and lower breath holding index (BHI) in relation to the control group. Changes in cerebral artery flow rate velocities indicate poor cerebral vasoreactivity in the group after SARS-CoV-2 infection in regard to the control group and suggest vascular endothelial damage by the SARS-CoV-2 virus.

Keywords: SARS-CoV-2; nonspecific neurological symptoms; transcranial color Doppler; vasoreactivity

Citation: Marcic, M.; Marcic, L.; Marcic, B.; Capkun, V.; Vukojevic, K. Cerebral Vasoreactivity Evaluated by Transcranial Color Doppler and Breath-Holding Test in Patients after SARS-CoV-2 Infection. *J. Pers. Med.* **2021**, *11*, 379. https://doi.org/10.3390/jpm11050379

Academic Editor: Franco M. Buonaguro

Received: 31 March 2021
Accepted: 4 May 2021
Published: 6 May 2021

Publisher's Note: MDPI stays neutral with regard to jurisdictional claims in published maps and institutional affiliations.

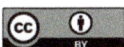

Copyright: © 2021 by the authors. Licensee MDPI, Basel, Switzerland. This article is an open access article distributed under the terms and conditions of the Creative Commons Attribution (CC BY) license (https://creativecommons.org/licenses/by/4.0/).

1. Introduction

Acute respiratory syndrome with coronavirus 2 (SARS-CoV-2) virus has been a major global health problem since 2020 year. As of March 2021, the SARS-CoV-2 pandemic has resulted in more than 125 million people worldwide infected and more than 2.8 million people have died (WHO COVID-19 Dashboard, March 2021). The SARS-CoV-2 virus has been known as a respiratory virus and the essential clinical feature is an acute respiratory infection [1], but from the beginning of the pandemic it has been clear that the virus is highly neurotrophic [2,3]. Patients with severe clinical manifestations of SARS-CoV-2 infection were more likely to experience neurological symptoms compared with those with mild disease [4]. The majority of these patients experienced prolonged headache, disturbance in consciousness, acute cerebrovascular disease (ischemic stroke, cerebral or subarachnoid hemorrhage), acute encephalopathy, encephalitis or meningitis, polyneuropathy, multiple sclerosis spectrum of disease and seizures. Milder forms of disease are often accompanied by nonspecific neurological complications such as headache, dizziness, ageusia (loss of taste), anosmia (loss of smell), myalgia and fatigue [5,6]. The SARS-CoV-2 virus membrane is characterized by the presence of the spike (S) glycoprotein which facilitates entry into neural, glial and endothelial cells which have angiotensin converting enzyme 2 (ACE2) receptors [7]. Several mechanisms may be involved in the pathophysiology of the virus as well as damage to the nervous system, but full mechanisms are still not fully understood. Neurological manifestations can be caused by non-specific complications of systemic infectious disease, inflammation of the nervous system or dysfunction of cerebral vasculature [8,9]. Vascular endothelial inflammation and SARS-CoV-2 complement-induced coagulopathy cause diffuse endothelial dysfunction, impaired vasoreactivity, in most severe cases associated with thrombus formation in the microcirculation [10,11]. As Hernadez-Fernandez et al. showed in their study, endothelial disruption is a basic mechanism of the virus pathophysiological process [12]. Hyperactivity of the host immune system and molecular mimicry may further aggravate brain damage and clinical picture [13] so as autoantibodies against heat shock proteins [14], prolonged hypoxia and electrolyte changes as a consequence of long-term respiratory disease also may contribute to the development of neurological complications. The involvement of the CNS may be related to poor prognosis and disease worsening, but even patients with mild respiratory symptoms can have some prolonged neurological symptoms. An increasing number of patients develop cerebrovascular disease after overcoming SARS-CoV-2 virus infection without having any risk factors prior to infection. Cerebrovascular disease is the second leading cause of death worldwide and some classic risk factors are well known, but new risk factors such as infectious agents have been documented recently [15]. Chronic infection, such as Chlamydia pneumonia, human cytomegalovirus, Helicobacter pylori, influenza virus, hepatitis C virus, etc., contribute to the development of cerebrovascular disease, causing changes in the small and large blood vessels of the brain [16]. Healthy brain arteries are capable of maintaining a constant cerebral blood supply via cerebral autoregulation mechanisms, despite changes in cerebral perfusion. A noninvasive, real-time, well tolerated and accurate method for the evaluation of main basal intracranial arteries, their flow rates and hemodynamic parameters is transcranial color Doppler (TCCD) [17,18] which provides useful information on peak systolic velocities (PSV), end diastolic velocities (EDV), mean velocities (MV), resistance index (RI) and pulsatility index (PI). In response to vasodilator stimulation such as CO_2 inhalation, the breath-holding test (BHT) or acetazolamide administration, we can estimate cerebral vasoreactivity by measuring flow velocities in cerebral arteries and flow velocity changes induced by hypercarbia [19]. Impaired vasoreactivity and reduced reserve capacity of brain arteries are predisposing conditions for cerebrovascular disease [20]. The aim of our study was to assess cerebrovascular reactivity in patients after SARS-CoV-2 infection with nonspecific neurological symptoms, using TCCD and the breath-holding test. The hypothesis of our study is that patients after mild SARS-CoV-2 infection have impaired cerebral vasoreactivity.

2. Materials and Methods

2.1. Population Study

Analyzing the electronic database of the University Hospital Canter Split, we found 456 patients who sought help at a neurology clinic, polyclinic department, for nonspecific neurological symptoms such as headache, loss of sense of smell and taste, dizziness, and weakness from January to March 2021. Among all of them, we found 185 patients who, according to available database, had SARS-CoV-2 infection, and 72 of them who had it in the last 60 days. Patients were classified as mild, moderate or severe based on WHO Criteria [21] and only 66 of them met the criteria for mild forms of COVID-19 disease. Only 54 patients of these were without a significant risk factors for cerebrovascular disease. Among them, only 49 were considered to be suitable for our study because they were neither older than 62 years nor younger than 32 years. We excluded the younger age group from the study due to the possible increased elasticity of blood vessels in the brain that gives high flow rates, while we excluded the older age group due to increased resistance and increased vessel stiffness. Just 34 patients agreed to participate in our study and signed informed consent. Among them, only 28 patients had a good insonation window through the right temporal bone so that TCDP could collect data on the flow velocity through the middle cerebral artery. Three patients withdrew from the study for personal reasons.

Within 2 weeks, subjects were contacted by phone. Before the collection of any data, all 25 remaining patients signed an individual informed consent form. Then, they were invited to attend a first interview when demographic data were collected, neurological examination performed, and somatic examination. Then, all subjects were measured by body weight and height, blood pressure, ECG and ultrasound of the blood vessels of the neck. A TCCD was then made according to the study protocol. We found a control group among healthcare professionals and post-graduate students. The basic condition was that they did not have SARS-CoV-2 infection, that they were negative on a real-time reverse PCR test and serological test for IgG and IgM antibodies to SARS-CoV-2 virus, and that they did not have significant risk factors for cerebrovascular disease. They also were measured for body weight, height, and blood pressure, and we recorded their ECG and ultrasound of the blood vessels of the neck, and TCCD as study protocol demanded.

2.2. Methods

We conducted a cross-sectional observational study. From each participant, written informed consent was obtained. The Ethics Committee of the University Hospital Split approved this study in March 2021 (class 500-03/21-01/39, NO 2181-147-01/06M.S-20-02). The test group was made up of 25 was patients who had mild respiratory symptoms of SARS-CoV-2 infection and a positive result of real-time reverse PCR test at the time of infection. They all had post-infection non-specific neurological symptoms such as smell and taste dysfunction, vertigo, headache, dizziness, myalgias or fatigue. All subjects overcame SARS-CoV infection from 28 to 50 days before TCCD recording. The control group was 25 healthy volunteers (postgraduate students or healthcare workers) who had no symptoms of infectious SARS-CoV-2 disease and who were negative for real-time reverse PCR test and seronegative for SARS-CoV IgG and IgM antibodies. All subjects were enrolled in March 2021. All participants were Caucasian adults, aged 33–62 years. Participant data include: age, gender, height, weight, body mass index, history of smoking, history of alcohol drinking, regular drugs use, amount of physical activity, hypertension, diabetes, hyperlipidemia, coronary heart disease, atrial fibrillation and prior cerebrovascular disease. The amount of physical activity was assessed using the International Physical Activity Questionnaire and are expressed as a minutes of moderate physical activity per week. None of the subjects from the SARS-CoV-2 group were hospitalized or treated on an outpatient basis for SARS-CoV-2 pneumonia, and they were treated exclusively with supportive therapy for SARS-CoV-2 infection (they did not use antibiotics, oxygen therapy, antiviral drugs or corticosteroids). We excluded all patients with a history of uncontrolled hypertension, unregulated diabetes mellitus, cerebrovascular disease, hematologic disease, atrial fibrillation, chronic heart disease or cancer, severe alcohol consumption (more than 10 alcoholic drinks per week), known occlusive disease of cerebral arteries, stenosis of the vertebral artery or external carotid artery more than 20%. We excluded all patients using anticoagulant or vasodilator drugs, hormone replacement therapy, β-blocking agents and calcium channel blockers (Table 1). The two groups of subjects were matched for age, gender, body mass index, systolic and diastolic blood pressure and amount of physical activity. All participants performed somatic and neurological status, electrocardiography testing, blood pressure testing, extra cranial carotid artery ultrasound, and transcranial Doppler ultrasonography with breath-holding test. We performed all ultrasonic measurements using the Hitachi Aloca Arietta 70 Ultrasound system (2.0 MHz frequency transducer). All tests were performed after working hours, in a quiet and peaceful room, possible sources of sound and light interference were excluded, and the patient was lying in supine position. Transcranial Doppler ultrasonography was performed first in the resting phase which lasted 5 min, after which, participants hold their breath as long as they could. After the breath-holding period, the subject would breathe normally for 5 min. We repeated the procedure three times for of each participant. Blood flow signals were detected using a 2.0 MHz pulse probe at a depth of 52–64 mm via right temporal bone window. We insonated arteries with special focus on the right middle cerebral artery (MCA). Measurements in our study included peak systolic velocity (PSV), end diastolic velocity (EDV) and mean velocity (MV), resistance index (RI) and pulsatility index (PI) of right middle cerebral artery (MCA). We measured PSV, EDV, MV, RI and PI values on right MCA continuously during the rest and after the breath-holding period. We particularly focused on velocities at beginning of respiratory arrest and at the very end of the respiratory arrest period. We recorded the velocities at rest as PSV rest, EDV rest, MV rest, RI rest and PI rest and at the end of breath-holding period as PSV max, EDV max, MV max, RI max and PI max. Furthermore, we also measured the length of time for each subject to stop breathing (time of breath-holding—BHT). We determined the mean values of each variable in all three measurements. Vascular reactivity was determined upon calculating the breath holding index (BHI) as the percent of velocity increase from resting baseline values (PSVmax/PSVrest) divided by breath holding time (BHT).

Table 1. Inclusion and exclusion criteria.

Inclusion Criteria	Exclusion Criteria
Age from 30 to 65 years	Age under 30 and over 65 years
Mild form of respiratory SARS-CoV-2 disease	Severe or critical form of SARS-CoV-2 pulmonary infection
Non-specific neurological symptoms such as smell and taste dysfunction, vertigo, headache, dizziness or fatigue	Disturbance in consciousness, acute cerebrovascular disease (ischemic stroke, cerebral hemorrhage, subarachnoid hemorrhage), acute encephalopathy, encephalitis or meningitis, polyneuropathy, demyelinating spectrum of disease and seizures.
SARS-CoV infection from 30 to 60 days before TCCD recording	More than 60 days from infection start and TCCD recording
Treated exclusively with supportive therapy	Use of antibiotics, corticosteroids, oxygen for SARS-CoV-2 infection
Diagnosis confirmed by a positive result of real-time reverse PCR test by nasal/pharyngeal swabs	History of uncontrolled hypertension, nonregulated diabetes mellitus, cerebrovascular disease, hematologic disease, atrial fibrillation, chronic heart disease or cancer
	Severe alcohol consumption (more than 10 drinks per week)
	Stenosis of extracranial vertebrobasilar artery > 20%
	Stenosis of extracranial carotid artery > 20%.
For control group negative real time reverese PCR test by nasal/pharyngeal swabs Negative serological IgM and IgG test on SARS-CoV-2 virus	Known occlusive disease of intracranial cerebral arteries
No SARS-CoV-2 symptoms at all	Using anticoagulant drug, vasodilatory drugs, hormone replacement therapy, β-blocking agents, calcium channel blockers

2.3. Statistical Analysis

Statistical significance was set to $p < 0.05$ and all confidence intervals were given at the 95% level. For numeric variables Shapiro–Wilk test was used to indicate deviation from normal distribution. Numeric variables were presented by median (Q1–Q3) or by mean ± SD. Statistical significance of the differences of categorical variables was calculated by the chi-square test. Analysis of differences of numeric variables between two groups was carried out by the independent-samples T-test or by the Mann–Whitney U test. Analysis of differences between two measurements of numeric variables was carried out by paired-samples T-test. Statistical analysis was carried out by SPSS 20.

3. Results

3.1. Patient Characteristics and Measured Variables

Our study included 25 subjects who had nonspecific neurological symptoms after SARS-CoV-2 infection and 25 subjects in the control group. For each subject, we measured blood flow velocities through the midbrain artery: peak systolic velocity (PSV), end diastolic velocity (EDV), mean velocity (MV), and resistance indices (RI) and pulsation rate (PI). Velocities were measured at rest (PSVrest, EDVrest, MVrest, RIrest, PIrest) and three times after the breath-holding test (BHT) as PSVmax, EDVmax, MVmax, RImax, PImax. All examined quantitative variables (blood flow velocities through the middle cerebral artery) had a normal distribution according to the Kolmogorov–Smirnov test ($p > 0.05$), both in the group of subjects after SARS-CoV-2 infection and in the control group. There were no clinical or statistically significant differences ($p > 0.05$) between three repeated measurements after the breath-holding test (BHT) in the group of subjects after SARS-CoV-2 infection and in the control group, so we made an arithmetic mean of three measurements after the breath-holding test (BHT) for each subject and we used it in further analysis. Groups were aligned by gender ($\chi^2 = 0.089$; $p = 0.765$), age ($T = 0.388$; $p = 0.699$), body mass index—BMI ($T = 0.717$; $p = 0.477$), systolic arterial pressure ($T = 1.7$; $p = 0.099$), diastolic arterial pressure ($T = 1.5$; $p = 0.129$) and physical activity ($T = 0.472$, $p = 0.639$).

There were only seven diabetics in both groups. Out of the total number, there were only three hypertensive subjects. One participant had elevated blood lipids. One subject from each group drank more than 10 alcoholic beverages per week. In both groups, a total of seven subjects regularly smoked cigars (Table 2 shows demographic data and some of clinical parameters).

Table 2. Display of the number (%) of subjects according to qualitative data and arithmetic mean ± SD and quantitative data in relation to the examined groups (subjects after SARS-CoV-2 infection and subjects of the control group).

		Subject Groups		
		after SARS-CoV-2 Infection	Control Group	p
gender	Male	16 (64)	17 (68)	0.765 *
	Female	9 (36)	8 (32)	
diabetes		4 (16)	3 (12)	
hypertension		3 (12)	1 (4)	
hyperlipidemia		1 (4)	0 (0)	
alcohol		1 (4)	1 (4)	
smoking		4 (16)	3 (12)	
age (years)		46.6 ± 8.5	45.7 ± 7.4	0.699 **
BMI (kg/m^2)		25.6 ± 2.9	25 ± 2.8	0.477 **
RR systolic (mmHg)		126.7 ± 11.6	120.8 ± 13.1	0.099 **
RR diastolic (mmHg)		78.4 ± 9.6	74.6 ± 7.9	0.129 **
Physical activity (minutes per week of moderate activity)		179.3 ± 25	182 ± 15	0.639 **

* χ^2 test; ** T test.

3.2. Disease Symptoms in a Group of Subjects after SARS-CoV-2 Infection

In the group of subjects after SARS-CoV-2 infection, according to nonspecific neurological symptoms, anosmic symptoms had 14 (56%) subjects, dysgeusia was present in 14 (56%) subjects, 10 (40%) subjects had dizziness, 17 (68%) of them had headaches, 18 (72%) had fatigue and myalgia was present in 14 (56%) of participants. None of the subjects had symptoms of stroke, epileptic seizures, signs of meningoencephalitis, narrowing of consciousness movement disorders, demyelinating disease or acute polyradiculoneuritis. According to the general symptoms of the disease, all subjects had fever (25, 100%), (80%)

20 of them had a cough, 10 subjects had sore throats (40%), 2 subjects had gastrointestinal symptoms (8%) and 4 (16%) had a rash. None of the subjects had dyspnea. None of the subjects were hospitalized for symptoms associated with SARS-CoV-2 virus infection.

3.3. Comparison of Flow Velocities through Middle Cerebral Artery at Rest and after Breath-holding Test between Test Groups

Table 3 shows the values of flow velocities through the middle cerebral artery in relation to the groups of subjects.

Table 3. Representation of arithmetic means of flow velocities through middle cerebral artery and standard deviations (±SD) (95% CI) of these parameters.

	Subject Groups		
	after SARS-CoV-2 Infection	Controls	p *
Subjects at rest			
PSV (cm/s)	107 ± 12.7 (102–112)	120 ± 5.5 (117–122)	<0.001
EDV (cm/s)	51.9 ± 4.6 (50–54)	56.5 ± 5.5 (54–59)	0.002
MV (cm/s)	72.1 ± 7.3 (69–75)	81.3 ± 7.5 (78–84)	<0.001
RI	0.53 ± 0.02 (0.50–0.53)	0.55 ± 0.04 (0.53–0.57)	0.003
PI	0.77 ± 0.07 (0.74–0.79)	0.78 ± 0.05 (0.78–0.76)	0.396
Subjects after breath-holding test			
PSV (cm/s)	122 ± 11.3 (117–127)	162 ± 7.8 (158–165)	<0.001
EDV (cm/s)	69.3 ± 3.5 (68–71)	81 ± 5.5 (79–84)	<0.001
MV (cm/s)	94.7 ± 8.6 (91–98)	110.1 ± 5 (108–112)	<0.001
RI	0.53 ± 0.02 (0.52–0.54)	0.51 ± 0.01 (0.51.0.52)	<0.001
PI	0.78 ± 0.08 (0.74–0.81)	0.76 ± 0.04 (0.74–0.77)	0.300

Legend: PSV—peak systolic velocity, EDV—end-diastolic velocity, MV—mean flow velocity, RI—resistance index, PI—pulsatility index, T test for independent samples. * T test for independent samples.

3.4. Comparison of Velocities in Middle Cerebral Artery at Rest between Group of Subjects after SARS-CoV-2 Infection and Control Group

At the rest period, subjects after SARS-CoV-2 infection had statistically significantly lower all measured velocities parameters compared to control group except PI:
-lower PSV (T = 4.5; p < 0.001), arithmetic mean difference was 12.5 (95%CI; 6.8 to 18).
-lower EDV (T = 3.2; p = 0.002), arithmetic mean difference was 4.6 (95%CI; 1.7 to 7.5).
-lower MV (T = 4.4; p < 0.001), arithmetic mean difference was 9.2 (95%CI; 5 to 13.5).
-lower RI (T = 3.1; p = 0.003), arithmetic mean difference was 0.03 (95%CI 0.01 do 0.05).
We did not prove statistically significant difference for PI values (T = 0.856; p = 0.396). (Table 4).

3.5. Comparison of Flow Velocities through Middle Cerebral Artery after a Breath-Holding Test between Group of Subjects after SARS-CoV-2 Infection and a Control Group

After the breath-holding test, velocity parameters were higher than at the rest period for both groups, but the group of subjects after SARS-CoV-2 infection had statistically significantly lower all measured velocity parameters compared to the control group, except PI:
-lower PSV max (T = 14.3; 0 < 0.001), arithmetic mean difference was 39.4 (95%CI; 34 to 45).
-lower EDV max (T = 9.1; p < 0.001), arithmetic mean difference was 12 (95%CI; 9 to 14.6)
-lower MV max (T = 7.7; p < 0.001), arithmetic mean difference was 15.4 (95%CI; 11 to 19).
-lower RI max (T = 3.6; p = 0.001), arithmetic mean difference was 0.015 (95%CI; 0.006 to 0.023).

Table 4. The frequency of nonspecific neurological and general symptoms in subjects who had mild form of SARS-CoV-2 infection.

	Symptoms in SARS-CoV-2 Group	
Neurological Symptoms	SARS-CoV-2	Control
	n	n
Anosmia	14 (56)	0 (0)
Dysgeusia	14 (56)	0 (0)
Dizziness	10 (40)	0 (0)
Headache	17 (68)	0 (0)
Fatigue	18 (72)	0 (0)
Myalgia	14 (56)	0 (0)
Symptoms of infective disease		
Fever	25 (100)	0 (0)
Cough	20 (80)	0 (0)
Sore throat	10 (40)	0 (0)
Gastrointestinal symptoms	2 (24)	0 (0)
Rash	4 (8)	0 (0)
Dyspnea	0 (0)	0 (0)

After the breath-holding test, there was no statistically significant difference of PI max value between the two groups (T = 1.05; $p < 0.300$) (Table 5).

Table 5. Median (Q1–Q3) presentation of changes in flow velocities rates through middle cerebral artery after breath-holding test and rest period in relation to groups of subjects.

	Subjects Groups		
	after SARS-CoV-2 Infection	Controls	p
Relative change of velocities parameters after breath-holding test compared to values at resting period (%)			
ΔPSV (%)	14 (11–19)	34 (32–39)	<0.001
ΔEDV (%)	36 (30–38)	42 (35–50)	0.010
ΔMV (%)	31 (26–38)	36 (25–41)	0.222
ΔRI (%)	1.4 (−0.6 to 3.9)	−5 (−12 to −2)	<0.001
ΔPI (%)	2.3 (0–3.3)	−4 (−6 to 1.4)	0.013
Breath holding index (BHI)	0.426 (0.28–0.57)	0.98 (0.81–1.12)	<0.001

Legend: PSV—peak systolic velocity, EDV—end-diastolic velocity, MV—mean flow velocity, RI—resistance index, PI—pulsatility index.

The mean value of breath holding time in both groups was 37 ± 4 s (minimum 29 to maximum 47); there was no statistically significant difference between the two groups of subjects (T = 0.951; $p = 0.346$) (Table 5).

3.6. Comparison of Changes in Flow Velocities through Middle Cerebral Artery after Breath-Holding Test and Rest Period between Two Examined Groups and Breath Holding Index (BHI)

Mann–Whitney U Test

After the breath-holding test, relative increases in flow velocities in the control group were statistically significantly greater than in the group of subjects after SARS-CoV-2 infection for PSV (2.4 times higher, median difference was 20 (95% CI: 15.4–23.04) (z = 6.01; $p < 0.001$) and EDV (1.2 times higher, median differences was 6 (95% CI: −0.38 to 13.54) (z = 2.6; $p = 0.010$). From these two parameters, we calculated the breath holding index, and that index was statistically significantly higher in control subjects compared to subjects who had SARS-CoV-2 infection. The median difference was 0.55 (95%CI; 0.41–0.69) (z = 6; $p < 0.001$).

3.7. Correlation of Flow Velocities through Middle Cerebral Artery with Age of the Subjects in Each Group

We did not prove a statistically significant correlation between examined flow velocities through the middle cerebral artery in relation to age of the subjects in both examined groups. Pearson's correlation coefficient for age was for RI $r = -0.031$, for PI, the correlation coefficient was $r = -0.075$, for PSV, the correlation coefficient was $r = -0.048$, for EDV, the correlation coefficient was $r = 0.115$, and for MV, the correlation coefficient was $r = -0.252$.

3.8. Correlation of Changes in Flow Velocities Parameters through Middle Cerebral Artery in Relation to Time from Onset of Symptoms

The median time from onset of symptoms of SARS-CoV-2 virus infection and TCCD measurements was 36 days (minimum–maximum: 28 to 50 days). We did not prove a statistically significant association of flow velocities parameters through the middle cerebral artery with time from onset of SARS-CoV-2 virus infection. All Spearman correlation coefficients were less than 0.4, $p > 0.05$.

3.9. Correlation of Flow Velocities through Middle Cerebral Artery with Gender of the Subjects after SARS-CoV-2 Infection

We did not prove a statistically significant correlation between the examined flow velocities through the middle cerebral artery in the rest period (PSV; $t = 1.19$, $p = 0.244$, EDV; $t = 0.082$, $p = 0.935$, MV; $t = 0.427$, $p = 0.673$, RI; $t = 0.154$, $p = 0.879$, PI; $t = 0.228$, $p = 0.822$) and after breath-holding test (PSV; $t = 1.151$, $p = 0.260$, EDV; $t = 0.104$, $p = 0.918$, MV; $t = 0.379$, $p = 0.708$, RI: $t = 0.347$, $p = 0.732$, PI; $t = 0.628$, $p = 0.536$) in relation to the gender of the subjects in SARS-CoV-2 group.

4. Discussion

To date, there has been no study investigating cerebral vasoreactivity in patients after SARS-CoV-2 infection. In our study, we showed that patients even after mild SARS-CoV-2 infection have impaired cerebral vasoreactivity. Values of flow velocities through the middle cerebral artery at the rest period and after breath-holding test were statistically significantly lower in subjects who had SARS-CoV-2 infection than in the control group. A smaller relative increase in PSV and EDV values in the group of subjects with SARS-CoV-2 infection leads to a consequent lower breath holding index (BHI) which directly indicates impaired vasoreactivity and weaker vasoconstriction response to hypercarbia in patients after SARS-CoV-2 infection. We did not prove a statistically significant correlation between examined flow velocities through the middle cerebral artery in relation to age, gender or with time from the onset of SARS-CoV-2 virus infection symptoms.

Romero-Sanchez et al. in their study showed that neurologic manifestations are very common in hospitalized patients with SARS-CoV-2 infection and more than half of them (57.4%) developed some form of neurologic symptom [22]. Nonspecific symptoms were present mostly in the early stages and in less severe cases, and anosmia and dysgeusia were common as a first clinical manifestation of SARS-CoV-2 disease. Serious neurologic complications were less frequent but can cause death in about 4.1% patients. In our study, we recruited subjects from the outpatient clinic's database so there were no serious neurological complications, no one was hospitalized, and due to mild and nonspecific neurological symptoms, examination was one month after the onset of infection. According to the data from this study, the most common nonspecific neurological symptoms in our study were dysgeusia (56%), anosmia (56%), headache (68%) and fatigue (72%).

Hernandez-Fernandez et al. showed in their study [12] that endothelial disruption is the primary mechanism of damage in SARS-CoV-2 patients who had cerebeovascular disease related to infection. Thrombotic microangiopathy, loss of vasoreactivity, increased bleeding predisposition and increased hypercoagulability along with systemic complications were the cause for poor clinical prognosis of these patients. SARS-CoV-2 patients who had cerebrovascular disease had an unfavorable clinical outcome (73.9% of them had modified Rankin score 4–6), and a high mortality rate (34.8%). Age was the only independent predictive factor of poor prognosis and it was a high incidence of large vessel occlusion (58.8%), and unexpectedly, many strokes were in the vertebrobasilar location (35.3%). As our subjects had mild symptoms of SARS-CoV-2 infection, both general and neurological, cerebral vasoreactivity disorder is an expression of SARS-CoV-2 virus neurotropicity and impaired endothelial function.

Chen et al. studied the frequency of neurological symptoms and complications in SARS-CoV-2 patients [23], and concluded that headache, dizziness, taste and smell dysfunctions were the most frequently reported neurological symptoms with an overall frequency of greater than 4% of the populations studied. In our study, it was not possible to determine the real prevalence of mild neurological symptoms because the database was outpatient clinic-based and did not necessarily reflect the incidence of neurologic complications of patients with SARS-CoV-2 in the community. However, the most common symptoms in the Chen et al. study were the most common also in our subjects.

The basic task of the cerebral arteries is to ensure a sufficient supply of nutrients and energy for the brain. The anatomical and functional organization of cerebral blood flow allows brain perfusion to be stable even in conditions of increased energy demand. The Willis circuit allows an anatomical and small vessel network system allows a functional aspect of physiological reserve. The basic principle of cerebral vasoreactivity is the dilatation of small blood vessels, which increase flow velocities through large basal arteries [24]. TCCD is a useful tool for the assessment of flow velocities in the large brain arteries [25] and to indirectly estimate cerebrovascular reserve capacity, as Widder showed in his book [26]. Flow velocities through large cerebral arteries increase after the breath-holding test, which induces hypercarbia and hypoxia [27]. The middle cerebral artery is suitable for examining these parameters, because most of the flow through the cerebral arteries goes through that large blood vessel.

SARS-CoV-2 virus binds to angiotensin converting enzyme 2 receptors for entry into cells, a receptor which can be found in numerous brain cells: neurons, glial cells, vascular endothelium and smooth muscle [28]. For example, in their study, Al-Ramadan et al. found that SARs-CoV-2 virus can cause both acute and long-term neurological complications in many patients [29]. Cerebrovascular disease in SARS-CoV-2 infection, according to Al-Ramadan et al., might be due to SARS-CoV-2 dysregulation of the renin–angiotensin system (RAS) by acting on ACE2 receptors, direct infection of the endothelial cell which can results in endothelial dysfunction and impaired cerebral vasoreactivity. Like other virus infections, the SARS-CoV-2 virus can cause severe endothelial dysfunction. Pavicic Ivelja et al. found that chronic hepatitis C patients have altered cerebrovascular reactivity and these negative effects on cerebrovascular hemodynamics could contribute to the increased risk of cerebrovascular disease [30]. Chow et al. found similar changes in patients with HIV infection and their cerebrovascular endothelial dysfunction may independently contribute to cognitive impairment [31]. Our study of SARS-CoV-2 subjects clearly showed impaired cerebrovascular reactivity, which had negative effects on cerebrovascular hemodynamics and can increase the risk of cerebrovascular disease. It is significant that subjects from the SARS-CoV-2 group did not have significant risk factors for cerebrovascular disease. Impaired vasoreactivity, and a weaker response to hypercarbia after the breath-holding test in patients after SARS-CoV-2 infection may lead to decreased vascular capacity and vascular reserve, especially in conditions of increased demand [32,33].

Transcranial color Doppler is a non-invasive, cheap and reproducible method, and it has been used for a long time in clinical practice for monitoring for cerebral vasospasm following subarachnoid hemorrhage, evaluation occlusive cerebrovascular disease and the detection of cerebral microembolic signals. It also can be used to identify patients with exhausted cerebrovascular reserve and for the assessment of cerebral autoregulation, as we showed in our study. In previous studies, TCCD has been shown to be a good method for assessing brain vasoreactivity in studies for patients with cerebrovascular disease, like Silvestrini et al. found in their study [33]. They concluded that alterations in cerebral hemodynamic function may play a relevant role in the occurrence of stroke in patients with carotid artery disease. Silvestrini et al. also concluded that the reduction in the BHI values strongly increases the probability of occurrence of a cerebrovascular ischemic event. All these studies have shown that the reduction in vasodilatatory capacity leads to the reduction in vascular adaptability and can be a precursor for the development of cerebrovascular disease [34–36]. Similar studies have not yet been published with SARS-CoV-2 patients and this is the first such study to occur during this pandemic. TCCD with the addition of the breath-holding test brings added value for these patients because induced hypercarbia increases the susceptibility to vasoreactivity disorder. There are no biological markers to accurately assess brain vasoreactivity and TCCD is a reliable method for assessing that. These patients, in the future, can be severely affected due to the inability to respond to conditions of increased cerebral perfusion demand, due to a lack of vascular reserve [37,38]. These patients are at increased risk of developing stroke [5,39], but also at increased risk that the ischemic zone is bigger than in patients with preserved vascular reserve [40,41]. Cerebral vasoreactivity can also be impaired in neurodegenerative diseases. Urbanova et al. in their study showed [42] that decreased cerebrovascular reserve capacity and altered vasoreactivity can be found in patients with Alzheimer's disease as a sign of microangiopathy even without severe underlying atherosclerosis and it can be identified using TCCD along with the breath-holding test (BHI). Shim et al. found in their study that underlying microangiopathy can be a mechanism in Alzheimer's disease patients and showed there was an association between the impaired function of cerebral microvessels and cognitive impairment [43]. Espino-Ojeda et al. in their study found that Parkinson's disease patients are prone to exhibit diminished cerebrovascular reserve and altered cerebral vasoreactivity in comparison with healthy individuals [44]. In the future, we need additional vasoreactivity studies, we need to monitor patients with impaired vasoreactivity, and we need rigorous and systematic longitudinal follow up. Time is our ally, and future studies should be performed on a larger number of patients if we want to prevent the possible numerous neurological complications of this pandemic.

The main limitation to this study is the small number of subjects included in both groups. The SARS-CoV-2 virus pandemic has significantly changed the work of the overall health care system, and also the neurological outpatient clinic, and there are certainly more patients who have nonspecific neurological symptoms and who need to be examined by a neurologist, but they were not registered in the hospital system at the time we recruited our subjects. Additionally, a short period of time had passed since the onset of the SARS-CoV-2 symptoms in our subjects, so the long-term consequences of impaired vasoreactivity have yet to be investigated through systematic longitudinal follow-up. One of the limiting factors of the study is TCCD itself as a method of assessing brain vasoreactivity, because the quality of the findings largely depends on the quality of the temporal bone window through which the middle cerebral artery is insonated. The hemodynamic effect of breath holding is lower than that of carbon dioxide inhalation or acetazolamide injection. All TCCD testing in our study was carried out by one examiner who has 15 years of experience working with TCCD, and thus we avoided a possible interpersonal difference depending on the experience of the examiner.

5. Conclusions

Neurological manifestations prior, during and after SARS-CoV-2 virus infection are increasingly diagnosed but pathophysiologically are not fully understood. The physicians must consider nonspecific neurological symptoms as a clear sign of virus neurotropism. The long-term effect of the neuroinvasive potential of the SARS-CoV-2 virus may increase the risk of cerebrovascular disease. In this study, we have showed that patients after SARS-CoV-2 virus infection had significantly lower average peak systolic, end-diastolic and mean velocity values at the end of the breath-holding procedure. Additionally, the breath holding index was significantly lower in the SARS-CoV-2 group than in the healthy control group. It is a direct expression of impaired cerebral artery vasoreactivity in patients with neurological symptoms after overcoming mild respiratory SARS-CoV-2 infection.

Cerebral vasoreactivity disorder points to a damaged mechanism of brain vasoregulation and indicates patients who without other risk factors will be predisposed for cerebrovascular disease. Such patients should be identified, properly selected and treated to reduce possible major health problems. Additional studies are needed to determine the association of neurological symptoms after SARS-CoV-2 infection and changes in cerebral artery vasoreactivity, as well as the impact of time on these changes.

Author Contributions: Conceptualization, M.M., L.M., B.M., V.C. and K.V.; formal analysis, M.M., L.M., B.M., V.C. and K.V.; methodology, M.M., L.M., B.M., V.C. and K.V.; writing—original draft, M.M., L.M., B.M., V.C. and K.V.; writing—review and editing, M.M., L.M., B.M., V.C. and K.V. All authors have read and agreed to the published version of the manuscript.

Funding: This research received no external funding.

Institutional Review Board Statement: The study was conducted according to the guidelines of the Declaration of Helsinki and approved by the Institutional Review Board (or Ethics Committee) of Ethics Committee of University Hospital Center Split (class 500-03/21-01/39, NO 2181-147-01/06M.S-20-02, March 2021). The study was conducted according to the guidelines of the Declaration of Helsinki, Patient Rights Protection Act (NN 169/04), Law on the Implementation of the General Regulation on Data Protection (NN42/18), Croatian Code of Medical Ethics and Deontology (NN55/08, 139/15).

Informed Consent Statement: Informed consent was obtained from all subjects involved in the study.

Conflicts of Interest: The authors declare no conflict of interest.

References

1. Desforges, M.; Le Coupanec, A.; Dubeau, P.; Bourgouin, A.; Lajoie, L.; Dubé, M.; Talbot, P.J. Human Coronaviruses and Other Respiratory Viruses: Underestimated Opportunistic Pathogens of the Central Nervous System? *Viruses* **2019**, *12*, 14. [CrossRef]
2. Shrestha, G.S.; Khanal, S.; Sharma, S.; Nepal, G. COVID-19: Current Understanding of Pathophysiology. *J. Nepal Health Res. Counc.* **2020**, *18*, 351–359. [CrossRef] [PubMed]
3. Yuki, K.; Fujiogi, M.; Koutsogiannaki, S. COVID-19 pathophysiology: A review. *Clin. Immunol.* **2020**, *215*, 108427. [CrossRef] [PubMed]
4. Helms, J.; Kremer, S.; Merdji, H.; Clere-Jehl, R.; Schenck, M.; Kummerlen, C.; Collange, O.; Boulay, C.; Fafi-Kremer, S.; Ohana, M.; et al. Neurologic Features in Severe SARS-CoV-2 Infection. *N. Engl. J. Med.* **2020**, *382*, 2268–2270. [CrossRef]
5. Mao, L.; Jin, H.; Wang, M.; Hu, Y.; Chen, S.; He, Q.; Chang, J.; Hong, C.; Zhou, Y.; Wang, D.; et al. Neurologic Manifestations of Hospitalized Patients With Coronavirus Disease 2019 in Wuhan, China. *JAMA Neurol.* **2020**, *77*, 683. [CrossRef]
6. Iadecola, C.; Anrather, J.; Kamel, H. Effects of COVID-19 on the Nervous System. *Cell* **2020**, *183*, 16–27.e1. [CrossRef]
7. Baig, A.M.; Khaleeq, A.; Ali, U.; Syeda, H. Evidence of the COVID-19 Virus Targeting the CNS: Tissue Distribution, Host–Virus Interaction, and Proposed Neurotropic Mechanisms. *ACS Chem. Neurosci.* **2020**, *11*, 995–998. [CrossRef]
8. Paterson, R.W.; Brown, R.L.; Benjamin, L.; Nortley, R.; Wiethoff, S.; Bharucha, T.; Jayaseelan, D.L.; Kumar, G.; Raftopoulos, R.; Zambreanu, L.; et al. The emerging spectrum of COVID-19 neurology: Clinical, radiological and laboratory findings. *Brain* **2020**, *143*, 3104–3120. [CrossRef]
9. Mohkhedkar, M.; Venigalla, S.S.K.; Janakiraman, V. Autoantigens That May Explain Postinfection Autoimmune Manifestations in Patients With Coronavirus Disease 2019 Displaying Neurological Conditions. *J. Infect. Dis.* **2021**, *223*, 536–537. [CrossRef]
10. Levi, M.; Thachil, J.; Iba, T.; Levy, J.H. Coagulation abnormalities and thrombosis in patients with COVID-19. *Lancet Haematol.* **2020**, *7*, e438–e440. [CrossRef]
11. Iba, T.; Connors, J.M.; Levy, J.H. The coagulopathy, endotheliopathy, and vasculitis of COVID-19. *Inflamm. Res.* **2020**, *69*, 1181–1189. [CrossRef]
12. Hernández-Fernández, F.; Valencia, H.S.; Barbella-Aponte, R.A.; Collado-Jiménez, R.; Ayo-Martín, Ó.; Barrena, C.; Molina-Nuevo, J.D.; García-García, J.; Lozano-Setién, E.; Alcahut-Rodriguez, C.; et al. Cerebrovascular disease in patients with COVID-19: Neuroimaging, histological and clinical description. *Brain* **2020**, *143*. [CrossRef] [PubMed]
13. Mehta, P.; McAuley, D.F.; Brown, M.; Sanchez, E.; Tattersall, R.S.; Manson, J.J. COVID-19: Consider cytokine storm syndromes and immunosuppression. *Lancet* **2020**, *395*, 1033–1034. [CrossRef]
14. Wang, E.Y.; Mao, T.; Klein, J.; Dai, Y.; Huck, J.D.; Liu, F.; Zheng, N.S.; Zhou, T.; Israelow, B.; Wong, P.; et al. Diverse Functional Autoantibodies in Patients with COVID-19. *medRxiv* **2020**. [CrossRef]
15. Garkowski, A.; Zajkowska, J.; Moniuszko, A.; Czupryna, P.; Pancewicz, S. Infectious causes of stroke. *Lancet Infect. Dis.* **2015**, *15*, 632. [CrossRef]

16. Staszewski, J.; Skrobowska, E.; Piusińska-Macoch, R.; Brodacki, B.; Stępień, A. Cerebral and Extracerebral Vasoreactivity in Patients with Different Clinical Manifestations of Cerebral Small-Vessel Disease: Data from the Significance of Hemodynamic and Hemostatic Factors in the Course of Different Manifestations of Cerebral Small-Vessel Disease Study. *J. Ultrasound Med.* **2019**, *38*, 975–987. [CrossRef]
17. Zavoreo, I.; Demarin, V. Breath holding index in the evaluation of cerebral vasoreactivity. *Acta Clin. Croat.* **2004**, *43*, 15–20.
18. Sam, K.; Peltenburg, B.; Conklin, J.; Sobczyk, O.; Poublanc, J.; Crawley, A.P.; Mandell, D.M.; Venkatraghavan, L.; Duffin, J.; Fisher, J.A.; et al. Cerebrovascular reactivity and white matter integrity. *Neurology* **2016**, *87*, 2333–2339. [CrossRef]
19. Markus, H.S.; Harrison, M.J. Estimation of cerebrovascular reactivity using transcranial Doppler, including the use of breath-holding as the vasodilatory stimulus. *Stroke* **1992**, *23*, 668–673. [CrossRef] [PubMed]
20. Lavi, S.; Gaitini, D.; Milloul, V.; Jacob, G. Impaired cerebral CO2 vasoreactivity: Association with endothelial dysfunction. *Am. J. Physiol. Circ. Physiol.* **2006**, *291*, H1856–H1861. [CrossRef]
21. World Health Organization. Clinical Management of COVID-19. Available online: https://www.who.int/publications/i/item/clinical-management-of-covid-19 (accessed on 22 June 2020).
22. Romero-Sánchez, C.M.; Díaz-Maroto, I.; Fernández-Díaz, E.; Sánchez-Larsen, Á.; Layos-Romero, A.; García-García, J.; González, E.; Redondo-Peñas, I.; Perona-Moratalla, A.B.; Del Valle-Pérez, J.A.; et al. Neurologic manifestations in hospitalized patients with COVID-19: The ALBACOVID registry. *Neurology* **2020**, *95*, e1060–e1070. [CrossRef] [PubMed]
23. Chen, X.; Laurent, S.; Onur, O.A.; Kleineberg, N.N.; Fink, G.R.; Schweitzer, F.; Warnke, C. A systematic review of neurological symptoms and complications of COVID-19. *J. Neurol.* **2021**, *268*, 392–402. [CrossRef] [PubMed]
24. Birns, J.; Jarosz, J.; Markus, H.S.; Kalra, L. Cerebrovascular reactivity and dynamic autoregulation in ischaemic subcortical white matter disease. *J. Neurol. Neurosurg. Psychiatry* **2009**, *80*, 1093–1098. [CrossRef] [PubMed]
25. Aaslid, R.; Markwalder, T.-M.; Nornes, H. Noninvasive transcranial Doppler ultrasound recording of flow velocity in basal cerebral arteries. *J. Neurosurg.* **1982**, *57*, 769–774. [CrossRef]
26. Widder, B. Cerebral vasoreactivity. In *Cerebrovascular Ultrasound: Theory, Practice and Future Developments*; Hennerici, M., Meairs, S., Eds.; Cambridge University Press: Cambridge, UK, 2001; pp. 324–334.
27. Settakis, G.; Lengyel, L.; Molnar, C.; Bereczki, D.; Csiba, L.; Fulesdi, B. Transcranial Doppler study of the cerebral hemodynamic changes during breath-holding and hyperventilation tests. *J. Neuroimaging* **2002**, *12*, 252–258. [CrossRef]
28. Xia, H.; Lazartigues, E. Angiotensin-converting enzyme 2 in the brain: Properties and future directions. *J. Neurochem.* **2008**, *107*, 1482–1494. [CrossRef]
29. Al-Ramadan, A.; Rabab'H, O.; Shah, J.; Gharaibeh, A. Acute and Post-Acute Neurological Complications of COVID-19. *Neurol. Int.* **2021**, *13*, 102–119. [CrossRef] [PubMed]
30. Ivelja, M.P.; Ivic, I.; Dolic, K.; Mestrovic, A.; Perkovic, N.; Jankovic, S. Evaluation of cerebrovascular reactivity in chronic hepatitis C patients using transcranial color Doppler. *PLoS ONE* **2019**, *14*, e0218206. [CrossRef]
31. Chow, F.C.; Boscardin, W.J.; Mills, C.; Ko, N.; Carroll, C.; Price, R.W.; Deeks, S.; Sorond, F.A.; Hsue, P.Y. Cerebral vasoreactivity is impaired in treated, virally suppressed HIV-infected individuals. *AIDS* **2016**, *30*, 45–55. [CrossRef]
32. Martinić-Popović, I.; Simundic, A.-M.; Dukic, L.; Lovrencic-Huzjan, A.; Popovic, A.; Šerić, V.; Basic-Kes, V.; Demarin, V. The association of inflammatory markers with cerebral vasoreactivity and carotid atherosclerosis in transient ischaemic attack. *Clin. Biochem.* **2014**, *47*, 182–186. [CrossRef] [PubMed]
33. Silvestrini, M.; Vernieri, F.; Pasqualetti, P.; Matteis, M.; Passarelli, F.; Troisi, E.; Caltagirone, C. Impaired Cerebral Vasoreactivity and Risk of Stroke in Patients With Asymptomatic Carotid Artery Stenosis. *JAMA* **2000**, *283*, 2122–2127. [CrossRef] [PubMed]
34. D'Andrea, A.; Conte, M.; Cavallaro, M.; Scarafile, R.; Riegler, L.; Cocchia, R.; Pezzullo, E.; Carbone, A.; Natale, F.; Santoro, G.; et al. Transcranial Doppler ultrasonography: From methodology to major clinical applications. *World J. Cardiol.* **2016**, *8*, 383–400. [CrossRef]
35. Pindzola, R.R.; Balzer, J.R.; Nemoto, E.M.; Goldstein, S.; Yonas, H. Cerebrovascular reserve in patients with carotid occlusive disease assessed by stable xenon-enhanced ct cerebral blood flow and transcranial Doppler. *Stroke* **2001**, *32*, 1811–1817. [CrossRef]
36. Schramm, P.; Klein, K.U.; Falkenberg, L.; Berres, M.; Closhen, D.; Werhahn, K.J.; David, M.; Werner, C.; Engelhard, K. Impaired cerebrovascular autoregulation in patients with severe sepsis and sepsis-associated delirium. *Crit. Care* **2012**, *16*, R181. [CrossRef] [PubMed]
37. Castro, P.; Azevedo, E.; Sorond, F. Cerebral Autoregulation in Stroke. *Curr. Atheroscler. Rep.* **2018**, *20*, 37. [CrossRef]
38. Diehl, R.R. Cerebral autoregulation studies in clinical practice. *Eur. J. Ultrasound* **2002**, *16*, 31–36. [CrossRef]
39. Xiong, L.; Liu, X.; Shang, T.; Smielewski, P.; Donnelly, J.; Guo, Z.-N.; Yang, Y.; Leung, T.; Czosnyka, M.; Zhang, R.; et al. Impaired cerebral autoregulation: Measurement and application to stroke. *J. Neurol. Neurosurg. Psychiatry* **2017**, *88*, 520–531. [CrossRef]
40. Li, Y.; Wang, M.; Zhou, Y.; Chang, J.; Xian, Y.; Mao, L.; Hong, C.; Chen, S.; Wang, Y.; Wang, H.; et al. Acute Cerebrovascular Disease Following COVID-19: A Single Center, Retrospective, Observational Study. *Stroke Vasc. Neurol.* **2020**, *5*, 279–284. [CrossRef] [PubMed]
41. Gupta, A.; Chazen, J.L.; Hartman, M.; Delgado, D.; Anumula, N.; Shao, H.; Mazumdar, M.; Segal, A.Z.; Kamel, H.; Leifer, D.; et al. Cerebrovascular reserve and stroke risk in patients with carotid stenosis or occlusion: A systematic review and meta-analysis. *Stroke* **2012**, *43*, 2884–2891. [CrossRef]

42. Urbanova, B.S.; Schwabova, J.P.; Magerova, H.; Jansky, P.; Markova, H.; Vyhnalek, M.; Laczo, J.; Hort, J.; Tomek, A. Reduced Cerebrovascular Reserve Capacity as a Biomarker of Microangiopathy in Alzheimer's Disease and Mild Cognitive Impairment. *J. Alzheimer's Dis.* **2018**, *63*, 465–477. [CrossRef]
43. Shim, Y.; Yoon, B.; Shim, D.S.; Kim, W.; An, J.-Y.; Yang, D.-W. Cognitive Correlates of Cerebral Vasoreactivity on Transcranial Doppler in Older Adults. *J. Stroke Cerebrovasc. Dis.* **2015**, *24*, 1262–1269. [CrossRef]
44. Espino-Ojeda, A.; Martínez-Rodríguez, H.; Escamilla-Garza, J.; Canfield-Medina, H.; Saldívar-Dávila, S.; Góngora-Rivera, F. Cerebral vasoreactivity in Parkinson's disease. *J. Neurol. Sci.* **2015**, *357* (Suppl. 1), e264. [CrossRef]

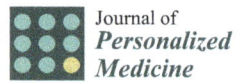

Article

Breast Cancer Screening during COVID-19 Emergency: Patients and Department Management in a Local Experience

Francesca Maio [1], Daniele Ugo Tari [2], Vincenza Granata [3], Roberta Fusco [3], Roberta Grassi [4], Antonella Petrillo [3,*] and Fabio Pinto [1]

[1] Department of Radiology, Marcianise Hospital, Caserta Local Health Authority, Viale Sossietta Scialla, 81025 Marcianise, Italy; francescamaio9@gmail.com (F.M.); fpinto1966@libero.it (F.P.)
[2] Department of Breast Radiology, Caserta Local Health Authority Dictrict 12, Viale Paul Harris 79, 81100 Caserta, Italy; medicina@danieletari.com
[3] Department of Radiology, Istituto Nazionale Tumori IRCCS Fondazione G.Pascale di Napoli, Via Mariano Semmola 53, 80131 Naples, Italy; v.granata@istitutotumori.na.it (V.G.); r.fusco@istitutotumori.na.it (R.F.)
[4] Department of Radiology, Università degli Studi della Campania "Luigi Vanvitelli", Piazza Miraglia, 80138 Naples, Italy; robertagrassi89@gmail.com
* Correspondence: a.petrillo@istitutotumori.na.it

Abstract: Background: During the COVID-19 public health emergency, our breast cancer screening activities have been interrupted. In June 2020, they resumed, calling for mandatory safe procedures to properly manage patients and staff. Methods: A protocol supporting medical activities in breast cancer screening was created, based on six relevant articles published in the literature and in the following National and International guidelines for COVID-19 prevention. The patient population, consisting of both screening and breast ambulatory patients, was classified into one of four categories: 1. Non-COVID-19 patient; 2. Confirmed COVID-19 in an asymptomatic screening patient; 3. suspected COVID-19 in symptomatic or confirmed breast cancer; 4. Confirmed COVID-19 in symptomatic or confirmed breast cancer. The day before the radiological exam, patients are screened for COVID-19 infection through a telephone questionnaire. At a subsequent in person appointment, the body temperature is checked and depending on the clinical scenario at stake, the scenario-specific procedures for medical and paramedical staff are adopted. Results: In total, 203 mammograms, 76 breast ultrasound exams, 4 core needle biopsies, and 6 vacuum-assisted breast biopsies were performed in one month. Neither medical nor paramedical staff were infected on any of these occasions. Conclusion: Our department organization model can represent a case of implementation of National and International guidelines applied in a breast cancer screening program, assisting hospital personnel into COVID-19 infection prevention.

Keywords: COVID-19; breast cancer screening; guideline; breast cancer; screening; pandemic

Citation: Maio, F.; Tari, D.U.; Granata, V.; Fusco, R.; Grassi, R.; Petrillo, A.; Pinto, F. Breast Cancer Screening during COVID-19 Emergency: Patients and Department Management in a Local Experience. J. Pers. Med. 2021, 11, 380. https://doi.org/10.3390/jpm11050380

Academic Editor: Franco M. Buonaguro

Received: 31 March 2021
Accepted: 4 May 2021
Published: 6 May 2021

Publisher's Note: MDPI stays neutral with regard to jurisdictional claims in published maps and institutional affiliations.

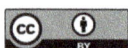

Copyright: © 2021 by the authors. Licensee MDPI, Basel, Switzerland. This article is an open access article distributed under the terms and conditions of the Creative Commons Attribution (CC BY) license (https://creativecommons.org/licenses/by/4.0/).

1. Introduction

On 30 January 2020, the World Health Organization (WHO) officially declared the COVID-19 (coronavirus disease '19) epidemic, caused by the virus SARS-CoV-2, a public health emergency and then, on 11 March 2020, officially declared the global situation as a pandemic [1,2]. WHO data report 83 million confirmed cases worldwide since the start of the outbreak and 1,8 million deaths (data as of 5 January 2021). As of 7 January 2021, 2,220,000 cases, including 77,291 deaths, had been confirmed in Italy and reported to the WHO [2,3]. One of the predominant transmission mechanisms of the virus is through droplet particles. Other transmission mechanisms include contact with infected surfaces touched by people who, without a sufficient disinfection of the hands, then touch their own mouth, nose or eyes [1]. People are often infectious 2–3 days before they exhibit symptoms [4], so the proportion of pre-symptomatic transmission ranges from 48% to

62% [4]. Spreading by asymptomatic carriers is estimated at 25% [5]. Moreover, the use of symptoms-based screening does not alone provide protection for all people [5].

At the same time, routine breast imaging, such as a mammogram or a breast ultrasound (US) examination, requires very close contact with patients with no chances for physical distancing. When performing these exams, the patient's face may be as close as 20–30 cm to the face of the radiologist and/or the radiographer performing the study [6]. Similarly, during US, stereotactic and MRI-guided breast procedures, including biopsies, drainages and clip placements, the interventional radiologist may be distanced at only 30 cm from the patient's face. In fact, it has been reported that the risk of infection with the novel coronavirus progressively increases with physical proximity and prolonged contact with people with COVID-19 [6,7].

Unfortunately, during the outbreak, breast screening activities were interrupted, whereas only emergency cancer-related medical activities were performed. Since June 2020, as the severity of the disease's infection rate reduced in our country, screening activities have been resumed. This raised the need for a protocol to guide specialists on measures to prevent COVID-19 infection and to optimize resources with the aim of ensuring the best service level in breast cancer screening. Accordingly, the aim of the present study was to propose a protocol for managing our daily screening activities in order to ward mitigate infection spread.

2. Methods

Our department operational plan was based on the master opinion of three radiologists, members of the Italian Society of Radiology and Interventional Radiology (SIRM), which are routinely involved into Italian National Healthcare Service. They identified two different categories of patients referred to the Radiology Breast Unit Department and depicted four possible clinical scenarios.

The department operational plan was drafted following both the national and international guidelines for COVID-19 prevention and those for breast unit organization. Moreover, the plan is supported by a comprehensive literature comprising relevant articles searched using the mesh terms "COVID-19 OR SARS-CoV 2" AND "Screening" AND "Management" AND "Breast Imaging".

Overall, 6 articles, published between March and July 2020, were selected based on their relevance with respect to the primary endpoint (Figure 1). A summary of key findings was created for each of the relevant articles.

According to the essential levels of care [9,10], these are the two kinds of patient categories which attend the radiology breast imaging department:

Outline of Patients Categories

1. Breast screening patients:
   (a) Asymptomatic patients who undergo mammography exam following the specific screening program, according to national regulations.
   (b) Patients with suspected breast lesion revealed through the mammographic exam, thus needing to complete the work-up with ultrasound and needle biopsy.
2. Breast ambulatory patients:
   (a) Patients who have to complete the mammography work-up with ultrasound, following the surgeon recommendation.
   (b) Symptomatic breast cancer patients (new onset palpable nodule; skin or nipple retraction; orange peel skin; unilateral secretion from the nipple).

During the COVID-19 emergency for each of the above categories of patients, the following clinical scenarios can be delineated:

Outline of Clinical Scenarios

- Non-COVID-19 patient;
- Confirmed COVID-19 in asymptomatic screening patient;
- Suspected COVID-19 in symptomatic or confirmed breast cancer patient;

• Confirmed COVID-19 in symptomatic or confirmed breast cancer patient.

```
                    PubMed Results
Items 1-6 of 6 (Display the 6 citations in PubMed)

1. Clinical course of coronavirus disease-2019 in pregnancy.
   Pereira A, Cruz-Melguizo S, Adrien M, Fuentes L, Marin E, Perez-
   Medina T.
   Acta Obstet Gynecol Scand. 2020 Jul;99(7):839-847. doi:
   10.1111/aogs.13921. Epub 2020 Jun 10.
   PMID: 32441332    Free PMC article.

2. Care of the pregnant woman with coronavirus disease 2019 in labor
   and delivery: anesthesia, emergency cesarean delivery, differential
   diagnosis in the acutely ill parturient, care of the newborn, and
   protection of the healthcare personnel.
   Ashokka B, Loh MH, Tan CH, Su LL, Young BE, Lye DC, Biswas A,
   Illanes SE, Choolani M.
   Am J Obstet Gynecol. 2020 Jul;223(1):66-74.e3. doi:
   10.1016/j.ajog.2020.04.005. Epub 2020 Apr 10.
   PMID: 32283073    Free PMC article.

3. [Breast cancer management during the COVID 19 pandemic: The
   CNGOF takes action].
   Mathelin C, Nisand I.
   Gynecol Obstet Fertil Senol. 2020 Jun;48(6):473-474. doi:
   10.1016/j.gofs.2020.04.008. Epub 2020 Apr 19.
   PMID: 32320812    Free PMC article.    French.
   No abstract available.

4. Tor Vergata University-Hospital in the Beginning of COVID-19-Era:
   Experience and Recommendation for Breast Cancer Patients.
   Buonomo OC, Materazzo M, Pellicciaro M, Caspi J, Piccione E, Vanni
   G.
   In Vivo. 2020 Jun;34(3 Suppl):1661-1665. doi: 10.21873/invivo.11958.
   PMID: 32503826

5. [Breast cancer screening and diagnosis at the end of the COVID-19
   confinement period, practical aspects and prioritization rules:
   recommendations of 6 French health professionals societies].
   Ceugnart L, Delaloge S, Balleyguier C, Deghaye M, Veron L,
   Kaufmanis A, Mailliez A, Poncelet E, Lenczner G, Verzaux L, Gligorov
   J, Thomassin-Naggara I.
   Bull Cancer. 2020 Jun;107(6):623-628. doi:
   10.1016/j.bulcan.2020.04.006. Epub 2020 May 7.
   PMID: 32416925    Free PMC article.    French.
   No abstract available.

6. Breast Cancer Surgery During the COVID-19 Pandemic: An
   Observational Clinical Study of the Breast Surgery Clinic at Ospedale
   Policlinico San Martino - Genoa, Italy.
   Fregatti P, Gipponi M, Giacchino M, Sparavigna M, Murelli F, Toni ML,
   Calabrò MT, Orsino L, Friedman D.
   In Vivo. 2020 Jun;34(3 Suppl):1667-1673. doi: 10.21873/invivo.11959.
   PMID: 32503827    Clinical Trial.
```

Figure 1. PubMed literature search using the mesh terms "COVID-19 OR SARS-CoV 2" AND "Screening" AND "Management" and "Breast Imaging" [8].

2.1. Practice Organization in the Radiology Breast Screening Department

Since the 3 June, when screening activities resumed, following the guidelines proposed by the SIRM Italian College of Breast Radiologists [11], the overall schedule of screening patients was split as follows: (1) patients who received a screening invitation before the COVID-19 pandemic onset within three months from the previous appointment were progressively scheduled; (2) symptomatic patients and those needing a needle biopsy for suspected cancer which were given an appointment with urgency (patients from group 1b and 2b, as shown above), were called back in order to complete the diagnostic pathway within 3 days; (3) ambulatory patients with previous appointments, were re-scheduled progressively for a dedicated day of the week. The time lapse between the exams was 30 min, with a total of 15 mammograms/ultrasounds per day. Moreover, a specific day per week was dedicated to ambulatory patients either for mammography or for breast ultrasound. Furthermore, a whole day was dedicated to breast interventional radiology, including core needle biopsy and vacuum-assisted breast biopsy. The "one-stop approach" was not applied in our department. The staff daily shift was organized as follows: 2 radiologists, 3 technicians and 1 nurse per shift, for a maximum of one shift (8 h) per day.

2.2. Infection Prevention in a Radiology Breast Screening Department

According to the recommendations of national legislation ISS COVID-19 n. 1/2020 [12] and the WHO recommendations set on February 2020 [2], which were properly adapted to our local requirements (refer to Figure 2), all patients had to undergo a telephone triage with a dedicated radiographer on the day before the radiologic exam. The pool of questions, fully reported in Table 1, was asked again and evaluated by the radiologist before the exam was performed. Body temperature measurement was performed for each patient before entering the hospital. Each appointment was scheduled every 30 min, in order to allow enough time for the exam execution, possible additional imaging (i.e., magnification views or spot views), and for the equipment's disinfection and air ventilation (10 min). Patient capacity in the waiting room was set at a maximum of two people. An entrance and an exit door were designated, so to optimize the use of spaces and avoid interaction with subsequent patients. Moreover, to prevent the infection by SARS-CoV-2 of both medical and paramedical staff and other patients, more procedures could be adopted, depending on the different clinical scenario below:

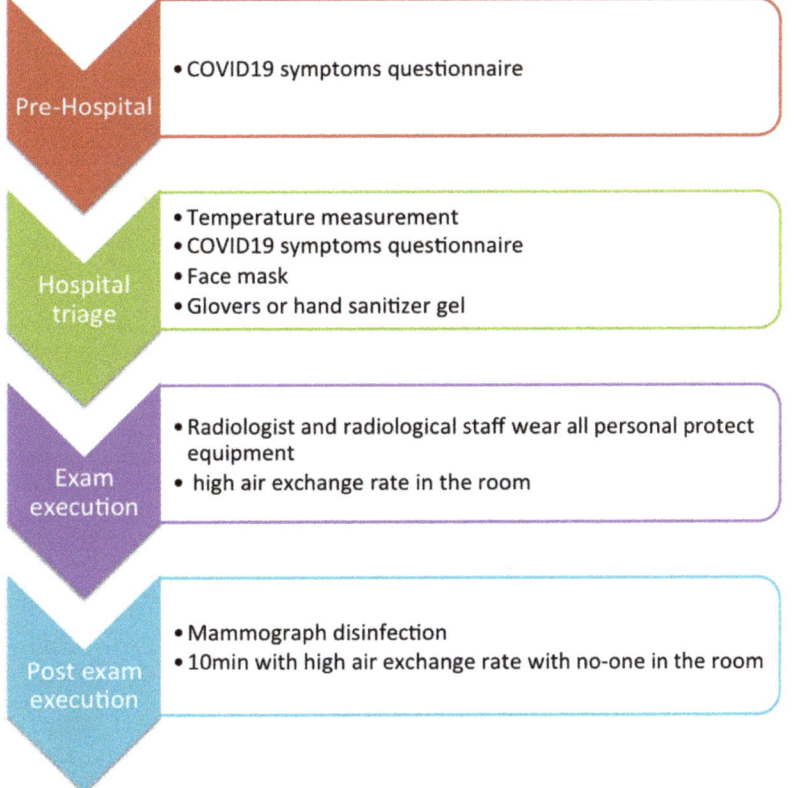

Figure 2. Patients and department management.

Table 1. Clinical assessment checklist the telephone questionnaire used to screen patients for COVID-19 infection before the radiological exam.

Questions	Yes	No
Do you have fever at the moment?		
Do you have cough?		
Did you have dyspnea or any respiratory disease, recently?		
Did you have anosmia or dysgeusia symptoms, recently?		
Did you have diarrhea, recently?		
Did you have unusual fatigue, recently?		
Did you have rash or ophthalmological disorders, recently?		
Have you done COVID-19 serology test?	If yes, ask for the test's result	
Have you performed nasopharyngeal swab for COVID-19?	If yes, ask for the test's result	

If any answer results positive, the patient will not be admitted to attend the radiological exam and rescheduled after a complete health evaluation made by his general practitioner doctor.

- *Non-COVID-19 patient:* Patients without COVID-19 infection, as laboratory-confirmed by a reverse transcriptase-polymerase chain reaction (RT-PCR) test, were defined as non-COVID-19 patients [13]. However, since the laboratory tests had not yet been used as a screening tool to identify COVID-19 patients and many people may be asymptomatic or pauci-symptomatic, it would be appropriate for health professionals to consider all patients as if they were infected [14]. Therefore, all patients must wear a surgical mask and maintain the minimum distance of 1 m from others while waiting for a radiological procedure. No one, including any accompanying person, is allowed to stay in the waiting room. The healthcare staff should a wear surgical mask, avoid direct contact with patient's oral and respiratory secretions, wear goggles or face shields and gloves and also wash hands before wearing and after removing gloves. A surgical cap and shoe covers are welcome. The ultrasound probe should be protected by a dedicated cover and disinfected after every single procedure [14–16]. After each radiological exam, the room and the radiological equipment must be cleaned and disinfected with chloro-derivate solutions and the room should be appropriately ventilated (>25 cycles/h) [14,17,18].
- *Confirmed COVID-19 in asymptomatic screening patient*: Considering the highly contagious nature of SARS-CoV-2, and taking count that this category of patients has no urgency to perform the mammographic exam, their appointments were rescheduled, as soon as was possible, after two negative nasopharyngeal swabs for SARS-CoV-2 RT-PCR test.
- *Suspected COVID-19 in symptomatic or confirmed breast cancer patient:* As in the first scenario, the patient must wear a surgical mask and follow the rules of social distancing in the waiting room. Radiological staff should wear an FFP2 mask (filtering face piece), goggles or face shield, gloves and cap. Ultrasound and mammographic machines must be covered by a plastic sheet and disinfected after the procedure with chloro-derivate solutions and the room should be appropriately ventilated (>25 cycles/h) [14,18].
- *Confirmed COVID-19 in symptomatic or confirmed breast cancer patient:* Considering the highly contagious nature of SARS-CoV-2, the patient wears a surgical mask and stays isolated from other people. Radiological staff must wear an FFP3 mask, eye protection, impermeable full-length long-sleeved gown, gloves and cap. Staff will pay maximum attention to the dressing and undressing procedures, as suggested by the Spallanzani Hospital [19]. Ultrasound and mammographic machines have to be covered by a plastic sheet and disinfected after the procedure with chloro-derivate solutions and the room should be appropriately ventilated (>25 cycles/h) [14,15,18].

Medical and paramedical staff were screened every month with a nasopharyngeal swab for SARS-CoV-2 RT-PCR test.

3. Results

Since 8 March 2020, 310 previously scheduled exams (267 breast screening and 43 breast ambulatory patients) were initially postponed because of the pandemic outbreak. Between 9 March and 29 May 2020, seven mammographic exams and two breast USs were performed for *ambulatory patients* identified as urgent/symptomatic for breast cancer. None of them resulted as confirmed breast cancer. One of them resulted as a suspected COVID-19 patient at the incoming triage.

Therefore, since the screening activities were resumed, those pending appointments were rescheduled, as soon as was possible, following the operational model above. In total, 205/267 previous appointments were rescheduled; 62/267 patients were no longer interested in having a screening appointment and were mostly scared by the SARS-CoV-2 infection risk. Some additional 50 new patients started regularly scheduling for breast cancer screening. In conclusion, 255 patients were screened in a month (3 June–3 July). Overall, 203 mammographic exams were performed, out of which 24/203 underwent a second-look US. In 52 cases, a breast US exam was performed as the first control. Moreover, four patients needed a core needle biopsy and six a vacuum-assisted breast biopsy: four patients were treated with subsequent surgery. No locally advanced breast cancer stage, such as: cancer >5 cm, or with skin/chest muscles infiltration, or multiple local lymph nodes invasion or a rapidly growing type [20], was revealed in the patients whose appointments had been postponed. All of the 255 patients who underwent breast cancer screening exams resulted as *non-COVID-19 patients* at the previous triage.

Until December 2020, 1479 *screening patients* received a mammographic exam. Of these patients, 163/1479 underwent a second-look US, 86 patients needed a core needle biopsy and 74 patients performed a vacuum-assisted breast biopsy. A total of 83 patients were treated with subsequent surgery. Overall, 15 *asymptomatic screening patients* resulted as *confirmed COVID-19 infections* at the telephone triage.

Moreover, in the same time interval, 174 *ambulatory patients* were screened by breast US. Among the 174 patients, 26 were symptomatic for breast cancer, out of which 9/26 received surgery for confirmed breast cancer. Among the 26, 5 symptomatic breast cancer patients were *suspected COVID-19* cases at previous triage. As of December 2020, no ambulatory patients were classified as *confirmed COVID-19* in symptomatic or confirmed breast cancer *patient*.

As for the matter of safety, a total of five radiologists, five technicians and one nurse were screened for SARS-CoV-2 between the beginning of March and the end of December, as described above. Each of them performed a total of 10 nasopharyngeal swabs. Nobody from the medical and paramedical staff resulted as positive to SARS-CoV-2 RT-PCR test.

4. Discussion

Our prospective study demonstrates efficacy in terms of continuity in the provision of an essential level of care in breast cancer screening. Furthermore, the absence of medical and paramedical staff SARS-CoV-2 infection is an additional fact that proofs the effectiveness of the infection prevention procedures adopted.

Due to the COVID-19 public health emergency outbreak, breast cancer units across the Italian territory have suffered significant restrictions and reductions in their clinical activities. Breast cancer is the first leading cause of cancer disease in the female population in Italy, with more than 50,000 breast cancer diagnosed every year and, out of which, 5000 are early breast cancer (infiltrating cancer <1 cm or ductal carcinoma in situ) [21]. The national screening program has improved the prognosis of patients with breast cancer by approximately 87% in 5 years, resulting in a lower number of tumors at the advanced stage (about 30%) [22]. The incidence rate reduction represents, also, a resource for our health system in terms of adjuvant therapy reduction, surgery duration, early return to work and improvement of the life quality standards. The estimated doubling time of breast cancer ranges between 45 and 260 days [23]. The latter growth rate variability did not allow us to estimate, precisely, the impact on not invited patients at breast cancer screening during the COVID-19 outbreak. A recent study compared breast unit activity in the first half of 2020 to the same time period on 2019 [24]. It reported an increased number of referrals either for diagnostic exams in suspected breast cancer patients (estimated around 28%) or for patients who received their first treatment for a breast cancer diagnosis (estimated around 16%) [24]. However, as reported in the literature [11], a short delay (e.g., 6–12 weeks) should not, in principle, affect the overall outcome. Furthermore, considering the periodical interruption/continuation of breast cancer screening activities, following the SARS-CoV-2 spread of infection in the population, these effects could be considerable on the female population. Vanni et al. [25] have estimated that 50% of the 11,000 cases will be identified with a delay of only 6 months, associated to a cancer stage progression. Moreover, they report that 8125 breast cancer diagnoses could be missed due to a screening interruption of 3 months [25]. This delayed diagnosis has several consequences, such as: an increase in the number of patients needing a diagnostic paths and treatments; a more invasive breast surgery or neoadjuvant or adjuvant therapy with a worse patient outcome; and an increase in healthcare costs. Therefore, some centers suggest a personalized screening program activity, which could be applied on urgent patients [22] or on patients with a high risk of breast cancer [26]. However, it is already known that its effectiveness in terms of incremental cost-effectiveness ratio (ICER) and quality adjusted life years (QALY) as well as its application during outbreaks could reduce their effect on women's health [27]. Consequently, an optimized and effective department organization, which allows continuing screening and preserves the regular breast cancer-related medical activities, is achievable, especially in consideration of the unpredictable COVID-19 pandemic evolution. Moreover, continuing breast cancer screening during a pandemic emergency will avoid having to raise assistance requests at the end of the lockdown period [28].

To the best of our knowledge, national and international guidelines on breast cancer treatment in patients with SARS-CoV-2 infection have not yet been updated. Thus, nowadays, breast cancer patients with confirmed COVID-19 have to wait 10 days and two negative nasopharyngeal swabs before surgery [29], which may result in a worsened situation.

Some centers [28] suggest PCR testing before breast interventional procedures in patient with a BIRADS 5 lesion, such as to reduce the waiting time before surgery. However, this would increase the cost of each procedure, and additionally, the waiting time (from 20 min to 2 h) before each interventional procedure [30–51]. Consequently, it would increase the time lapse between the exams with a reduced number of procedures accomplished per day.

In our experience, our proposed model has proven a contraction of the waiting lists in a few weeks and also, has not been reported cases of advanced breast cancer stage.

Furthermore, a well standardized and SARS-CoV-2-free model is desirable to reduce the time lapse between the diagnoses and the treatment, avoiding the lengthening of waiting lists.

In conclusion, as little is known about the pandemic evolution, especially of its duration, the impact on screening breast cancer could be worse than reported. Therefore, our protocol, used to manage patients and radiological staff, could serve as a best practice in the application of national and international guidelines in the domain of the breast cancer screening program. If largely disseminated, it could assist specialists in preventing COVID-19 infection and in optimizing resources for breast cancer screening diagnosis.

Author Contributions: Conceptualization: F.M., V.G. and A.P. Investigation: F.M. and R.G. Methodology: F.M., V.G and A.P. Validation: D.U.T. and F.P. Visualization: D.U.T., R.F. and F.M. Data curation: R.F. Writing—original draft: F.M. Project administration: F.P. Writing—review: F.P. Supervision: F.P. All authors have read and agreed to the published version of the manuscript.

Funding: This research received no external funding.

Institutional Review Board Statement: Institutional Review Institute (IRB) is not applicable considering the retrospective nature of the study without patient data.

Informed Consent Statement: Written informed consent has been obtained from the patient(s) to publish this paper before any radiological exam either mammography or US and before any interventional procedure.

Data Availability Statement: The reported data come from SANIARP.it, the ASL Caserta reporting database and from the register of our daily activities.

Acknowledgments: This research and its authors did not receive any specific grant neither from funding agencies in the public, commercial, nor from not-for-profit sectors or any other provider.

Conflicts of Interest: The authors declare no conflict of interest.

Abbreviations

WHO	World Health Organization
COVID-19	coronavirus disease '19
SARS-CoV-2	severe acute respiratory syndrome coronavirus 2
US	ultrasound
SIRM	Italian Society of Radiology and Interventional Radiology
MRI	magnetic resonance imaging
RT-PCR	reverse transcriptase-polymerase chain reaction
FFP	filtering face piece
BIRADS	breast imaging reporting and data system

References

1. Lake, M.A. What we know so far: COVID-19 current clinical knowledge and research. *Clin. Med.* **2020**, *20*, 124–127. [CrossRef] [PubMed]
2. World Health Organization. Coronavirus Disease (COVID-19) Pandemic. 2020. Available online: https://www.who.int/emergencies/diseases/novel-coronavirus-2019 (accessed on 26 November 2020).
3. Salute M della. Ministero della Salute. Available online: http://www.salute.gov.it/portale/home.html (accessed on 26 November 2020).
4. He, X.; Lau, E.H.Y.; Wu, P.; Deng, X.; Wang, J.; Hao, X.; Lau, Y.C.; Wong, J.Y.; Guan, Y.; Tan, X.; et al. Temporal dynamics in viral shedding and transmissibility of COVID-19. *Nat. Med.* **2020**, *26*, 672–675. [CrossRef]
5. Kimball, A.; Hatfield, K.M.; Arons, M.; James, A.; Taylor, J.; Spicer, K.; Bardossy, A.C.; Oakley, L.P.; Tanwar, S.; Chisty, Z.; et al. Asymptomatic and Presymptomatic SARS-CoV-2 Infections in Residents of a Long-Term Care Skilled Nursing Facility—King County, Washington, March 2020. *MMWR. Morb. Mortal. Wkly. Rep.* **2020**, *69*, 377–381. [CrossRef] [PubMed]
6. Lu, M. The Front Line: Visualizing the Occupations with the Highest COVID-19 Risk. Visual Capitalist 2020. Available online: https://www.visualcapitalist.com/the-front-line-visualizing-the-occupations-with-the-highest-covid-19-risk/ (accessed on 15 April 2020).
7. Granata, V.; Fusco, R.; Izzo, F.; Setola, S.V.; Coppola, M.; Grassi, R.; Reginelli, A.; Cappabianca, S.; Petrillo, A. Covid-19 infection in cancer patients: The management in a diagnostic unit. *Radiol. Oncol.* **2021**, *1*, 1–9. [CrossRef]
8. National Library of Medicine. PubMed.gov. Available online: https://pubmed.ncbi.nlm.nih.gov/ (accessed on 26 June 2020).
9. Torbica, A.; Fattore, G. The "Essential Levels of Care" in Italy: When being explicit serves the devolution of powers. *Eur. J. Heal. Econ.* **2005**, *6*, 46–52. [CrossRef] [PubMed]
10. Salute M della. Screening per il Tumore della Mammella. Available online: http://www.salute.gov.it/portale/salute/p1_5.jsp?lingua=italiano&id=23&area=Screening (accessed on 21 April 2020).
11. Pediconi, F.; Galati, F.; Bernardi, D.; Belli, P.; Brancato, B.; Calabrese, M.; Camera, L.; Carbonaro, L.A.; Caumo, F.; Clauser, P.; et al. Breast imaging and cancer diagnosis during the COVID-19 pandemic: Recommendations from the Italian College of Breast Radiologists by SIRM. *Radiol. Med.* **2020**, *125*, 926–930. [CrossRef] [PubMed]
12. Salute M della. Nuovo Coronavirus. Available online: http://www.salute.gov.it/nuovocoronavirus?gclid=EAIaIQobChMIz_rmnZPP6gIVgrTtCh0M6wYPEAAYASAAEgKY0fD_BwE (accessed on 21 April 2020).
13. Cozzi, D.; Albanesi, M.; Cavigli, E.; Moroni, C.; Bindi, A.; Luvarà, S.; Lucarini, S.; Busoni, S.; Mazzoni, L.N.; Miele, V. Chest X-ray in new Coronavirus Disease 2019 (COVID-19) infection: Findings and correlation with clinical outcome. *Radiol. Med.* **2020**, *125*, 730–737. [CrossRef]
14. Too, C.W.; Wen, D.W.; Patel, A.; Syafiq, A.R.A.; Liu, J.; Leong, S.; Gogna, A.; Lo, R.H.G.; Tashi, S.; Lee, K.A.; et al. Interventional Radiology Procedures for COVID-19 Patients: How we Do it. *Cardiovasc. Interv. Radiol.* **2020**, *43*, 827–836. [CrossRef]
15. Checklist for Preparing Your IR Service for COVID-19. Available online: https://www.cirse.org/wp-content/uploads/2020/04/cirse_APSCVIR_Checklist_COVID19_prod.pdf (accessed on 27 March 2020).

16. Modalità di Comportamento per L'effettuazione di un Esame Ecografico in Questo Momento Pandemico Su. Available online: https://www.sirm.org/wp-content/uploads/2020/03/Modalita%CC%80-di-comportamento-per-l%E2%80%99effettuazione-di-un-esame-ecografico-.pdf.pdf (accessed on 22 March 2020).
17. Jin, Y.-H.; Cai, L.; Cheng, Z.-S.; Cheng, H.; Deng, T.; Fan, Y.-P.; Fang, C.; Huang, D.; Huang, L.-Q.; Huang, Q.; et al. A rapid advice guideline for the diagnosis and treatment of 2019 novel coronavirus (2019-nCoV) infected pneumonia (standard version). *Mil. Med. Res.* **2020**, *7*, 4. [CrossRef]
18. Coccolini, F.; Perrone, G.; Chiarugi, M.; Di Marzo, F.; Ansaloni, L.; Scandroglio, I.; Marini, P.; Zago, M.; De Paolis, P.; Forfori, F.; et al. Surgery in COVID-19 patients: Operational directives. *World J. Emerg. Surg.* **2020**, *15*, 1–7. [CrossRef]
19. Pianura, E.; Stefano, F.D.; Cristofaro, M.; Petrone, A.; Albarello, F.; Fusco, N.; Schininà, V. COVID-19: A review of the literature and the experience of INMI Lazzaro Spallanzani two months after the epidemic outbreak. *J. Radiol. Rev.* **2020**, *7*, 196–207. [CrossRef]
20. Yeh, E.D.; Jacene, H.A.; Bellon, J.R.; Nakhlis, F.; Birdwell, R.L.; Georgian-Smith, D.; Giess, C.S.; Hirshfield-Bartek, J.; Overmoyer, B.; van den Abbeele, A.D.; et al. What Radiologists Need to Know about Diagnosis and Treatment of Inflammatory. Breast Cancer: A Multidisciplinary Approach. *RadioGraphics* **2013**, *33*, 2003–2017. [CrossRef] [PubMed]
21. I 5 Tumori Più Frequenti in Italia Nel 2019. Available online: http://www.salute.gov.it/imgs/C_17_notizie_3897_4_file.pdf (accessed on 21 January 2020).
22. Buonomo, O.C.; Materazzo, M.; Pellicciaro, M.; Caspi, J.; Piccione, E.; Vanni, G. Tor Vergata University-Hospital in the Beginning of COVID-19-Era: Experience and Recommendation for Breast Cancer Patients. *In Vivo* **2020**, *34*, 1661–1665. [CrossRef] [PubMed]
23. Bleicher, R.J. Timing and Delays in Breast Cancer Evaluation and Treatment. *Ann. Surg. Oncol.* **2018**, *25*, 2829–2838. [CrossRef]
24. Gathani, T.; Clayton, G.; MacInnes, E.; Horgan, K. The COVID-19 pandemic and impact on breast cancer diagnoses: What happened in England in the first half of 2020. *Br. J. Cancer* **2021**, *124*, 710–712. [CrossRef]
25. Vanni, G.; Pellicciaro, M.; Materazzo, M.; Bruno, V.; Oldani, C.; Pistolese, C.A.; Buonomo, C.; Caspi, J.; Gualtieri, P.; Chiaravalloti, A.; et al. Lockdown of Breast Cancer Screening for COVID-19: Possible Scenario. *In Vivo* **2020**, *34*, 3047–3053. [CrossRef]
26. Cancino, R.S.; Su, P.; Mesa, R.E.; Tomlinson, G.; Wang, J. The Impact of COVID-19 on Cancer Screening: Challenges and Opportunities. *JMIR Cancer* **2020**, *6*, e21697. [CrossRef]
27. Román, M.; Sala, M.; Domingo, L.; Posso, M.; Louro, J.; Castells, X. Personalized breast cancer screening strategies: A systematic review and quality assessment. *PLoS ONE* **2019**, *14*, e0226352. [CrossRef]
28. Salem, C.; Hajj, M.-A.; Kourié, H.; Haddad, A.; Khaddage, A.; Ayoub, E.N.; Jabbour, K.; Moubarak, M.; Atallah, D. Radiology management of a 'breast unit' during COVID-19 pandemic: A single institution experience. *Future Oncol.* **2020**, *16*, 2917–2922. [CrossRef]
29. Rocco, N.; Montagna, G.; Di Micco, R.; Benson, J.; Criscitiello, C.; Chen, L.; Di Pace, B.; Colmenarejo, A.J.E.; Harder, Y.; Karakatsanis, A.; et al. The Impact of the COVID-19 Pandemic on Surgical Management of Breast Cancer: Global Trends and Future Perspectives. *Oncologist* **2021**, *26*, 66–67. [CrossRef]
30. Mantellini, P.; Battisti, F.; Armaroli, P.; Giubilato, P.; Ventura, L.; Zorzi, M.; Battagello, J.; de Bianchi, P.S.; Senore, C.; Zappa, M. Ritardati maturati dai programmi di screening oncologici ai tempi del COVID-19 in Italia, velocità della ripartenza e sti-ma dei possibili ritardi diagnostici [Oncological organized screening programmes in the COVID-19 era: An Italian survey on accrued delays, reboot velocity, and diagnostic delay estimates]. *Epidemiol. Prev.* **2020**, *44*, 344–352.
31. Carotti, M.; Salaffi, F.; Sarzi-Puttini, P.; Agostini, A.; Borgheresi, A.; Minorati, D.; Galli, M.; Marotto, D.; Giovagnoni, A. Chest CT features of coronavirus disease 2019 (COVID-19) pneumonia: Key points for radiologists. *Radiol. Med.* **2020**, *125*, 636–646. [CrossRef]
32. Shaw, B.; Daskareh, M.; Gholamrezanezhad, A. The lingering manifestations of COVID-19 during and after convalescence: Update on long-term pulmonary consequences of coronavirus disease 2019 (COVID-19). *Radiol. Med.* **2021**, *126*, 40–46. [CrossRef] [PubMed]
33. Belfiore, M.P.; Urraro, F.; Grassi, R.; Giacobbe, G.; Patelli, G.; Cappabianca, S.; Reginelli, A. Artificial intelligence to codify lung CT in Covid-19 patients. *Radiol. Med.* **2020**, *125*, 500–504. [CrossRef] [PubMed]
34. Borghesi, A.; Maroldi, R. COVID-19 outbreak in Italy: Experimental chest X-ray scoring system for quantifying and monitoring disease progression. *Radiol. Med.* **2020**, *125*, 509–513. [CrossRef] [PubMed]
35. Di Serafino, M.; Notaro, M.; Rea, G.; Iacobellis, F.; Paoli, V.D.; Acampora, C.; Ianniello, S.; Brunese, L.; Romano, L.; Vallone, G. The lung ultrasound: Facts or artifacts? In the era of COVID-19 outbreak. *Radiol. Med.* **2020**, *125*, 738–753. [CrossRef]
36. Giovagnoni, A. Facing the COVID-19 emergency: We can and we do. *Radiol. Med.* **2020**, *125*, 337–338. [CrossRef]
37. Brogna, B.; Bignardi, E.; Brogna, C.; Volpe, M.; Lombardi, G.; Rosa, A.; Gagliardi, G.; Capasso, P.; Gravino, E.; Maio, F.; et al. A Pictorial Review of the Role of Imaging in the Detection, Management, Histopathological Correlations, and Complications of COVID-19 Pneumonia. *Diagnostics* **2021**, *11*, 437. [CrossRef]
38. Neri, E.; Miele, V.; Coppola, F.; Grassi, R. Use of CT and artificial intelligence in suspected or COVID-19 positive patients: Statement of the Italian Society of Medical and Interventional Radiology. *Radiol. Med.* **2020**, *125*, 505–508. [CrossRef]
39. Borghesi, A.; Zigliani, A.; Masciullo, R.; Golemi, S.; Maculotti, P.; Farina, D.; Maroldi, R. Radiographic severity index in COVID-19 pneumonia: Relationship to age and sex in 783 Italian patients. *Radiol. Med.* **2020**, *125*, 461–464. [CrossRef]

40. Gatti, M.; Calandri, M.; Barba, M.; Biondo, A.; Geninatti, C.; Gentile, S.; Greco, M.; Morrone, V.; Piatti, C.; Santonocito, A.; et al. Baseline chest X-ray in coronavirus disease 19 (COVID-19) patients: Association with clinical and laboratory data. *Radiol. Med.* **2020**, *125*, 1271–1279. [CrossRef]
41. Agostini, A.; Floridi, C.; Borgheresi, A.; Badaloni, M.; Pirani, P.E.; Terilli, F.; Ottaviani, L.; Giovagnoni, A. Proposal of a low-dose, long-pitch, dual-source chest CT protocol on third-generation dual-source CT using a tin filter for spectral shaping at 100 kVp for CoronaVirus Disease 2019 (COVID-19) patients: A feasibility study. *Radiol. Med.* **2020**, *125*, 365–373. [CrossRef]
42. Caruso, D.; Polici, M.; Zerunian, M.; Pucciarelli, F.; Polidori, T.; Guido, G.; Rucci, C.; Bracci, B.; Muscogiuri, E.; De Dominicis, C.; et al. Quantitative Chest CT analysis in discriminating COVID-19 from non-COVID-19 patients. *Radiol. Med.* **2021**, *126*, 243–249. [CrossRef]
43. Palmisano, A.; Scotti, G.M.; Ippolito, D.; Morelli, M.J.; Vignale, D.; Gandola, D.; Sironi, S.; De Cobelli, F.; Ferrante, L.; Spessot, M.; et al. Chest CT in the emergency department for suspected COVID-19 pneumonia. *Radiol. Med.* **2021**, *126*, 498–502. [CrossRef]
44. Grassi, R.; Belfiore, M.P.; Montanelli, A.; Patelli, G.; Urraro, F.; Giacobbe, G.; Fusco, R.; Granata, V.; Petrillo, A.; Sacco, P.; et al. COVID-19 pneumonia: Computer-aided quantification of healthy lung parenchyma, emphysema, ground glass and consolidation on chest computed tomography (CT). *Radiol. Med.* **2020**. [CrossRef]
45. Cappabianca, S.; Fusco, R.; De Lisio, A.; Paura, C.; Clemente, A.; Gagliardi, G.; Lombardi, G.; Giacobbe, G.; Russo, G.M.; Belfiore, M.P.; et al. Correction to: Clinical and laboratory data, radiological structured report findings and quantitative evaluation of lung involvement on baseline chest CT in COVID-19 patients to predict prognosis. *Radiol. Med.* **2021**, *126*, 29–39. [CrossRef]
46. Giannitto, C.; Sposta, F.M.; Repici, A.; Vatteroni, G.; Casiraghi, E.; Casari, E.; Ferraroli, G.M.; Fugazza, A.; Sandri, M.T.; Chiti, A.; et al. Chest CT in patients with a moderate or high pretest probability of COVID-19 and negative swab. *Radiol. Med.* **2020**, *125*, 1260–1270. [CrossRef]
47. Lombardi, A.F.; Afsahi, A.M.; Gupta, A.; Gholamrezanezhad, A. Severe acute respiratory syndrome (SARS), Middle East respiratory syndrome (MERS), influenza, and COVID-19, beyond the lungs: A review article. *Radiol. Med.* **2021**, *126*, 561–569. [CrossRef]
48. Ierardi, A.M.; Wood, B.J.; Arrichiello, A.; Bottino, N.; Bracchi, L.; Forzenigo, L.; Andrisani, M.C.; Vespro, V.; Bonelli, C.; Amalou, A.; et al. Preparation of a radiology department in an Italian hospital dedicated to COVID-19 patients. *Radiol. Med.* **2020**, *125*, 894–901. [CrossRef]
49. Fichera, G.; Stramare, R.; De Conti, G.; Motta, R.; Giraudo, C. It's not over until it's over: The chameleonic behavior of COVID-19 over a six-day period. *Radiol. Med.* **2020**, *125*, 514–516. [CrossRef]
50. Reginelli, A.; Grassi, R.; Feragalli, B.; Belfiore, M.; Montanelli, A.; Patelli, G.; La Porta, M.; Urraro, F.; Fusco, R.; Granata, V.; et al. Coronavirus Disease 2019 (COVID-19) in Italy: Double Reading of Chest CT Examination. *Biology* **2021**, *10*, 89. [CrossRef]
51. Grassi, R.; Fusco, R.; Belfiore, M.P.; Montanelli, A.; Patelli, G.; Urraro, F.; Petrillo, A.; Granata, V.; Sacco, P.; Mazzei, M.A.; et al. Coronavirus disease 2019 (COVID-19) in Italy: Features on chest computed tomography using a structured report system. *Sci. Rep.* **2020**, *10*, 1–11. [CrossRef]

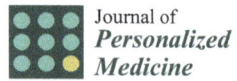

Article

Special Attention to Physical Activity in Breast Cancer Patients during the First Wave of COVID-19 Pandemic in Italy: The DianaWeb Cohort

Valentina Natalucci [1], Milena Villarini [2,*], Rita Emili [3], Mattia Acito [2], Luciana Vallorani [1], Elena Barbieri [1,*] and Anna Villarini [4]

1. Department of Biomolecular Sciences, University of Urbino Carlo Bo, 61029 Urbino, Italy; valentina.natalucci@uniurb.it (V.N.); luciana.vallorani@uniurb.it (L.V.)
2. Department of Pharmaceutical Sciences, University of Perugia, 06122 Perugia, Italy; mattia.acito@studenti.unipg.it
3. U.O.C. Oncologia Medica, ASUR Area Vasta 1, Ospedale Santa Maria della Misericordia di Urbino, 61029 Urbino, Italy; rita.emili@sanita.marche.it
4. Department of Research, Epidemiology Unit, Fondazione IRCCS Istituto Nazionale dei Tumori, 20133 Milano, Italy; anna.villarini@istitutotumori.mi.it
* Correspondence: milena.villarini@unipg.it (M.V.); elena.barbieri@uniurb.it (E.B.); Tel.: +39-075-5857419 (M.V.); +39-0722-303417 (E.B.)

Citation: Natalucci, V.; Villarini, M.; Emili, R.; Acito, M.; Vallorani, L.; Barbieri, E.; Villarini, A. Special Attention to Physical Activity in Breast Cancer Patients during the First Wave of COVID-19 Pandemic in Italy: The DianaWeb Cohort. *J. Pers. Med.* **2021**, *11*, 381. https://doi.org/10.3390/jpm11050381

Academic Editor: Franco M. Buonaguro

Received: 11 April 2021
Accepted: 4 May 2021
Published: 6 May 2021

Publisher's Note: MDPI stays neutral with regard to jurisdictional claims in published maps and institutional affiliations.

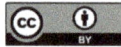

Copyright: © 2021 by the authors. Licensee MDPI, Basel, Switzerland. This article is an open access article distributed under the terms and conditions of the Creative Commons Attribution (CC BY) license (https://creativecommons.org/licenses/by/4.0/).

Abstract: Recent evidence highlights that physical activity (PA) is associated with decreased recurrence risk, improved survival and quality of life for breast cancer (BC) patients. Our study aimed to explore patterns of increased/decreased PA, and sedentary behaviors among BC women of the DianaWeb cohort during the first wave of COVID-19 pandemic, and examined the association with residential locations, work changes, different modality used to increase PA, and quality of life. The study analyzed the questionnaires completed by the 781 BC women (age 54.68 ± 8.75 years on both December 2019 and June 2020. Results showed a decrease of 22%, 57%, and 26% for walking activity, vigorous activity, and total PA, respectively. Sitting/lying time increased up to 54.2% of the subjects recruited. High quality of life was associated with lower odds of being sedentary ($p = 0.003$). Our findings suggest that innovative health management fostering compliance with current guidelines for PA and active behavior should be implemented, especially in unpredictable emergency conditions.

Keywords: breast cancer; COVID-19 pandemic; health management; physical activity; DianaWeb; epidemiology

1. Introduction

Physical activity (PA) and exercise for breast cancer (BC) patients and survivors are emerging key elements in the oncological prevention spectrum. In this regard, exercise oncology (i.e., exercise medicine in the management of cancer) represents an important option for patients during rehabilitation, aftercare, and survival [1], with the aim of making the patient more active in everyday life. A growing body of literature shows the positive influence of PA and exercise on the reduction of recurrence and mortality [2,3]. Additionally, exercise can have a favorable impact on cancer- and treatment-related side effects (including fatigue, depression, and physical functioning) and quality of life (QoL) of cancer survivors. However, there are differences in outcomes depending on clinical setting of the BC patients and functional factors related to exercise, such as type, intensity, and activity level. Indeed, there is a positive correlation between high level of cardiorespiratory fitness and probability of survival [4], however, a high level of activity is not necessarily associated with the best QoL [5]. Ultimately, it is important to meet the stated American College of Sports Medicine (ACSM) recommendations on the basis of BC patient's health status [6]. Indeed, current guidelines recommend people who have been treated for cancer to "avoid inactivity" and suggest that an effective exercise prescription includes moderate-intensity aerobic exercise at least three times per week. Moreover, the exercise program should add resistance-training activities, at least two times per week, using two sets of 8–15 repetitions at least 60% of one maximum repetition [6]. Unfortunately, population-based studies showed a general poor adherence to the PA guidelines in both the general population and cancer survivors, and data highlight that only 9–20% of the oncological patients meet both aerobic and resistance exercise guidelines, only 22–44% meet aerobic guidelines, and only 10–34% meet resistance guidelines [7].

The outbreak of the novel 2019 Coronavirus Disease (COVID-19) pandemic has represented a global public health emergency and routine cancer care, including health and supportive care interventions, was completely altered and movement behaviors have been impacted as well. Italy was the first European nation to be affected by COVID-19 which is, to date, a major global health issue. At the beginning of March 2020, the Italian Government adopted stringent containment measures on the entire national territory, which included lockdown and social distancing, to contain the spread of the virus SARS-CoV-2. The stringency of such measures has continuously varied [8], and also within the same country, according to the current diffusion of the disease and the burden on the healthcare system. In Italy, when the strictest measures have been adopted, the imperative was "stay at home", to better control disease transmission, even at the cost of increasing risk factors for non-communicable diseases [9]. The policies and guidelines to implement physical distancing have significantly affected how people living with and beyond cancer spend their active time and receive cancer treatment. While the focus was mainly centered on cancer care and conventional standards in BC patients [10–12], little attention was paid to exercise oncology, although low levels of PA are recognized as an important risk factor.

The closure of common indoor and outdoor places to stay active, such as gyms, stadiums, pools, dance and fitness studios, physiotherapy centers, and parks and playgrounds, has undoubtedly had a negative impact on physiologic and psychosocial response of the general population [13], especially in people who have been diagnosed with BC and people who are at high risk for BC [14].

In this emergency context, it is possible that some BC women have altered their behaviors by facing additional barriers to PA, beyond those already documented [15]. Despite the challenges faced during this pandemic, we believe that it is important for BC women to continue to benefit from an active lifestyle in a safe environment.

The DianaWeb Project is a community-based participatory research that uses a specific interactive website which contributes to the growth of knowledge about lifestyles to be adopted by sharing recipes, movement strategies, and how to manage the change in daily practice involving Italian women with a BC diagnosis [16]. In this new scenario, understanding the barriers that may have influenced an active lifestyle could allow the development of further supportive strategies for oncological exercise.

In this study: (i) we described PA behavior of the DianaWeb cohort during the first wave of the COVID-19 pandemic, (ii) we made a comparison with data collected prior to lockdown, and (iii) we explored some factors that should be considered as moderators of PA, such as residential locations, living in an apartment building or in a dense living environment, BC clinical characteristics, or QoL, through private chat created for the study. Finally, we discussed the importance of identifying detrimental and positive lifestyle changes and the importance of developing possible interventions as an implementation of the DianaWeb platform for future PA coaching programs for women with BC.

2. Materials and Methods

DianaWeb protocol was previously detailed [17] and was approved by the ethics Committee of the Fondazione IRCCS Istituto Nazionale dei Tumori di Milano (Approval INT 24/16). Briefly, patients are recruited on a voluntary basis and, after having signed an informed consensus form, they are enrolled in the study. Once registered, all participants are requested to complete—twice a year—on-line questionnaires including: (a) the self-reported questionnaires on PA levels assessed by International Physical Activity Questionnaire Short Form (IPAQ-SF) [18,19], and (b) medical history. Participants also provided demographic information, anthropometric data (body weight, body height, and waist circumference), results of routine biochemical analysis, and clinical information (histology report and hospital discharge letters, and any other subsequent diagnosis). Volunteers can also make use of a private chat, supervised daily by researchers. Although dietary lifestyle habits are included in the DianaWeb platform, they are not a specific focus of this study.

2.1. Study Populations

Data was collected via an internet platform (http://www.dianaweb.org, accessed on July 2020). The DianaWeb is an open cohort established in September 2016. All Italian BC patients, whatever the disease stage at diagnosis, histological diagnosis, time elapsed since diagnosis, with or without metastasis, local recurrence or second cancers, and with in situ or invasive cancer, are eligible to join the cohort.

In particular, this study uses data collected on both December 2019 and June 2020. In December 2019, the DianaWeb cohort was composed of 1527 breast cancer women. Overall, we selected BC patients (n = 781) that completed the questionnaires in December 2019 and immediately after the first Italian lockdown (June 2020).

2.2. Questionnaires

The questionnaire areas are accessible only with patient ID and password. The questionnaires considered for this study provided the following data:

(i) general information, such as sociodemographic characteristics (age, education level, marital status, region of residence, and residential density);
(ii) anthropometric parameters (body weight, body height, and waist circumference);
(iii) information about medical history (lymphedema arms, use of drugs, tumor metastasis, secondary tumor, etc.) and other health issues (from this section we collected information on SARS-CoV-2 positive swab);
(iv) results of the last routine blood tests;
(v) physical activity level, through the IPAQ-SF, whose reliability and validity are documented [18,19]: subjects reported the frequency (days/week) and duration (minutes/day) of different types of activity: vigorous (e.g., intense home or gardening activity, performing intense aerobic exercises, and using bike or treadmill); moderate (e.g., moderate home activity, work out in the garden, carrying light loads, and bicycling at a steady pace); and walking activities, as well as the average time spent sitting on a day; and
(vi) lifestyle habits on QoL, through the question on one-dimension present in EORTC QLQ-C30 questionnaire [20]: global health-status/quality of life. The global health-status/quality of life scale has response options ranging from (1) "very poor" to (7) "excellent".

In May 2020, participants freely provided information through the chat about: (a) different modality used to increase physical activity [technology-based interventions (e.g., apps, Facebook®, or Instagram); technology-based interventions with a personal trainer (e.g., video-conference, Skype, Zoom video communications including phone conversations, and FaceTime); non-technology interventions (autonomously, without technology support)]; (b) house dwelling floor space (e.g., <50 m^2, 50–90 m^2, and >90 m^2) and private outdoor spaces (e.g., presence or absence of balcony and/or garden); (c) number of family members; and (d) working activity during quarantine.

2.3. Statistical Analysis

Frequency and percentage were provided for categorical data, whereas arithmetic means and standard deviation (SD) were provided for continuous variables. The patients were classified for residence as living in Northern, Central, or Southern Italy. Furthermore, by extending the analysis to residential density, the subjects were classified for living in cities, suburbs, or countryside cities. The education variable was dichotomized into high school or some college ($\leq$13 years) and college graduates or higher (>13 years). The number of family members variable was trichotomized (1, 2, 3, or more members) as well as the dwelling floor space (<50 m^2, 50–90 m^2, and >90 m^2).

PA levels were calculated from IPAQ-SF, converting questionnaire data in metabolic equivalent minutes per week (MET-min/week): each exercise intensity was associated with the metabolic equivalent of the task (MET): MET = 8 for vigorous, MET = 4 for moderate, MET = 3.3 for walking [21].

The BMI (kg/m^2) was calculated using self-reported height and weight data. The degrees of obesity were established according to the World Health Organization's (WHO) criteria: BMI: 18.5–24.9 kg/m^2, normal weight; BMI: 25.0–29.9 kg/m^2, overweight; BMI: 30.0–34.9 kg/m^2, grade I obesity; BMI: 35.0–39.9 kg/m^2, grade II obesity; and BMI $\geq$ 40.0 kg/m^2, grade III obesity [22].

The χ^2 test was used to compare qualitative data, whereas ANOVA was used to compare means of normally distributed quantitative data. In the case of statistically significant F-statistics, ANOVA was followed by a Dunnet post-hoc analysis. Pearson's correlation coefficient was calculated to assess the strength and direction of the linear relationships between pairs of variables normally distributed. For non-ordinal variables, the Spearman correlation coefficient was calculated.

A linear multiple regression (LMR, block-wise) method was computed for PA levels (METs for moderate PA, vigorous PA, walking, and total PA) and sitting/lying time as dependent variables. Three blocks of variables were processed. Being the primary purpose of our LMR analysis was to explore the relationship between environment characteristics and PA, the first block consisted in area of residence, residential density, dwelling floor space, and private outdoor spaces. The second block contained socio-demographic variables (age, marital status, number of family members, level of education, and working activity). The third block was made up with health status variables (BMI, waist circumference, lymphedema, health perceptions, QoL, use of psychotropic drugs, and strategies to increase PA).

The independent variables that were relevant and significantly associated with PA from each block ($p < 0.05$) were included in the logistic regression analysis. Odds ratios values (OR = eβ), showing how the odds change with a one-unit increase in the independent variables, were also reported. All statistical analyses were carried out with SPSS software for Windows (version 20.0; SPSS Inc., Chicago, IL, USA) and p-values <0.05 were considered as statistically significant.

3. Results

Sample Characteristics

Among the 1527 subjects enrolled in the DianaWeb cohort, 781 (51.5%) completed IPAQ-SF and EORTC-QLQ-C30 questionnaires on both December 2019 and June 2020.

Table 1 shows the main sociodemographic characteristics of women enrolled until December 2019 in the DianaWeb study, in particular, the whole cohort and subjects included (Group A) or not in the surveillance study (Group B).

Patients in the two sub-cohorts were similar for age (in both groups the enrolled women were in their 50s), marital status (most of the women were married), level of education, and Italian region of residence.

Table 2 presents the distribution of the study population also considering the presence of some barriers or facilitators for PA, as well as referring to the environment (population density, building design, and greenness), family (number of family members), working and clinical characteristics (lymphedema, and SARS-CoV-2 positive swab).

Table 1. Main sociodemographic characteristics of the DianaWeb cohort, and surveillance study participants.

Characteristic	Whole DianaWeb Cohort (n = 1527)	Group A (n = 781)	Group B (n = 746)	p
Age in years [a]	54.14 (±8.80)	54.68 (± 8.75)	53.58 (±8.83)	0.014 [d]
Young adults (aged 21–40) [b]	85 (5.6)	37 (4.7)	48 (6.4)	0.170 [e]
Adults (aged 41–60) [b]	1.108 (72.6)	562 (72.0)	546 (73.2)	
Over 60 age [b]	334 (21.9)	182 (23.3)	152 (20.4)	
Marital status [b]				
Married	987 (64.6)	526 (67.3)	461 (61.8)	0.053 [e]
Separated/divorced	177 (11.6)	92 (11.8)	85 (11.4)	
Widowed	44 (2.9)	21 (2.7)	23 (3.1)	
Never married	319 (20.9)	142 (18.2)	177 (23.7)	
Level of education [b]				
High school or some college ($\leq$13 years)	810 (53.0)	392 (50.2)	418 (56.0)	0.022 [e]
College graduates or higher (>13 years)	717 (47.0)	389 (49.8)	328 (44.0)	
Region of residence [b,c]				
Northern Italy	1033 (67.6)	576 (73.8)	457 (61.3)	0.000 [e]
Central Italy	331 (21.7)	128 (16.4)	203 (27.2)	
Southern Italy	163 (10.7)	77 (9.9)	86 (11.5)	

[a] Results expressed as the mean ± SD. [b] Results expressed as the number of subjects, percentage between brackets. [c] Northern Italy: Valle d'Aosta, Emilia-Romagna, Friuli-Venezia Giulia, Liguria, Lombardia, Piemonte, Trentino-Alto Adige, and Veneto. Central Italy: Lazio, Marche, Toscana, and Umbria. Southern Italy: Abruzzo, Puglia, Basilicata, Calabria, Campania, Molise, Sardegna, and Sicilia. [d] Group A vs. Group B, Student t-test. [e] Group A vs. Group B χ^2 test.

Table 2. Facilitators or barriers to physical activity in subjects included in the surveillance study.

Facilitators or Barriers	Number of Subjects (%)
Residential density	
Cities	373 (57.7)
Suburbs	235 (30.1)
Countryside	173 (22.2)
House dwelling floor space	
<50 m^2	45 (5.8)
50–90 m^2	306 (39.2)
>90 m^2	430 (55.1)
Private outdoor spaces	
None	48 (6.1)
Balcony	451 (57.7)
Garden	282 (36.1)
Number of family members	
1	224 (28.7)
2	248 (31.8)
3 or more	309 (39.6)
Working activity during quarantine	
Retired or laid off	215 (27.5)
Remote working	352 (45.1)
Normal working activity	72 (9.2)
Other	142 (18.2)
Lymphedema	
No	695 (89.0)
Yes	86 (11.0)
SARS-CoV-2 diagnostic test	
Positive	4 (0.5)
Negative	204 (26.1)
Not tested	573 (73.4)

Almost half of the sample lived in cities with high population densities and in houses $\geq$ 90 m^2 (55.1%) with one or more balconies (57.7%). Throughout the period covered by the study, only 9.2% of women worked outside of their homes; most of the women (45.1%) worked remotely.

From March until May 2020, 208 women (26.6%) of the DianaWeb surveillance were tested for SARS-CoV-2 infection and four of them resulted positive.

The anthropometric data after and before quarantine in subjects included in the surveillance study are presented in Table 3. Mean body weight, waist circumference (WC), and BMI were lower before than during quarantine. When individuals were categorized according to their WC ($\leq$80 cm) or BMI (<18.5, 18.5–24.9 and $\geq$25.0), we did not observe any significant differences before and during quarantine.

Table 3. Anthropometric parameters in subjects included in the surveillance study.

	Before Quarantine	During Quarantine	p
Body Weight [a]	61.46 ± 11.50	61.57 ± 11.03	0.525 [c]
Waist circumference [a]	80.52 ± 10.33	80.91 ± 11.03	0.101 [c]
Normal [b]	449 (57.5)	446 (57.1)	0.459 [d]
Abdominal obesity [b]	332 (42.5)	335 (42.9)	
Body mass index (BMI) [a]	23.08 ± 4.00	23.13 ± 3.87	0.390 [c]
Underweight [b]	54 (6.9)	53 (6.8)	
Normal weight [b]	542 (69.4)	528 (67.6)	0.678 [d]
Overweight and obese [b]	185 (23.7)	200 (5.6)	

[a] Results expressed as the mean ± SD. [b] Results expressed as the number of subjects, percentage between brackets. [c] Before vs. during quarantine, student t-test. [d] Before vs. during quarantine, χ^2 test.

In Table 4, results about QoL and health perception are reported. The analysis showed statistically significant differences between before and during quarantine for both parameters.

Table 4. Quality of life and health perception in the studied population.

	Before Quarantine	During Quarantine	p [b]
Quality of life [a]			
Very poor	10 (1.3)	27 (3.5)	<0.001
Poor	44 (5.6)	146 (18.7)	
Neither poor nor good	238 (30.5)	306 (39.2)	
Good	421 (53.9)	275 (35.2)	
Very good	68 (8.7)	27 (3.5)	
Health perception [a]			
Very poor	5 (0.6)	8 (1.0)	<0.001
Poor	37 (4.7)	113 (14.5)	
Neither poor nor good	253 (32.4)	273 (35.0)	
Good	423 (54.2)	341 (43.7)	
Very good	63 (8.1)	46 (5.9)	
Psychotropic drugs [a]	123 (15.7)	128 (16.4)	0.391

[a] Results expressed as the number of subjects, percentage between brackets. [b] Before vs. during quarantine, χ^2 test.

Stressful events may impact significantly on the initiation of psychotropic drug use. As Table 4 shows, the prevalence of psychotropic drugs use (such as anxiolytics, sedatives, and antidepressants) among participants was, during social isolation, about 16%.

In Table 5, the results about the PA section are reported. METs of walking, vigorous intensity, and total PA were significantly lower during quarantine, compared with before quarantine. The decreases during home confinement were about 22%, 57%, and 26%, respectively. Additionally, an increase was observed in sedentary behavior: daily sitting/lying time increased significantly from about 5 to 7 h/day, and during lockdown over 54% of women were high sitting (sitting more than 6 h/day).

Table 5. Level (MET-min/week assessed with IPAQ-SF score) and time sitting/lying (h/day) before and during nearly two months of quarantine.

	Before Quarantine	During Quarantine	Δ [a]	p
Vigorous PA [a]	361.95 ± 793.62	117.70 ± 468.78	−244.25 ± 685.82	<0.001 [b]
Moderate PA [a]	909.71 ± 902.68	888.53 ± 940.88	−21.18 ± 754.87	0.433 [b]
Walking [a]	941.22 ± 841.80	331.44 ± 590.33	−609.78 ± 801.77	<0.001 [b]
Total PA [a]	2212.87 ± 1696.11	1337.66 ± 1305.51	−875.20 ± 1361.51	<0.001 [b]
Sitting time ≤ 6 h/day [c]	480 (61.5)	358 (45.8)		<0.001 [d]
Sitting time > 6 h/day [c]	301 (38.5)	423 (54.2)		

[a] Results expressed as the mean ± SD. [b] Before vs. during quarantine, student's t-test. [c] Results expressed as the number of subjects, percentage between brackets. [d] Before vs. during quarantine, χ^2 test. *Notes:* PA = Physical Activity.

The proportion of women who did vigorous PA or walking decreased significantly (Figure 1a). The proportion of women who were physically active (a combination of vigorous/moderate PA, and walking) decreased from 98.5% before quarantine to 93.7% during quarantine.

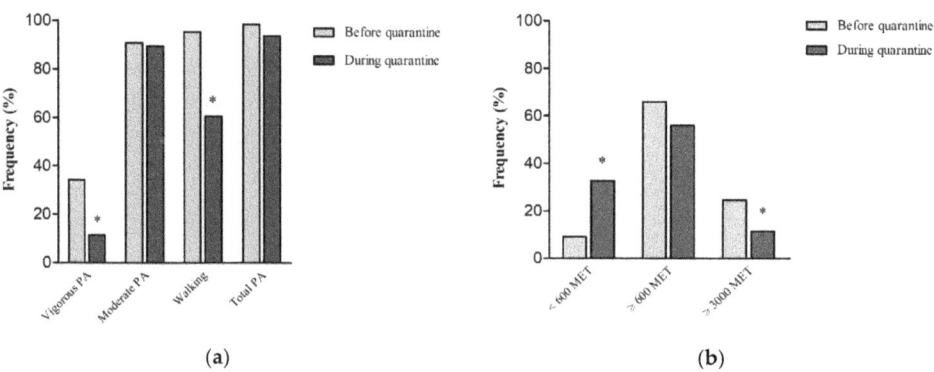

Figure 1. (a) Proportion of total and domain-specific physical activity of women before and during COVID-19 home confinement; (b) Proportion of low active (MET < 600), moderate active (MET ≥ 600), and high active (MET ≥ 3000) women before and during COVID-19 home confinement. * Before vs. during quarantine, χ^2 test, $p < 0.05$; *Notes:* IPAQ score is expressed as MET-min/week; PA = Physical Activity.

In addition, the IPAQ score expressed as MET-min/week was used as a general indicator of low active (MET < 600), moderate active (MET ≥ 600), and high active (MET ≥ 3000) people. We found an increase of low active women (<600 MET-min/week) from 9.3% before quarantine to 32.7% during quarantine, with a concurrent and significant reduction of high active women (≥3000 MET-min/week) from 24.7% to 11.4% (Figure 1b).

Participants most frequently indicated that they did PA without a gym instructor, and only 19.8% did PA with remote personal training (Figure 2).

The PA level and sitting/lying time, according to sociodemographic characteristics, barriers or facilitators to PA, self-reported PA strategies, anthropometric parameters, QoL, and health perception of the study population during quarantine are presented in Table S1. A higher prevalence of physically active women was found among individuals which were 21–40 years old, separated or divorced, worked remotely, lived in Central Italy or in a large house with garden, did not use strategies to do PA, were underweight, did not suffer from lymphedema, and perceived their QoL and health as good.

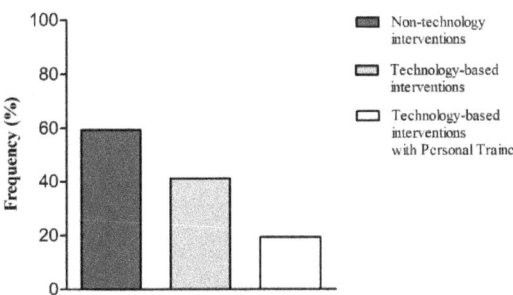

Figure 2. Proportion of self-reported physical activity modality of women before and during COVID-19 home confinement.

In the multiple regression analysis (Table 6), block 1 showed that macroregion of residence and dwelling floor space were significant predictors of moderate PA. Based on our analysis, women living in Northern Italy or owning a house of 90 m² or more resulted being facilitated in performing moderate PA. As reported in block 2, age and working activity were also significant predictors of moderate PA. METs from moderate PA were positively associated with age and with time spent at home (women who are retired or working at home increased their moderate PA). Age and number of family members had an inverse association with sitting or lying time. In block 3, BMI was negatively associated with walking, thus indicating that an increase in BMI may be associated with difficulty in walking. QoL had a negative association with sitting or lying time and a positive association with vigorous and total PA, showing that QoL is a key motivator of PA.

Table 6. LMR between possible independent predictors and physical activity level (MET-min/week) or sitting/lying time (h/day) in the DianaWeb cohort during quarantine.

	Vigorous PA		Moderate PA		Walking		Total PA		Sitting/Lying	
	β	p	β	p	β	p	β	p	β	p
Block 1										
Region of residence	−0.032	0.380	0.076	0.032	0.031	0.392	0.057	0.107	0.004	0.905
Residential density	0.042	0.294	0.035	0.381	0.074	0.064	0.074	0.064	−0.043	0.280
Dwelling floor space	−0.011	0.780	0.092	0.015	−0.032	0.397	0.048	0.209	−0.060	0.115
Private outdoor spaces	−0.024	0.574	0.073	0.083	0.031	0.463	0.058	0.169	−0.068	0.105
Block 2										
Age	−0.074	0.070	0.097	0.017	0.058	0.155	0.070	0.090	−0.173	0.000
Marital status	−0.022	0.587	0.071	0.079	−0.008	0.837	0.039	0.334	0.038	0.349
Level of education	0.013	0.735	−0.031	0.407	0.073	0.052	0.015	0.681	0.045	0.221
Working activity	0.023	0.543	0.086	0.024	−0.024	0.523	0.059	0.122	−0.016	0.676
Family members	−0.011	0.788	0.072	0.082	0.008	0.846	0.052	0.218	−0.093	0.025
Block 3										
Body Mass Index	−0.046	0.402	0.039	0.484	−0.146	0.008	−0.055	0.322	0.067	0.227
Waist circumference	−0.024	0.666	0.010	0.860	0.074	0.174	0.032	0.561	−0.050	0.363
Lymphedema	0.012	0.731	−0.021	0.554	−0.030	0.401	−0.024	0.495	−0.037	0.302
Quality of life	0.098	0.034	0.070	0.135	0.217	0.000	0.184	0.000	−0.136	0.003
Health perception	−0.012	0.792	−0.017	0.715	−0.059	0.205	−0.044	0.352	0.028	0.559
Psychotropic drugs	−0.031	0.394	0.033	0.372	0.005	0.885	0.015	0.685	−0.011	0.772
Physical activity strategies	−0.003	0.931	−0.011	0.759	−0.025	0.486	−0.020	0.571	−0.004	0.912

After identification of patterns involved in movement behavior changes during the first wave of the COVID-19 pandemic in Italy, we conducted logistic regression analysis (Table 7) including two built environment variables (microregion of residence and dwelling floor space), three socio-demographic variables (age, working activity, and number of family members), and one health status variable (QoL). Logistic regression models identified in QoL the independent variable that increased PA. The results indicated that women with higher values of QoL were more likely to increase vigorous PA (OR = 1.429; 95% CI 1.092–1.870), moderate PA (OR = 1.415; 95% CI 1.093–1.831), walking (OR = 1.432; 95% CI 1.211–1.693), and total PA (OR = 1.649; 95% CI 1.191–2.284). The logistic analysis showed that there were about 22% lower odds of sedentary (OR = 0.779; 95% CI 0.659–0.920; $p = 0.003$) for participants with high QoL, and 4% lower odds of sedentary (OR = 0.961; 95% CI 0.943–0.979; $p = 0.001$) for aged women.

Table 7. Logistic regression analysis between possible independent predictors and physical activity level (MET-min/week) or sitting/lying time (h/day) in the DianaWeb cohort during quarantine.

	B	p	OR	95% CI
Vigorous PA				
Region of residence	−0.176	0.335	0.839	0.587–1.199
Dwelling floor space	0.201	0.336	1.222	0.812–1.840
Age	−0.045	0.002	0.956	0.929–0.983
Working activity	−0.125	0.302	0.883	0.696–1.119
Family members	−0.040	0.796	0.961	0.710–1.301
Quality of life	0.357	0.009	1.429	1.092–1.870
Moderate PA				
Region of residence	0.033	0.861	1.033	0.714–1.495
Dwelling floor space	−0.010	0.962	0.990	0.655–1.496
Age	−0.006	0.674	0.994	0.965–1.024
Working activity	0.064	0.607	1.066	0.836–1.359
Family members	−0.138	0.392	0.871	0.636–1.194
Quality of life	0.347	0.008	1.415	1.093–1.831
Walking				
Region of residence	0.031	0.789	1.032	0.822–1.294
Dwelling floor space	−0.137	0.300	0.872	0.673–1.130
Age	0.017	0.081	1.017	0.998–1.036
Working activity	0.034	0.661	1.034	0.890–1.201
Family members	−0.032	0.747	0.968	0.796–1.178
Quality of life	0.359	0.000	1.432	1.211–1.693
Total PA				
Region of residence	0.017	0.945	1.017	0.637–1.624
Dwelling floor space	0.227	0.384	1.255	0.753–2.093
Age	−0.008	0.699	0.993	0.955–1.031
Working activity	−0.009	0.954	0.991	0.733–1.340
Family members	−0.255	0.217	0.775	0.517–1.162
Quality of life	0.500	0.003	1.649	1.191–2.284
Sitting/lying time				
Region of residence	−0.059	0.609	0.943	0.753–1.181
Dwelling floor space	−0.230	0.078	0.794	0.615–1.026
Age	−0.040	0.001	0.961	0.943–0.979
Working activity	0.029	0.704	1.029	0.887–1.193
Family members	−0.047	0.636	0.954	0.786–1.159
Quality of life	−0.250	0.003	0.779	0.659–0.920

Notes: PA = Physical Activity.

4. Discussion

The DianaWeb study responds to the pressing request of patients diagnosed with BC to know the most advanced point of scientific research on the improvement of prognosis and to have a virtual space to meet, where to obtain evidence-based information about a healthy lifestyle [23]. The DianaWeb page can be effectively used to increase access to accurate information and to monitor participants' lifestyles and health status over time in a very inexpensive way.

It has been observed that COVID-19 quarantine measures could have reduced PA and exercise in different subclasses of population [24–26], potentially causing various health side effects. Previous research has demonstrated that compared with individuals without a history of cancer, BC survivors are significantly more likely to develop unhealthy behaviors [27].

Our survey with 781 BC Italian women revealed that most of the participants reduced their PA level during the quarantine period, in which strict lockdown measures were adopted.

The results showed that MET-min/week of walking, vigorous intensity, and total PA were significantly lower during quarantine compared with before quarantine. In particular, the strongest differences were found in the percentage of high active women (from 24.7% before quarantine to 11.4% during quarantine) and sedentary women (from 9.3% before quarantine to 32.7% during quarantine). Our study also showed that during the pandemic, the daily sitting time significantly increased from about 5 to 7 h/day. Given that previous studies pointed out the detrimental effects of both sedentary behavior and PA on physical and psychological health [28], BC women of the whole lockdown sample were classified by time sitting/lying (h/day) (Table 5). During lockdown, more than 54% of the surveyed sample spent more than 6 h/day sitting. This phenomenon could be due to a radical change in everyday schedules and habits. However, to mitigate the deleterious effects of inactivity and social isolation, there are many creative ways to be physically active that do not require specialized technology and equipment. In this regard, our data showed that about 60% of the participants did PA autonomously, with non-technological interventions; about 40% had made use of technology-based interventions and only 20% had made use of technology-based interventions with a personal trainer. Although many suggestions and recommendations already exist [29] to PA practice, the COVID-19 pandemic highlighted the importance of understanding common barriers to PA practice and contrasting sedentary lifestyle, creating effective strategies in women with BC diagnosis. About that, this study showed that an emergency context influenced negatively the women's PA behavior with an increase of 25% in inactive time and a decrease of 26% in active time, highlighting the importance of implementing cancer-management strategies.

Our survey agrees with other early reports on lifestyle habits during a pandemic and confirms that the quarantine restrictions were making people more sedentary than ever. In particular, an Italian study [30] highlighted that people who did not practice sports before the quarantine did not take advantage of this period as an opportunity to start and training frequency has increased only among those who already took part in sports. *Meyer et al.* [31] observed that in a sample of about 3000 American adults, people who were meeting exercise guidelines before the pandemic reported an average 32% reduction in PA level during the emergency and, interestingly, those who were sedentary before were inclined to keep their inactive condition [31].

The same behavior was observed in previously active BC survivors who reduced their PA, increased weight and sedentary behavior [32].

Intriguingly, the greatest prevalence of physically active women was among those aged 21 to 40, underweight, who did not suffer from lymphedema, and perceived their QoL and health as good. In multiple regression analyses, QoL was the only significant predictor for vigorous PA. Instead, macroregion of residence, dwelling floor space, age, and working activity were significant predictors of moderate PA. On the other side, age and number of family members had an inverse association with sitting or lying time. Notwithstanding, there were significant negative associations between sitting/lying time and age and QoL. We observed a slight increase in the use of psychotropic drugs (15.7% before vs. 16% during the quarantine) and, in accordance with our data, women with higher QoL values were more likely to increase total PA. These data support the positive association between exercise and improved physical/psychological health that has been well-established and demonstrated in people with cancer. In this regard, clinical evidence of exercise medicine efficacy in cancer management includes diminished symptomatology, enhanced functional capacity, and improved physical/psychological well-being, as well as a potential contribution to BC-specific mortality reduction, and possibly BC non-recurrence [33–37].

Efforts should be made to promote physical activity in BC patients. In this context, the implementation of the DianaWeb platform with specific coaching programs to overcome barriers, set realistic goals, and provide personalized advice adapted to BC patients can increase the proportion of women that meet the basic daily recommendation for the level of PA.

Strengths and Limitations

The DianaWeb platform itself, centered on an interactive website (http://www.dianaweb.org, accessed on July 2020) designed to supervise the lifestyle habits and health status of BC patients and provide recommendations and suggestions for sustainable lifestyle changes, is considered an important strength. As a community-based participatory research, it is based on the collaborative involvement of all partners in all phases of the research, resulting in high compliance and an incisive knowledge dissemination process.

A limitation is the use of single items for unhealthy behaviors instead of more extensive measurement, e.g., devices to measure PA, which could have given a more precise estimate of the risk, as well as the self-reported questionnaire, which may lead to the actual misreporting of data.

One general limitation attributed to survey research is the oversimplification of social reality and the inconsistency of some collected data such as the percentage of COVID-19 infection within the DianaWeb Italian cohort.

5. Conclusions

This study showed that COVID-19 emergency increased the unhealthy behaviors in BC patients, indicative of a possible higher risk of worse prognosis. This observation was crucial to support our research group in improving the DianaWeb platform strategy.

In this context, the DianaWeb platform could help women with BC to maintain correct lifestyles based on continuous scientific information easily accessible through the internet, especially in those situations where it is harder to find and obtain conventional forms of professional communication. This tool might support clinical practice also through the development of smartphone apps that are more feasible and faster to use. Fitness applications for smartphones have enjoyed increasing popularity in recent years because of their ease of use. We intend to develop an app to track women's dietary habits, how long they sleep, and how long they perform physical activity. This would be an intriguing way to collect data more objectively, in order to minimize memory bias related to self-compilation of questionnaires. Furthermore, in the future, tumor progression and/or survival data of the DianaWeb study participants will be traced to evaluate whether PA is able to reduce recurrence and mortality for BC. We have established a five-year follow-up to estimate the survival rate in the DianaWeb cohort and to compare it with BC survival rate in the Italian population.

Supplementary Materials: The following are available online at https://www.mdpi.com/article/10.3390/jpm11050381/s1, Table S1: PA levels (MET-min/week) and sitting/lying time (h:min/day) by sociodemographic characteristics, region of residence, number of family members, dwelling floor space, private outdoor spaces, residential density, self-reported PA strategies, anthropometric parameters, quality of life, and health perception and use of psychotropic drugs of the study population during quarantine. Data are expressed as the means ± SD and percent of respondents engaged in PA or in sitting/lying.

Author Contributions: Conceptualization, V.N. Writing—original draft, review and editing, V.N., M.V., L.V., E.B. and A.V. Methodology, V.N. and M.V. Data curation, V.N., M.V., M.A. and A.V. Formal analysis V.N., M.V. and M.A. Funding acquisition, R.E. and A.V. Supervision, L.V. and E.B. All authors have read and agreed to the published version of the manuscript.

Funding: This study was supported by Golden Brain ETS Cultural Association.

Institutional Review Board Statement: Not applicable.

Informed Consent Statement: Informed consent was obtained from all subjects involved in the study.

Data Availability Statement: The data presented in this study are available on request from the corresponding author.

Acknowledgments: The authors wish to thank the women participating in the DianaWeb study for their effort and time spent to help with this research.

Conflicts of Interest: The authors declare no conflict of interest.

References

1. Wirtz, P.; Baumann, F.T. Physical Activity, Exercise and Breast Cancer—What is the Evidence for Rehabilitation, Aftercare, and Survival? A Review. *Breast Care* **2018**, *13*, 93–101.
2. Cormie, P.; Zopf, E.M.; Zhang, X.; Schmitz, K.H. The Impact of Exercise on Cancer Mortality, Re-currence, and Treatment-Related Adverse Effects. *Epidemiol. Rev.* **2017**, *39*, 71–92. [CrossRef] [PubMed]
3. Liu, L.; Shi, Y.; Li, T.; Qin, Q.; Yin, J.; Pang, S.; Nie, S.; Wei, S. Leisure time physical activity and cancer risk: Evaluation of the WHO's recommendation based on 126 high-quality epidemiological studies. *Br. J. Sports Med.* **2016**, *50*, 372–378. [CrossRef]
4. Vainshelboim, B.; Lima, R.M.; Myers, J. Cardiorespiratory fitness and cancer in women: A prospective pilot study. *J. Sport Health Sci.* **2019**, *8*, 457–462. [CrossRef] [PubMed]
5. Adamo, R.; Klika, R.J.; Ballard, T.M. How Does Physical Activity Prior to Breast Cancer Diagnosis Effect Rehabilitation Outcomes? Southern California Conferences for Undergraduate Research. November 2016. Available online: https://www.sccur.org/sccur/fall_2016_conference/posters/220/ (accessed on 12 November 2016).
6. Campbell, K.L.; Winters-Stone, K.M.; Wiskemann, J.; May, A.M.; Schwartz, A.L.; Courneya, K.S.; Zucker, D.S.; Matthews, C.E.; Ligibel, J.A.; Gerber, L.H.; et al. Exercise guidelines for cancer survivors: Consensus statement from international multidisciplinary roundtable. *Med. Sci. Sports Exerc.* **2019**, *51*, 2375–2390. [CrossRef]
7. Coletta, A.M.; Marquez, G.; Thomas, P.; Thoman, W.; Bevers, T.; Brewster, A.M.; Hawk, E.; Basen-Engquist, K.; Gilchrist, S.C. Clinical factors associated with adherence to aerobic and resistance physical activity guidelines among cancer prevention patients and survivors. *PLoS ONE.* **2019**, *14*, e0220814. [CrossRef] [PubMed]
8. Gibney, E. Coronavirus lockdowns have changed the way Earth moves. *Nature* **2020**, *580*, 176–177. [CrossRef]
9. Lee, I.M.; Shiroma, E.J.; Lobelo, F.; Puska, P.; Blair, S.N.; Katzmarzyk, P.T. Lancet Physical Activity Series Working Group. Effect of physical inactivity on major non-communicable diseases worldwide: An analysis of burden of disease and life expectancy. *Lancet* **2012**, *380*, 219–229. [CrossRef]
10. American Society of Clinical Oncology (ASCO). COVID-19 Clinical Oncology Frequently Asked Questions (FAQs). 2020. Available online: https://www.asco.org/sites/new-www.asco.org/files/content-files/blog-release/pdf/COVID-19-Clinical%20Oncology-FAQs-3-12-2020.pdf (accessed on 12 March 2021).
11. Battershill, P.M. Influenza pandemic planning for cancer patients. *Curr. Oncol.* **2006**, *13*, 119–120. [CrossRef]
12. World Health Organization (WHO). Coronavirus Disease (COVID-19) Pandemic. 2020. Available online: https://www.who.int/emergencies/diseases/novel-coronavirus-2019 (accessed on 10 February 2021).
13. Violant-Holz, V.; Gallego-Jiménez, M.G.; González-González, C.S.; Muñoz-Violant, S.; Rodríguez, M.J.; Sansano-Nadal, O.; Guerra-Balic, M. Psychological Health and Physical Activity Levels during the COVID-19 Pandemic: A Systematic Review. *Int. J. Environ. Res. Public Health* **2020**, *17*, 9419. [CrossRef]
14. Breastcancer.org. Available online: https://www.breastcancer.org/treatment/covid-19-and-breast-cancer-care (accessed on 10 February 2021).
15. Brunet, J.; Taran, S.; Burke, S.; Sabiston, C.M. A qualitative exploration of barriers and motivators to physical activity participation in women treated for breast cancer. *Disabil. Rehabil.* **2013**, *35*, 2038–2045. [CrossRef] [PubMed]
16. Gianfredi, V.; Nucci, D.; Balzarini, M.; Acito, M.; Moretti, M.; Villarini, A.; Villarini, M. E-Coaching: The DianaWeb study to prevent breast cancer recurrences. *Clin. Ter.* **2020**, *170*, e59–e65. [PubMed]
17. Villarini, M.; Lanari, C.; Nucci, D.; Gianfredi, V.; Marzulli, T.; Berrino, F.; Borgo, A.; Bruno, E.; Gargano, G.; Moretti, M.; et al. Community-based participatory research to improve life quality and clinical outcomes of patients with breast cancer (DianaWeb in Umbria pilot study). *BMJ Open* **2016**, *6*, e009707. [CrossRef] [PubMed]
18. Lee, P.H.; Macfarlane, D.J.; Lam, T.; Stewart, S.M. Validity of the international physical activity questionnaire short form (IPAQ-SF): A systematic review. *Int. J. Behav. Nutr. Phys. Act.* **2011**, *8*, 115. [CrossRef] [PubMed]
19. Craig, C.L.; Marshall, A.L.; Sjöström, M.; Bauman, A.E.; Booth, M.L.; Ainsworth, B.E.; Pratt, M.; Ekelund, U.; Yngve, A.; Sallis, J.F.; et al. International physical activity questionnaire: 12-country reliability and validity. *Med. Sci. Sports Exerc.* **2003**, *35*, 1381–1395. [CrossRef]
20. Aaronson, N.K.; Ahmedzai, S.; Bergman, B.; Bullinger, M.; Cull, A.; Duez, N.J.; Filiberti, A.; Flechtner, H.; Fleishman, S.B.; de Haes, J.C.; et al. The European Organization for Research and Treatment of Cancer QLQ-C30: A quality-of-life instrument for use in international clinical trials in oncology. *J. Natl. Cancer Inst.* **1993**, *85*, 365–376. [CrossRef] [PubMed]
21. Cheng, H.L. A simple, easy-to-use spreadsheet for automatic scoring of the International Physical Activity Questionnaire (IPAQ) Short Form. *ResearchGate* **2016**. [CrossRef]

22. World Health Organization. Available online: https://www.euro.who.int/en/health-topics/disease-prevention/nutrition/a-healthy-lifestyle/body-mass-index-bmi (accessed on 4 March 2021).
23. Villarini, A.; Villarini, M.; Gargano, G.; Moretti, M.; Berrino, F. DianaWeb: Un progetto dimostrativo per migliorare la prognosi in donne con carcinoma mammario attraverso gli stili di vita [DianaWeb: A demonstration project to improve breast cancer prognosis through lifestyles]. *Epidemiol. Prev.* **2015**, *39*, 402–405.
24. Chen, P.; Mao, L.; Nassis, G.P.; Harmer, P.; Ainsworth, B.E.; Li, F. Coronavirus disease (COVID-19): The need to maintain regular physical activity while taking precautions. *J. Sport Health Sci.* **2020**, *9*, 103–104. [CrossRef]
25. Narici, M.; De Vito, G.; Franchi, M.; Paoli, A.; Moro, T.; Marcolin, G.; Grassi, B.; Baldassarre, G.; Zuccarelli, L.; Biolo, G.; et al. Impact of sedentarism due to the COVID-19 home confinement on neuromuscular, cardiovascular and metabolic health: Physiological and pathophysiological implications and recommendations for physical and nutritional countermeasures. *Eur. J. Sport Sci.* **2020**, *12*, 1–22. [CrossRef]
26. Luciano, F.; Cenacchi, V.; Vegro, V.; Pavei, G. COVID-19 lockdown: Physical activity, sedentary behaviour and sleep in Italian medicine students. *Eur. J. Sport Sci.* **2020**, *6*, 1–10. [CrossRef] [PubMed]
27. Kanera, I.M.; Bolman, C.A.; Mesters, I.; Willems, R.A.; Beaulen, A.A.; Lechner, L. Prevalence and correlates of healthy lifestyle behaviors among early cancer survivors. *BMC Cancer* **2016**, *5*, 4. [CrossRef]
28. Trinh, L.; Amireault, S.; Lacombe, J.; Sabiston, C.M. Physical and psychological health among breast cancer survivors: Interactions with sedentary behavior and physical activity. *Psychooncology* **2015**, *24*, 1279–1285. [CrossRef] [PubMed]
29. Newton, R.U.; Hart, N.H.; Clay, T. Keeping Patients with Cancer Exercising in the Age of COVID-19. *JCO Oncol. Pract.* **2020**, *16*, 656–664. [CrossRef] [PubMed]
30. Di Renzo, L.; Gualtieri, P.; Pivari, F.; Soldati, L.; Attinà, A.; Cinelli, G.; Leggeri, C.; Caparello, G.; Barrea, L.; Scerbo, F.; et al. Eating habits and lifestyle changes during COVID-19 lockdown: An Italian survey. *J. Transl. Med.* **2020**, *18*, 229. [CrossRef]
31. Meyer, J.; McDowell, C.; Lansing, J.; Brower, C.; Smith, L.; Tully, M.; Herring, M. Changes in Physical Activity and Sedentary Behavior in Response to COVID-19 and Their Associations with Mental Health in 3052 US Adults. *Int. J. Environ. Res. Public Health* **2020**, *17*, 6469. [CrossRef]
32. Gurgel, A.R.B.; Mingroni-Netto, P.; Farah, J.C.; de Brito, C.M.M.; Levin, A.S.; Brum, P.C. Determinants of Health and Physical Activity Levels Among Breast Cancer Survivors During the COVID-19 Pandemic: A Cross-Sectional Study. *Front. Physiol.* **2021**, *12*, 624169. [CrossRef]
33. Kang, D.W.; Lee, J.; Suh, S.H.; Ligibel, J.; Courneya, K.S.; Jeon, J.Y. Effects of Exercise on Insulin, IGF Axis, Adipocytokines, and Inflammatory Markers in Breast Cancer Survivors: A Systematic Review and Meta-analysis. *Cancer Epidemiol. Biomark. Prev. Publ. Am. Assoc. Cancer Res. Am. Soc. Prev. Oncol.* **2017**, *26*, 355–365. [CrossRef]
34. Newton, R.U. Overwhelming research and clinical evidence of exercise medicine efficacy in cancer management-translation into practice is the challenge before us. *Current oncology* **2018**, *25*, 117–118. [CrossRef]
35. Patsou, E.D.; Alexias, G.D.; Anagnostopoulos, F.G.; Karamouzis, M.V. Effects of physical activity on depressive symptoms during breast cancer survivorship: A meta-analysis of randomised control trials. *ESMO Open* **2017**, *2*, e000271. [CrossRef]
36. Spei, M.E.; Samoli, E.; Bravi, F.; La Vecchia, C.; Bamia, C.; Benetou, V. Physical activity in breast cancer survivors: A systematic review and meta-analysis on overall and breast cancer survival. *Breast* **2019**, *44*, 144–152. [CrossRef] [PubMed]
37. Naughton, M.J.; Weaver, K.E. Physical and mental health among cancer survivors: Considerations for long-term care and quality of life. *N. C. Med. J.* **2014**, *75*, 283–286. [CrossRef] [PubMed]

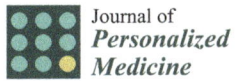

Case Report

A Rare Case of Cerebral Venous Thrombosis and Disseminated Intravascular Coagulation Temporally Associated to the COVID-19 Vaccine Administration

Vincenzo D'Agostino [1], Ferdinando Caranci [2,*], Alberto Negro [1], Valeria Piscitelli [1], Bernardino Tuccillo [3], Fabrizio Fasano [1], Giovanni Sirabella [1], Ines Marano [4], Vincenza Granata [5], Roberta Grassi [2], Davide Pupo [2] and Roberto Grassi [2,3,4,5,6]

[1] Neuroradiology Unit, PO Ospedale del Mare, ASL NA1, via Enrico Russo, 80147 Naples, Italy; vincenzo-dagostino@libero.it (V.D.); alberto.negro@hotmail.it (A.N.); valeria.piscitelli@libero.it (V.P.); fabriziodoc@gmail.com (F.F.); gianni.sirabella6@gmail.com (G.S.)

[2] Department of Medicine of Precision, School of Medicine, "Luigi Vanvitelli" University of Campania, 80147 Naples, Italy; roberta.grassi89@gmail.com (R.G.); dave.dp93@gmail.com (D.P.); roberto.grassi@unicampania.it (R.G.)

[3] Cardiology Unit, PO Ospedale del Mare, ASL NA1, via Enrico Russo, 80147 Naples, Italy; bernardino.tuccillo@aslnapoli1centro.it

[4] Radiology Unit, PO Ospedale del Mare, ASL NA1, via Enrico Russo, 80147 Naples, Italy; ines.marano@tiscali.it

[5] Division of Radiology, "Istituto Nazionale Tumori IRCCS Fondazione Pascale—IRCCS di Napoli", I-80131 Naples, Italy; v.granata@istitutotumori.na.it

[6] Italian Society of Medical and Interventional Radiology (SIRM), SIRM Foundation, 20122 Milan, Italy

* Correspondence: ferdinando.caranci@unicampania.it

Citation: D'Agostino, V.; Caranci, F.; Negro, A.; Piscitelli, V.; Tuccillo, B.; Fasano, F.; Sirabella, G.; Marano, I.; Granata, V.; Grassi, R.; et al. A Rare Case of Cerebral Venous Thrombosis and Disseminated Intravascular Coagulation Temporally Associated to the COVID-19 Vaccine Administration. *J. Pers. Med.* **2021**, *11*, 285. https://doi.org/10.3390/jpm11040285

Academic Editor: Franco M. Buonaguro

Received: 25 March 2021
Accepted: 8 April 2021
Published: 8 April 2021

Publisher's Note: MDPI stays neutral with regard to jurisdictional claims in published maps and institutional affiliations.

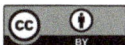

Copyright: © 2021 by the authors. Licensee MDPI, Basel, Switzerland. This article is an open access article distributed under the terms and conditions of the Creative Commons Attribution (CC BY) license (https://creativecommons.org/licenses/by/4.0/).

Abstract: Globally, at the time of writing (20 March 2021), 121.759.109 confirmed COVID-19 cases have been reported to the WHO, including 2.690.731 deaths. Globally, on 18 March 2021, a total of 364.184.603 vaccine doses have been administered. In Italy, 3.306.711 confirmed COVID-19 cases with 103.855 deaths have been reported to WHO. In Italy, on 9 March 2021, a total of 6.634.450 vaccine doses have been administered. On 15 March 2021, Italian Medicines Agency (AIFA) decided to temporarily suspend the use of the AstraZeneca COVID-19 vaccine throughout the country as a precaution, pending the rulings of the European Medicines Agency (EMA). This decision was taken in line with similar measures adopted by other European countries due to the death of vaccinated people. On 18 March 2021, EMA's safety committee concluded its preliminary review about thromboembolic events in people vaccinated with COVID-19 Vaccine AstraZeneca at its extraordinary meeting, confirming the benefits of the vaccine continue to outweigh the risk of side effects, however, the vaccine may be associated with very rare cases of blood clots associated with thrombocytopenia, i.e., low levels of blood platelets with or without bleeding, including rare cases of cerebral venous thrombosis (CVT). We report the case of a 54-year-old woman who developed disseminated intravascular coagulation (DIC) with multi-district thrombosis 12 days after the AstraZeneca COVID-19 vaccine administration. A brain computed tomography (CT) scan showed multiple subacute intra-axial hemorrhages in atypical locations, including the right frontal and the temporal lobes. A plain old balloon angioplasty (POBA) of the right coronary artery was performed, without stent implantation, with restoration of distal flow, but with persistence of extensive thrombosis of the vessel. A successive thorax angio-CT added the findings of multiple contrast filling defects with multi-vessel involvement: at the level of the left upper lobe segmental branches, of left interlobar artery, of the right middle lobe segmental branches and of the right interlobar artery. A brain magnetic resonance imaging (MRI) in the same day showed the presence of an acute basilar thrombosis associated with the superior sagittal sinus thrombosis. An abdomen angio-CT showed filling defects at the level of left portal branch and at the level of right suprahepatic vein. Bilaterally, it was adrenal hemorrhage and blood in the pelvis. An evaluation of coagulation factors did not show genetic alterations so as the nasopharyngeal swab ruled out a COVID-19 infection. The patient died after 5 days of hospitalization in intensive care.

Keywords: COVID-19; cerebral venous thrombosis; intravascular coagulation; vaccine

1. Introduction

In December 2019, health Chinese authorities recognized a cluster of acute respiratory disease of unknown etiology [1]. Afterwards, a new viral agent, SARS-CoV-2, was isolated as responsible for the heart of an epidemic located in Hubei. On 30 January 2020, the World Health Organization (WHO) defined the COVID-19 epidemic as a public health emergency and on 11 March 2020 as a pandemic in the world [1,2]. Currently, a valuable therapy has not yet been improved so that mechanical respiratory support is the only treatment in critically ill patients [3–5]. In this scenario, it was essential to develop a vaccine as soon as possible, to prevent SARS-CoV-2 and to protect persons who are at high risk for complications. At the time of writing three vaccines have been approved in Italy: the mRNA-1273 vaccine Moderna [6], the mRNA BNT162b2 Pfizer drug [7], and the ChAdOx1 nCoV-19 vaccine (AZD1222), that consists of a replication-deficient chimpanzee adenoviral vector ChAdOx1, containing the SARS-CoV-2 structural surface glycoprotein antigen (spike protein; nCoV-19) gene [8]. Globally, at the time of writing (20 March 2021), 121.759.109 confirmed COVID-19 cases have been reported to WHO, including 2.690.731 deaths. Globally, on 18 March 2021, a total of 364.184.603 vaccine doses have been administered. In Italy, 3.306.711 confirmed COVID-19 cases with 103.855 deaths have been reported to WHO. In Italy, on 9 March 2021, a total of 6.634.450 vaccine doses have been administered [2].

The Italian authorities have used the following vaccination strategy, reserving the mRNA vaccines for health personnel and the population over 80 years old, and the administration of the COVID-19 Vaccine AstraZeneca for law enforcement personnel, school personnel and the population between 70 and 80 years old [9]. A strategy for monitoring adverse events of vaccines is based on the collaboration of local and national health structures, assisted by Italian Medicines Agency (AIFA) [10,11]. On 15 March 2021, AIFA has decided to suspend temporarily the use of the AstraZeneca Covid19 vaccine throughout the country as a precaution, pending the rulings of the European Medicines Agency (EMA). This decision was taken in line with similar measures adopted by other European countries due to the death of some vaccinated people [10]. On 18 March 2021, EMA's safety committee concluded its preliminary review about thromboembolic events in people vaccinated with COVID-19 Vaccine AstraZeneca at its extraordinary meeting [12]. The Committee confirmed that:

- the benefits of the vaccine in combating the still widespread threat of COVID-19 (which itself results in clotting problems and may be fatal) continue to outweigh the risk of side effects;
- the vaccine is not associated with an increase in the overall risk of blood clots (thromboembolic events) in those who receive it;
- there is no evidence of a problem related to specific batches of the vaccine or to particular manufacturing sites;
- however, the vaccine may be associated with very rare cases of blood clots associated with thrombocytopenia, i.e., low levels of blood platelets with or without bleeding, including rare cases of cerebral venous thrombosis (CVT).

Rare cases—around 20 million people in the UK and European Economic Area (EEA) received the vaccine until 16 March and the EMA reviewed only 7 cases of blood clots in multiple blood vessels (disseminated intravascular coagulation (DIC)) and 18 cases of CVT. A causal link with the vaccine is not proven but is possible and it deserves further analysis [12].

We report the case of a woman who developed DIC with multi-district thrombosis 12 days after the AstraZeneca COVID-19 vaccine administration.

2. Case

The study was conducted according to the guidelines of the Declaration of Helsinki. Approval by the Institutional Review Board was not needed considering the nature of the study: the findings description of a single case report. Informed consent was obtained by the patient. On 13 March 2021, a 54-year-old woman patient arrived at the emergency room at 10.00 a.m. because of an acute cerebrovascular accident. In anamnesis a Meniere's disease and recent administration of the AstraZeneca vaccine (12 days ago) was reported, without any kind of drug therapy. At clinical evaluation left side signs were found, with a Glasgow Coma Score (GCS) 13; the lower limbs were normothermic and normoconformed, with the preserved femoral, popliteal, and posterior tibial wrist bilaterally. Laboratory tests showed elevated cardiac enzymes, PT 51%, PTT 41 sec, elevated D dimers and normal fibrinogen with blood count, normocytic anemia (HB 8.7 g/dL) and thrombocytopenia, signs of DIC. ECG showed signs of myocardial infarction. Ecocolordoppler examination excluded deep vein thrombosis (DVT) in the explored vessels, with patency of the distal popliteal femoral arterial axis with normal flows.

Clinical and laboratory tests excluded sepsis, various infections, malignancy, vascular diseases, toxic and immunological reactions.

Evaluation of coagulation factors did not show genetic alterations so as the nasopharyngeal swab ruled out a COVID-19 infection.

No severe trauma was reported.

A brain computed tomography (CT) scan showed multiple subacute intra-axial hemorrhages in atypical locations, including the right frontal and the temporal lobes (Figure 1), with ipsilateral hemorrhagic subarachnoid suffusion, raising the suspicion of Labbè/superior longitudinal sinus thrombosis, even if brain angio-CT demonstrated only a non-occlusive thrombosis of the vein of Galen (Figure 2a), but also a floating thrombus within the aortic arch (Figure 2b).

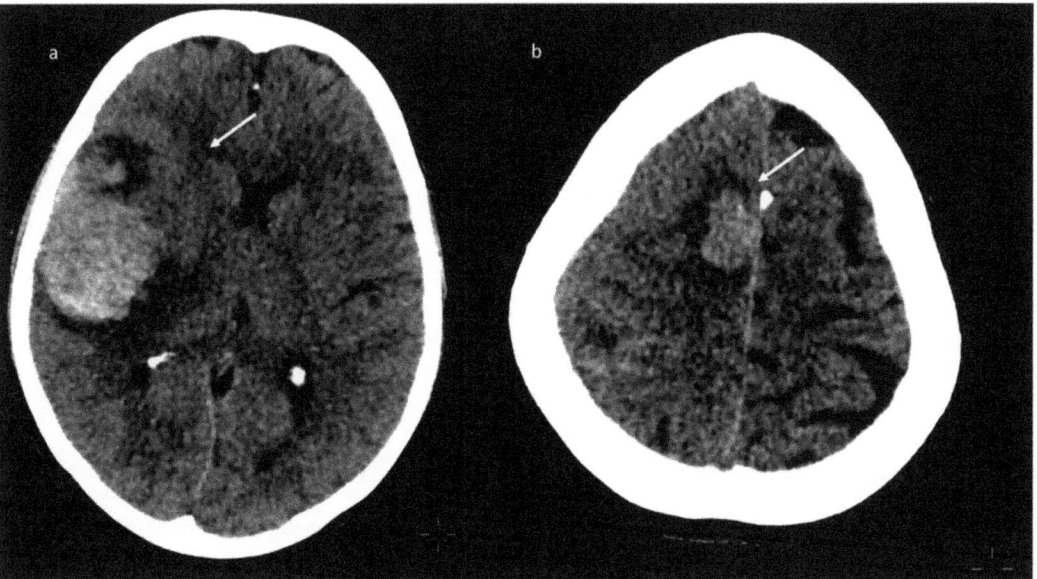

Figure 1. Brain computed tomography (CT) scan: presence of multiple subacute intra-axial hemorrhages in atypical locations (**a**,**b**).

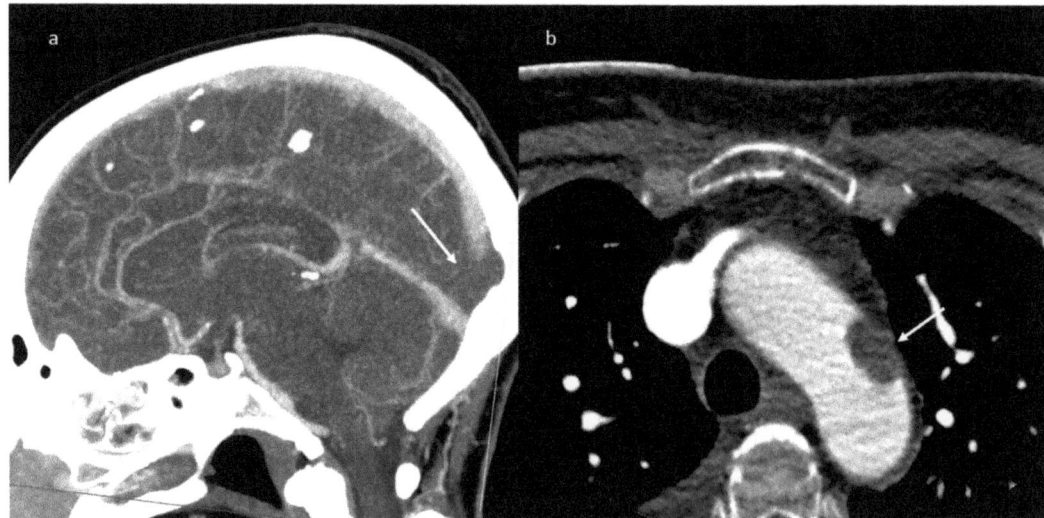

Figure 2. CT-angiography: partial thrombosis of the vein of Galen (**a**); presence of a floating thrombus within the aortic arch (**b**).

The patient was transferred to the Hemodynamics room at 1.00 p.m. a plain old balloon angioplasty (POBA) of the right coronary artery was performed, without stent implantation, with restoration of distal flow, but with persistence of extensive thrombosis of the vessel (Figure 3) with a theoretic indication for administration of intracoronary antiplatelet agents (Aggrastat). However, given the hematological and neurological status, such therapy was not performed. A progressive worsening of the neurological state was observed until a comatose status (GCS 6) started during the procedure. The patient was transferred to the Intensive Care Unit.

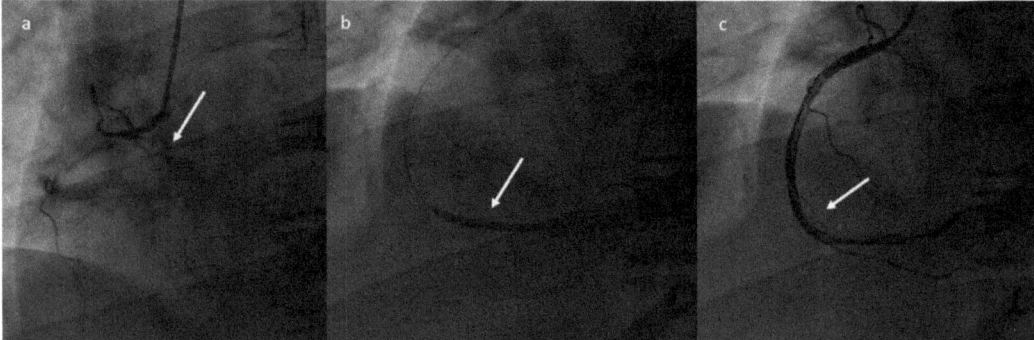

Figure 3. Plain Old Balloon Angioplasty (POBA) of the right coronary artery (**a–c**): restoration of the distal flow, with persistence of extensive thrombosis.

A successive thorax angio-CT added the findings of multiple contrast filling defect with multi-vessel involvement: at the level of the left upper lobe segmental branches, of left interlobar artery, of the right middle lobe segmental branches and of the right interlobar artery (Figure 4).

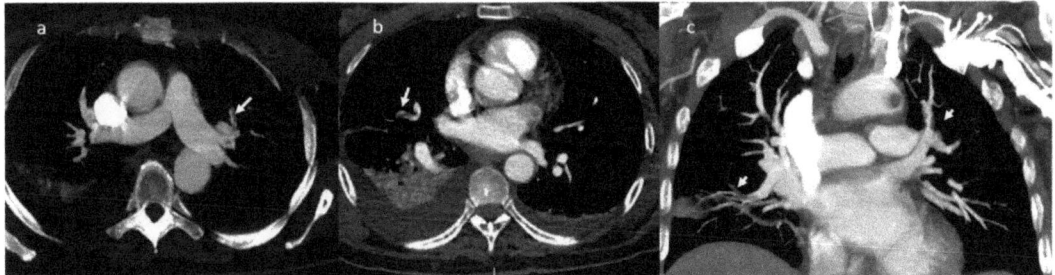

Figure 4. CT-angiography: presence of multiple contrast filling defects involving the left upper lobe segmental branches (**a**), the right segmental artery (**b**); MPR coronal plane in (**c**).

Brain magnetic resonance imaging (MRI) in the same day showed the presence of an acute basilar thrombosis (Figure 5a) associated with the superior sagittal sinus thrombosis (Figure 5b) with the delineation of hyperacute ischemic lesions in the vascular territory of the right posterior cerebral artery and of the perforating pontine branches (Figure 6).

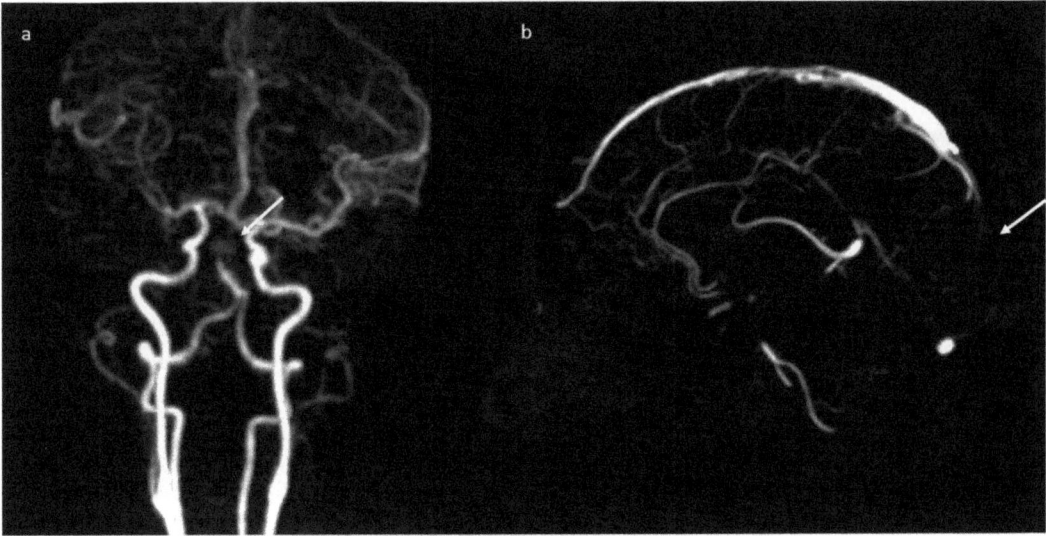

Figure 5. MR-angiography: acute basilar thrombosis associated with superior coronal (**a**) and sagittal (**b**) sinus thrombosis.

An abdomen angio-CT showed filling defects at the level of left portal branch (Figure 7) and at the level of right suprahepatic vein (7). Bilaterally, it was adrenal hemorrhage (Figure 8) and blood in the pelvis.

A brain CT performed one day later showed a diffuse ischemic hypodensity involving the right occipito-temporal and the superior cerebellar regions, the right thalamic and internal capsula regions, pons, and mesencephalon (Figure 9), conditioning edema-based mass effect and contralateral shift of the midline structures.

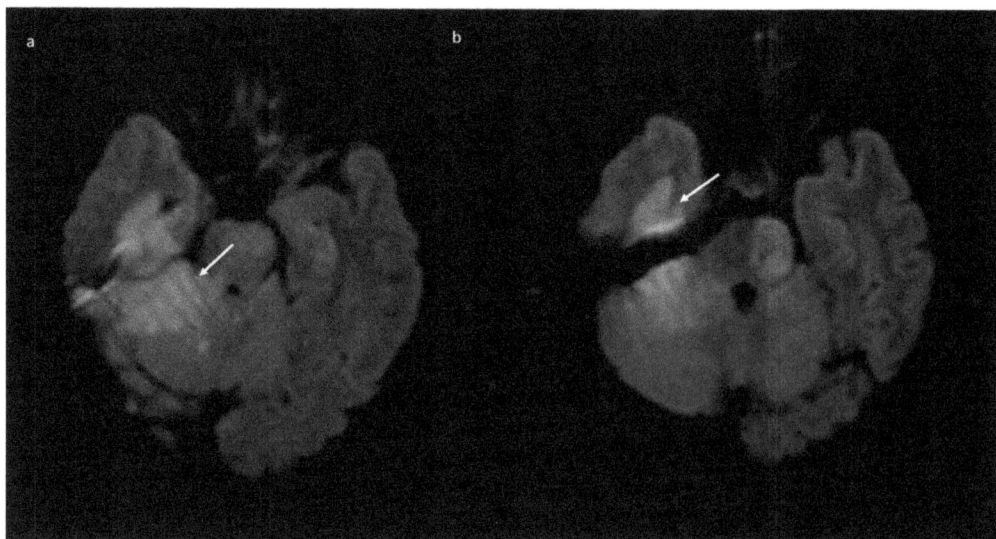

Figure 6. Brain MRI (DWI): acute ischemic lesion with restricted diffusion involving the pons, mesencephalon, the right superior cerebellar hemisphere with the vermis (**a**), and the right posterior temporal lobe (**b**).

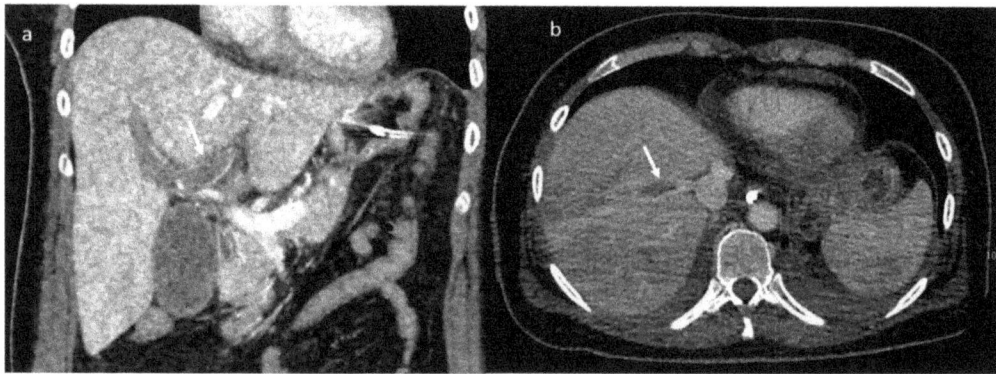

Figure 7. CT scan; in (**a**) MPR (arrow shows thrombosis of the left portal branch) and in (**b**) axial plain during portal phase arrow shows thrombosis if the right (Figuer suprahepatic vein).

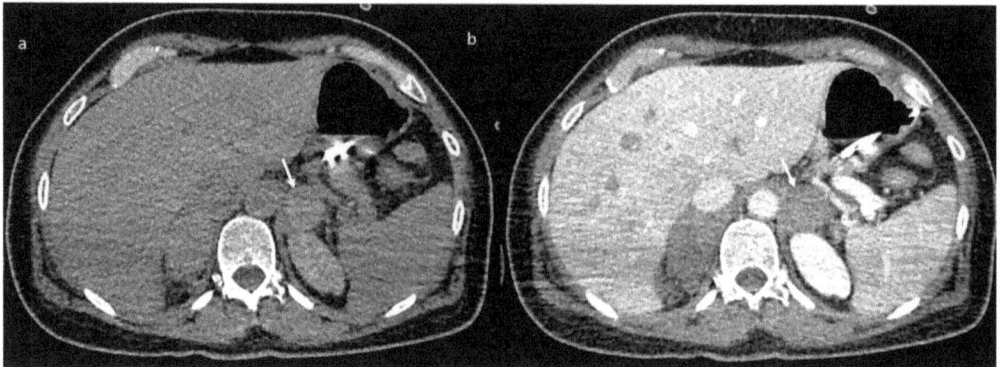

Figure 8. CT scan without (**a**) and with contrast (**b**) shows adrenal hemorrhage (arrow).

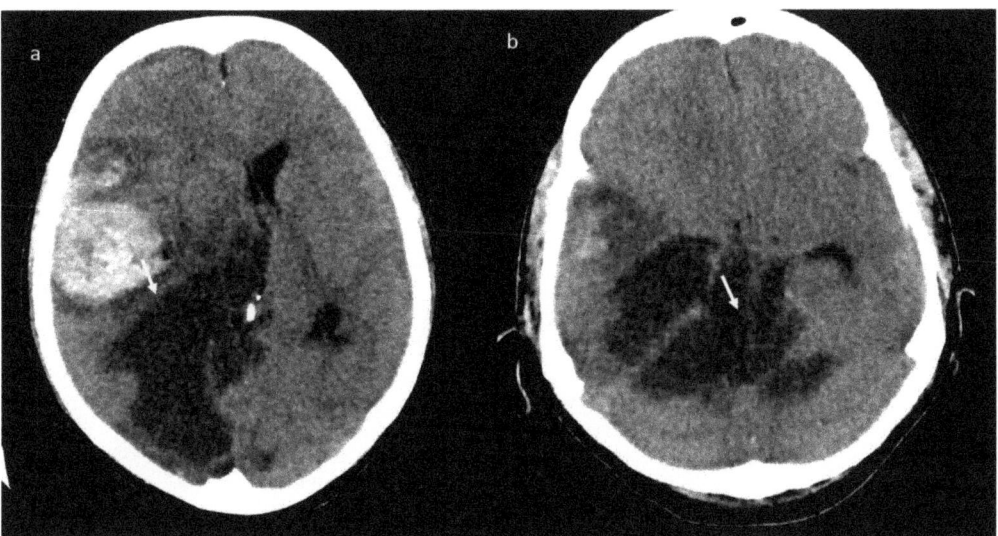

Figure 9. Brain CT scan: diffuse ischemic hypodensity involving the right occipito-temporal (**a**) and the superior cerebellar regions, the right thalamic and internal capsula regions, pons and mesencephalon (**b**).

The patient died after 5 days of hospitalization in intensive care.

3. Discussion

The efficacy and safety of the ChAdOx1 nCoV-19 vaccine includes data from four ongoing blinded, randomized, controlled trials done across three countries: COV001 (phase 1/2; UK), COV002 (phase 2/3; UK), COV003 (phase 3; Brazil), and COV005 (phase 1/2; South Africa). The interim efficacy is assessed by a prespecified global pooled analysis combining data from COV002 and COV003. The safety of the vaccine is assessed using data from all four studies [8]. Three of the studies are single blind and one is double blind (COV005). Primary efficacy was assessed in participants who received two doses of the vaccine. All four studies included participants who received two doses, with a booster dose incorporated into the three trials, that were initially designed to assess a single-dose of ChAdOx1 nCoV-19 compared with control (COV001, COV002, and COV003) after review of the antibody response data from COV001 [8]. All four studies stated that the vaccine has a good safety profile with serious adverse events and adverse events of special interest balanced across the study arms. Serious adverse events occurred in 168 participants, 79 of whom received ChAdOx1 nCoV-19 and 89 of whom received MenACWY or saline control [8]. A total of 175 events were reported (84 in the ChAdOx1 nCoV-19 group and 91 in the control group), three of which were considered possibly related to either the experimental or a control vaccine. A case of transverse myelitis was reported 14 days after ChAdOx1 nCoV-19 booster vaccination possibly related to vaccination. A potentially vaccine-related serious adverse event was reported 2 days after vaccination in South Africa in an individual who recorded fever higher than 40 °C, but who recovered rapidly without an alternative diagnosis and was not admitted to the hospital. Four non-COVID-19 deaths were reported from the studies (three in the control arm and one in the ChAdOx1 nCoV-19 arm), all considered unrelated to the vaccine [8]. Nevertheless, due to the occurrence of some episodes of DIC and CVT, on 15 March 2021, European countries decided to suspend temporarily the use of the AstraZeneca Covid19 vaccine throughout the country as a precaution, pending the rulings of the EMA. According to the EMA data, around 20 million people in the UK and EEA had received the ChAdOx1 nCoV-19 vaccine as of March 16 and EMA had reviewed only 7 cases of blood clots in multiple blood vessels (disseminated intravascular coagulation, DIC) and 18 cases of CVST. A causal link with the vaccine is not proven but is possible and deserves further analysis [12]. The EMA Pharmacovigilance Risk Assessment Committee (PRAC) involved experts in blood disorders in its review and worked closely with other health authorities including the UK's MHRA which has experience with administration of this vaccine to around 11 million people. Overall, the number of thromboembolic events reported after vaccination, both in studies before licensing and in reports after rollout of vaccination campaigns (469 reports, 191 of them from the EEA), was lower than that expected in the general population [8]. This allows the PRAC to confirm that there is no increase in overall risk of blood clots. However, in younger patients there remain some concerns, related in particular to these rare cases. The Committee's experts looked in extreme detail at records of DIC and CVST reported from Member States, 9 of which resulted in death. Most of these occurred in people under 55 and the majority were women [12]. Because these events are rare, and COVID-19 itself often causes blood clotting disorders in patients, it is difficult to estimate a background rate for these events in people who have not had the vaccine. In fact, besides the respiratory manifestations with severe disabling complications, another major concern is represented by evidence of consistent hemostatic changes in patients with severe or critical COVID-19, likely related to a pro-thrombotic switch [13–32]. Among COVID-19 patients, it is reasonable to assume that those with a very severe disease could exhibit high risk of venous thromboembolism (VTE), including deep vein thrombosis (DVT) and/or pulmonary embolism (PE) [31]. In recently published studies, the incidence of PE in patients with coronavirus disease 2019 (COVID-19) who underwent pulmonary CT angiography was reported to be between 23% and 30% [14,15] and the severity of COVID-19 infection should be an important feature in the onset of PE in critically ill patients [14,15]. However, based on pre-COVID-19 figures, it was calculated that less than 1 reported case of DIC might have been expected by 16 March among people under 50 within 14 days of receiving the vaccine, whereas 5 cases had been reported. Similarly, on average 1.35 cases of CVST might have been expected among this age group whereas by the same cut-off date there had been [12]. A similar imbalance was not visible in the older population given the vaccine [12].

We reported the case of a woman who developed a multidistrict thrombotic condition 12 days after AstraZeneca COVID-19 vaccine administration. Although it is not possible to establish the causal link with the vaccine, it should nevertheless be emphasized that the patient had no concomitant cause of DIC.

DIC is defined as a condition characterized by systemic intravascular activation of coagulation, leading to the widespread deposition of fibrin, with formation of widespread microvascular thrombosis. During the coagulation process, consumption of coagulation factors and aggregation of platelets occur resulting in reduced levels of both procoagulant and anticoagulant clotting proteins. Therefore, thromboembolic events and hemorrhage may coexist [32,33]. The uniqueness of the case herein reported relies on the widespread arterial and venous large vessel involvement, with polidistrict organ dysfunction related to the predominance of thrombus formation. To the best of our knowledge this is the first case described in the literature in which a temporal relationship with the administration of a vaccine is found. DIC is not a disease by itself, but always secondary to an existing disease. It may occur especially after sepsis, various infections, malignancy, obstetric and vascular diseases, severe trauma, toxic and immunological reactions [34–36]. Severe anaphylaxis and hemolytic transfusion reaction are associated to DIC [34]. A variety of relevant mechanisms contributing to the derangement of coagulation in DIC have been elucidated. Initiation and propagation of coagulation with concurrent impairment of physiological anticoagulant pathways and a deficit of endogenous fibrinolysis, all as a result of systemic inflammatory activation, are resulting in platelet activation and fibrin deposition. Important inflammatory mediators that govern these processes include tumor necrosis factor (TNF)-α and interleukin (IL)-1 and IL-6. In addition, recent work indicates that intravascular webs ("neutrophil extracellular traps") composed of denatured DNA from destructed cells and entangling neutrophils, platelets, fibrin, and cationic proteins, such as histones, may play a crucial role in the development of thrombus deposition [34].

In this reported case there is no evidence of sepsis, as well as no genetic alterations of coagulation or recent trauma or malignancy. The only factor showing a temporal association was vaccine administration.

4. Conclusions

According to the EMA Committee, the vaccine's proven efficacy in preventing hospitalization and death from COVID-19 outweighs the extremely small likelihood of developing thromboembolic events. However, we should be aware of the remote possibility of such events. In case of suggestive symptoms immediate medical attention is needed, informing healthcare professionals of the recent vaccination. Close safety monitoring of reports of blood clotting disorders will continue, and further studies are being instituted to provide more laboratory data as well as real-world evidence.

Author Contributions: Each author have participated sufficiently in any submission to take public responsibility for its content: cnceptualization; Data curation; Formal analysis; Investigation; Methodology; Supervision; Validation; Visualization; Roles/Writing-original draft; Writing-review & editing. All authors have read and agreed to the published version of the manuscript.

Funding: This research received no external funding.

Institutional Review Board Statement: The study was conducted according to the guidelines of the Declaration of Helsinki. Approval by the Institutional Review Board was not needed considering the nature of the study: the findings description of a single case report.

Informed Consent Statement: Informed consent was obtained by the patient.

Data Availability Statement: All data are presented in the manuscript.

Conflicts of Interest: The authors have no conflict of interest to be disclosed. The authors confirm that the article is not under consideration for publication elsewhere. Each author has participated sufficiently in any part of the manuscript and submission to take public responsibility for its content.

References

1. Granata, V.; Fusco, R.; Izzo, F.; Setola, V.; Coppola, M.; Grassi, R.; Reginelli, A.; Cappabianca, S.; Grassi, R.; Petrillo, A. Covid-19 infection in cancer patients: The management in a diagnostic unit. *Radiol. Oncol.* **2021**. [CrossRef] [PubMed]
2. World Health Organization (WHO). Available online: https://www.who.int/emergencies/diseases/novel-coronavirus-2019/events-as-they-happen (accessed on 10 March 2021).
3. Chaudhary, S.; Benzaquen, S.; Woo, J.G.; Rubinstein, J.; Matta, A.; Albano, J.; De Joy, R., III; Lo, K.B.; Patarroyo-Aponte, G. Clinical Characteristics, Respiratory Mechanics and Outcomes in Critically Ill Subjects with COVID-19 Infection in an Underserved Urban Population. *Respir. Care* **2021**. [CrossRef] [PubMed]
4. Zhou, S.; Xu, J.; Sun, W.; Zhang, J.; Zhang, F.; Zhao, X.; Wang, X.; Zhang, W.; Li, Y.; Ning, K.; et al. Clinical Features for Severely and Critically Ill Patients with COVID-19 in Shandong: A Retrospective Cohort Study. *Ther. Clin. Risk Manag.* **2021**, *17*, 9–21. [CrossRef]
5. Bagherzade, M.; Parham, M.; Zohali, S.; Molaei, S.; Vafaeimanesh, J. Plasmapheresis with corticosteroids and antiviral: A life-saving treatment for severe cases of Covid 19. *Casp. J. Intern. Med.* **2020**, *11*, 572–576.
6. Baden, L.R.; El Sahly, H.M.; Essink, B.; Kotloff, K.; Frey, S.; Novak, R.; Diemert, D.; Spector, S.A.; Rouphael, N.; Creech, C.B.; et al. COVE Study Group. Efficacy and Safety of the mRNA-1273 SARS-CoV-2 Vaccine. *N. Engl. J. Med.* **2020**, *384*, 403–416. [CrossRef]
7. Polack, F.P.; Thomas, S.J.; Kitchin, N.; Absalon, J.; Gurtman, A.; Lockhart, S.; Perez, J.L.; Pérez Marc, G.; Moreira, E.D.; Zerbini, C.; et al. C4591001 Clinical Trial Group. Safety and Efficacy of the BNT162b2 mRNA Covid-19 Vaccine. *N. Engl. J. Med.* **2020**, *383*, 2603–2615. [CrossRef] [PubMed]
8. Voysey, M.; Clemens, S.A.C.; Madhi, S.A.; Weckx, L.Y.; Folegatti, P.M.; Aley, P.K.; Angus, B.; Baillie, V.L.; Barnabas, S.L.; Bhorat, Q.E.; et al. Safety and efficacy of the ChAdOx1 nCoV-19 vaccine (AZD1222) against SARS-CoV-2: An interim analysis of four randomised controlled trials in Brazil, South Africa, and the UK. *Lancet* **2021**, *397*, 99–111, Epub 8 December 2020; Erratum in Lancet. 9 January 2021, 397, 98. [CrossRef]
9. Covid-19-Situazione in Italia. Available online: http://www.salute.gov.it/portale/nuovocoronavirus/dettaglioContenutiNuovoCoronavirus.jsp?area=nuovoCoronavirus&id=5351&lingua=italiano&menu=vuoto (accessed on 10 March 2021).
10. Available online: https://www.aifa.gov.it/ (accessed on 10 March 2021).
11. Granata, V.; Fusco, R.; Setola, S.V.; Galdiero, R.; Picone, C.; Izzo, F.; D'Aniello, R.; Miele, V.; Grassi, R.; Grassi, R.; et al. Lymphadenopathy after BNT162b2 Covid-19 Vaccine: Preliminary Ultrasound Findings. *Biology* **2021**, *10*, 214. [CrossRef]

12. COVID-19 Vaccine AstraZeneca: Benefits Still Outweigh the Risks Despite Possible Link to Rare Blood Clots with Low Blood Platelets. Available online: https://www.ema.europa.eu/en/news/covid-19-vaccine-astrazeneca-benefits-still-outweigh-risks-despite-possible-link-rare-blood-clots (accessed on 10 March 2021).
13. Wu, C.; Chen, X.; Cai, Y.; Xia, J.; Zhou, X.; Xu, S.; Huang, H.; Zhang, L.; Zhou, X.; Du, C.; et al. Risk factors associated with acute respiratory distress syndrome and death in patients with coronavirus disease 2019 pneumonia in Wuhan, China. *JAMA Intern. Med.* **2020**, *180*, 934–943. [CrossRef]
14. Di Minno, A.; Ambrosino, P.; Calcaterra, I.; Di Minno, M.N.D. COVID-19 and Venous Thromboembolism: A Meta-analysis of Literature Studies. *Semin. Thromb. Hemost.* **2020**, *46*, 763–771. [CrossRef]
15. Grillet, F.; Behr, J.; Calame, P.; Aubry, S.; Delabrousse, E. Acute Pulmonary Embolism Associated with COVID-19 Pneumonia Detected with Pulmonary CT Angiography. *Radiology* **2020**, *296*, E186–E188. [CrossRef]
16. Belfiore, M.P.; Urraro, F.; Grassi, R.; Giacobbe, G.; Patelli, G.; Cappabianca, S.; Reginelli, A. Artificial intelligence to codify lung CT in Covid-19 patients. *Radiol. Med.* **2020**, *125*, 500–504. [CrossRef]
17. Borghesi, A.; Zigliani, A.; Masciullo, R.; Golemi, S.; Maculotti, P.; Farina, D.; Maroldi, R. Radiographic severity index in COVID-19 pneumonia: Relationship to age and sex in 783 Italian patients. *Radiol. Med.* **2020**, *125*, 461–464. [CrossRef]
18. Borghesi, A.; Maroldi, R. COVID-19 outbreak in Italy: Experimental chest X-ray scoring system for quantifying and monitoring disease progression. *Radiol. Med.* **2020**, *125*, 509–513. [CrossRef]
19. Fichera, G.; Stramare, R.; De Conti, G.; Motta, R.; Giraudo, C. It's not over until it's over: The chameleonic behavior of COVID-19 over a six-day period. *Radiol. Med.* **2020**, *125*, 514–516. [CrossRef] [PubMed]
20. Neri, E.; Miele, V.; Coppola, F.; Grassi, R. Use of CT and artificial intelligence in suspected or COVID-19 positive patients: Statement of the Italian Society of Medical and Interventional Radiology. *Radiol. Med.* **2020**, *125*, 505–508. [CrossRef] [PubMed]
21. Agostini, A.; Floridi, C.; Borgheresi, A.; Badaloni, M.; Pirani, P.E.; Terilli, F.; Ottaviani, L.; Giovagnoni, A. Proposal of a low-dose, long-pitch, dual-source chest CT protocol on third-generation dual-source CT using a tin filter for spectral shaping at 100 kVp for CoronaVirus Disease 2019 (COVID-19) patients: A feasibility study. *Radiol. Med.* **2020**, *125*, 365–373. [CrossRef]
22. Giovagnoni, A. Facing the COVID-19 emergency: We can and we do. *Radiol. Med.* **2020**, *125*, 337–338. [CrossRef] [PubMed]
23. Grassi, R.; Fusc, R.; Belfiore, M.P.; Montanelli, A.; Patelli, G.; Urraro, F.; Petrillo, A.; Granata, V.; Sacco, P.; Mazzei, M.A.; et al. Cappabianca S. Coronavirus disease 2019 (COVID-19) in Italy: Features on chest computed tomography using a structured report system. *Sci Rep.* **2020**, *10*, 17236; Erratum in *Sci. Rep.* **2021**, *11*, 4231. [CrossRef]
24. Di Serafino, M.; Notaro, M.; Rea, G.; Iacobellis, F.; Paoli, V.D.; Acampora, C.; Ianniello, S.; Brunese, L.; Romano, L.; Vallone, G. The lung ultrasound: Facts or artifacts? In the era of COVID-19 outbreak. *Radiol. Med.* **2020**, *125*, 738–753. [CrossRef]
25. Reginelli, A.; Grassi, R.; Feragalli, B.; Belfiore, M.; Montanelli, A.; Patelli, G.; La Porta, M.; Urraro, F.; Fusco, R.; Granata, V.; et al. Coronavirus Disease 2019 (COVID-19) in Italy: Double Reading of Chest CT Examination. *Biology* **2021**, *10*, 89. [CrossRef] [PubMed]
26. Grassi, R.; Belfiore, M.P.; Montanelli, A.; Patelli, G.; Urraro, F.; Giacobbe, G.; Fusco, R.; Granata, V.; Petrillo, A.; Sacco, P.; et al. COVID-19 pneumonia: Computer-aided quantification of healthy lung parenchyma, emphysema, ground glass and consolidation on chest computed tomography (CT). *Radiol. Med.* **2020**. [CrossRef] [PubMed]
27. Özel, M.; Aslan, A.; Araç, S. Use of the COVID-19 Reporting and Data System (CO-RADS) classification and chest computed tomography involvement score (CT-IS) in COVID-19 pneumonia. *Radiol. Med.* **2021**, *12*, 1–9. [CrossRef]
28. Ierardi, A.M.; Gaibazzi, N.; Tuttolomondo, D.; Fusco, S.; La Mura, V.; Peyvandi, F.; Aliberti, S.; Blasi, F.; Cozzi, D.; Carrafiello, G.; et al. Deep vein thrombosis in COVID-19 patients in general wards: Prevalence and association with clinical and laboratory variables. *Radiol. Med.* **2021**, 1–7. [CrossRef]
29. Ippolito, D.; Giandola, T.; Maino, C.; Pecorelli, A.; Capodaglio, C.; Ragusi, M.; Porta, M.; Gandola, D.; Masetto, A.; Drago, S.; et al. Acute pulmonary embolism in hospitalized patients with SARS-CoV-2-related pneumonia: Multicentric experience from Italian endemic area. *Radiol. Med.* **2021**, 1–10. [CrossRef]
30. Moroni, C.; Cozzi, D.; Albanesi, M.; Cavigli, E.; Bindi, A.; Luvarà, S.; Busoni, S.; Mazzoni, L.N.; Grifoni, S.; Nazerian, P.; et al. Chest X-ray in the emergency department during COVID-19 pandemic descending phase in Italy: Correlation with patients' outcome. *Radiol. Med.* **2021**, 1–8. [CrossRef]
31. Cereser, L.; Girometti, R.; Da Re, J.; Marchesini, F.; Como, G.; Zuiani, C. Inter-reader agreement of high-resolution computed tomography findings in patients with COVID-19 pneumonia: A multi-reader study. *Radiol. Med.* **2021**, 1–8. [CrossRef]
32. Disseminated IntravascularCoagulation (DIC). Available online: https://www.esicm.org/wp-content/uploads/2020/04/Disseminated-Intravascular-Coagulation-_.pdf (accessed on 10 March 2021).
33. Levi, M.; Ten Cate, H. Disseminated intravascular coagulation. *N. Engl. J. Med.* **1999**, *341*, 586–592. [CrossRef]
34. Levi, M. Pathogenesis and diagnosis of disseminated intravascular coagulation. *Int. J. Lab. Hematol.* **2018**, *40* (Suppl. 1), 15–20. [CrossRef]
35. Nardone, V.; Reginelli, A.; Guida, C.; Belfiore, M.P.; Biondi, M.; Mormile, M.; Buonamici, F.B.; Di Giorgio, E.; Spadafora, M.; Tini, P.; et al. Delta-radiomics increases multicentre reproducibility: A phantom study. *Med. Oncol.* **2020**, *37*, 1–7. [CrossRef]
36. Reginelli, A.; Capasso, R.; Petrillo, M.; Rossi, C.; Faella, P.; Grassi, R.; Belfiore, M.P.; Rossi, G.; Muto, M.; Muto, P.; et al. Looking for Lepidic Component inside Invasive Adenocarcinomas Appearing as CT Solid Solitary Pulmonary Nodules (SPNs): CT Morpho-Densitometric Features and 18-FDG PET Findings. *BioMed Res. Int.* **2019**, *2019*, 1–9. [CrossRef] [PubMed]

MDPI
St. Alban-Anlage 66
4052 Basel
Switzerland
www.mdpi.com

Journal of Personalized Medicine Editorial Office
E-mail: jpm@mdpi.com
www.mdpi.com/journal/jpm

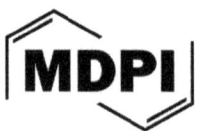

Disclaimer/Publisher's Note: The statements, opinions and data contained in all publications are solely those of the individual author(s) and contributor(s) and not of MDPI and/or the editor(s). MDPI and/or the editor(s) disclaim responsibility for any injury to people or property resulting from any ideas, methods, instructions or products referred to in the content.

www.ingramcontent.com/pod-product-compliance
Lightning Source LLC
LaVergne TN
LVHW070618100526
838202LV00012B/679